AN INTRODUCTION TO HUMAN SERVICES

SIXTH EDITION

Marianne Woodside
University of Tennessee

Tricia McClam
University of Tennessee

The authors contributed equally to the writing of this book.

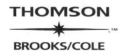
THOMSON

BROOKS/COLE

Australia • Brazil • Canada • Mexico • Singapore • Spain
United Kingdom • United States

THOMSON

BROOKS/COLE

An Introduction to Human Services, Sixth Edition
Marianne Woodside, Tricia McClam

Senior Acquisitions Editor: Marquita Flemming
Assistant Editor: Christina Ganim
Editorial Assistant: Ashley Cronin
Technology Project Manager: Andrew Keay
Marketing Manager: Karin Sandberg
Marketing Communications Manager: Shemika Britt
Project Manager, Editorial Production: Rita Jaramillo
Production Technology Analyst: Greg Shepherd
Creative Director: Rob Hugel

Art Director: Vernon Boes
Print Buyer: Linda Hsu
Permissions Editor: Bob Kauser
Production Service: Matrix Productions
Photo Researcher: Terri Wright
Copy Editor: Ann Whetstone
Cover Designer: Ross Carron
Cover Image: Farida Zaman/Images.com
Compositor: International Typesetting and Composition

Printed in the United States of America
1 2 3 4 5 6 7 11 10 09 08

ExamView® and ExamView Pro® are registered trademarks of FSCreations, Inc. Windows is a registered trademark of the Microsoft Corporation used herein under license. Macintosh and Power Macintosh are registered trademarks of Apple Computer, Inc. Used herein under license.

Library of Congress Control Number: 2007939119

ISBN-13: 978-0-495-50336-1
ISBN-10: 0-49550336-3

Thomson Higher Education
10 Davis Drive
Belmont, CA 94002-3098
USA

For more information about our products, contact us at:
Thomson Learning Academic Resource Center
1-800-423-0563
For permission to use material from this text or product, submit a request online at
http://www.thomsonrights.com.
Any additional questions about permissions can be submitted by e-mail to **thomsonrights@thomson.com.**

CONTENTS

PREFACE ix

ABOUT THE AUTHORS xii

PART I | DEFINING HUMAN SERVICES 1

CHAPTER 1 **An Introduction to Human Services** 3

Themes and Purposes of Human Services 5
Problems in Living 5
The Growing Number of Problems in the Modern World 7
Self-Sufficiency 7
BOX 1.1: INTERNATIONAL FOCUS: TEEN PREGNANCY 8
Social Care, Social Control, and Rehabilitation 9
The Interdisciplinary Nature of Human Services 10
BOX 1.2: WEB SOURCES: FIND OUT MORE ABOUT MEETING ALMEADA'S NEEDS 12
The Relationship Between Client and Helper 13
The Client and the Client's Environment 14
Management Principles in Human Service Delivery 15
BOX 1.3: A PIONEER IN HUMAN SERVICES 16
Networking to Develop a Human Service Umbrella 16
Forming Teams and Partnerships to Provide Services 17
Case Management 19
Roles and Activities of the Human Service Professional 21
The Generalist 21
Activities of the Human Service Professional 22
BOX 1.4: CLASSIFIED ADS 23

CHAPTER 2   **A History of Helping**   27

Early History: A Summary   28
   BOX 2.1: ELIZABETHAN POOR LAWS   31
Human Services in the United States: Colonial America   32
The 19th Century: A Time of Change   33
   Social Philosophies   34
   Probation   35
   Treatment of People with Mental Illness   36
   Child Welfare   37
   Reform Movements   37
   BOX 2.2: INTERNATIONAL FOCUS: MENTAL HEALTH IN DEVELOPING
         COUNTRIES   38
Early 20th Century: New Directions   39
   Seeds of the Mental Health Movement   40
   BOX 2.3: AN ASYLUM IN 1902   41
   Increased Federal Involvement   42
   Mid-20th Century: Focus on Mental Health   43
   Serving Those in Need   44
   The Human Service Movement   46
Late-20th Century: Revising the Social Welfare System   47
   Dismantling the Welfare System   48
Welfare Reform   50
   BOX 2.4: HIGHLIGHTS OF THE NEW LAW   51
   Policies and Procedures   51
   BOX 2.5: WEB SOURCES: WELFARE REFORM   52
   The Faces of Welfare to Work   52
   Evaluation of Welfare Reform   53
   Significant Challenges   53
Legislative Changes in the 21st-century   54
A Final Thought   56

CHAPTER 3   **Human Services Today**   60

New Settings for Human Service Delivery   61
   Institutional and Community-Based Services   61
   BOX 3.1: YOUTH IN NEED   62
   Human Services in Rural Areas   63
   Human Services in Industry and the Military   64
The Impact of Technology   66
   Communication   66
   Information Management   68
   Providing Services to Clients   68
   BOX 3.2: WEB SOURCES: FIND OUT MORE ABOUT HUMAN SERVICES ON THE
         INTERNET   69
   Professional Development   70
Managed Care   71

The Influence of Managed Care 71
Managed Care and the Human Service Professional 74
The International Dimension 75
Challenges in International Human Services 76
BOX 3.3: INTERNATIONAL FOCUS: A LIBERIAN REFUGEE 78
Influences on the United States 78
Trends in Human Services 79
BOX 3.4: INTERNATIONAL FOCUS: KEVIN BURNS—A PEACE CORPS
EXPERIENCE 80
Aging in America 81
An Emphasis on Diversity 83
BOX 3.5: WEB SOURCES: FIND OUT MORE ABOUT OLDER ADULTS 84
Terrorism 86
BOX 3.6: WEB SOURCES: RESOURCES FOR COPING WITH TRAUMATIC
EVENTS 88
New Roles and Skills for Clients and Helpers 88
Conservatism 90

CHAPTER 4   **Models of Service Delivery** 95

The Medical Model   97
Definition 97
BOX 4.1: INTERNATIONAL FOCUS: MODELS OF SERVICE DESIGN 98
History 98
BOX 4.2: PHILIPPE PINEL 100
BOX 4.3: WEB SOURCES: FIND OUT MORE ABOUT PSYCHOTROPIC
MEDICATIONS 103
Case Studies 104
The Public Health Model 107
Definition 107
History 108
BOX 4.4: PUBLIC HEALTH SERVICES 110
Case Studies 111
Remote Area Medical Volunteer Corps 113
The Human Service Model 114
Definition 114
Philosophy 116
Case Study 118

PART II | CLIENTS AND HELPERS IN HUMAN SERVICES 125

CHAPTER 5   **The Client** 127

The Whole Person 129
Perceptions of Client Problems 131

Defining Problems 131

Understanding Client Problems 132

BOX 5.1: WEB SOURCES: FIND OUT MORE ABOUT CLIENT PROBLEMS 134

BOX 5.2: INTERNATIONAL FOCUS: COMMUNITIES IN CRISIS—REACHING
THE VULNERABLE 140

Case Studies 143

Clients As Individuals, Groups, and Populations 145

BOX 5.3: WEB SOURCES: FIND OUT MORE ABOUT GANGS 147

Getting Help 147

Ways of Getting Help 148

BOX 5.4: GETTING HELP: LOCATE SERVICES 150

Barriers to Seeking Help 151

The Client's Perspective 153

Client Expectations 153

BOX 5.5: GETTING HELP: ONE CLIENT'S PERSPECTIVE 154

Client Evaluations of Services 154

BOX 5.6: A CLIENT SPEAKS 155

CHAPTER 6 **The Human Service Professional** 159

Who Is the Helper? 160

Motivations for Choosing a Helping Profession 161

Values and Helping 162

BOX 6.1: MY WORK AS A HUMAN SERVICE PROFESSIONAL 164

Characteristics of the Helper 166

BOX 6.2: MASLOW'S VIEW OF HELPING 167

Typology of Human Service Professionals 170

Categories of Workers 170

The Human Service Professional 171

Other Professional Helpers 172

Human Service Roles 175

Providing Direct Service 176

Performing Administrative Work 177

Working with the Community 179

Frontline Helper or Administrator 181

BOX 6.3: WEB SOURCES: FIND OUT MORE ABOUT HELPER ROLES 183

Case Study 183

PART III | THE PRACTICE OF HUMAN SERVICES 187

CHAPTER 7 **The Helping Process** 189

The Nature of the Helping Process 191

The Helping Relationship 191

Stages of the Helping Process 192

BOX 7.1: INTERNATIONAL FOCUS: MOTHER TERESA AND THE MISSIONARIES OF CHARITY **193**

BOX 7.2: CARL ROGERS AND CLIENT-CENTERED THERAPY **195**

An Introduction to Helping Skills **197**

Nonverbal Messages **198**

Verbal Messages **199**

Listening and Responding **200**

Working with Groups **205**

BOX 7.3: A CLIENT SPEAKS **207**

Skills for Challenging Clients **207**

Culturally Different Clients **208**

The Reluctant or Resistant Client **210**

The Silent Client **211**

The Overly Demanding Client **212**

The Unmotivated Client **213**

Intervention Strategies **213**

Crisis Intervention **213**

BOX 7.4: WEB SOURCES: FIND OUT MORE ABOUT CRISIS INTERVENTION **214**

Resolution-Focused Brief Therapy **218**

CHAPTER 8 **Working Within a System** **222**

The Agency Environment **223**

Mission and Goals **224**

Structure **225**

BOX 8.1: HELP WANTED: A CASE MANAGER **226**

Resources **227**

The Community Context **228**

Using Available Services **229**

Referral **230**

BOX 8.2: HOME HEALTH SERVICES **232**

Building an Information Network **232**

Knowing the Formal and Informal Networks **234**

Challenges in Day-to-Day Human Service Work **235**

Allocation of Resources **235**

Paperwork Blues **237**

Turf Issues **238**

Encapsulation and Burnout **240**

Professional Development **243**

Promoting Change in a Dynamic World **244**

Developing Services in Response to Human Needs **244**

BOX 8.3: INTERNATIONAL FOCUS: WORLD BANK: GENDER EQUITY AS SMART ECONOMICS **246**

Organizing to Promote Community Change **247**

BOX 8.4: WEB SOURCES: FIND OUT MORE ABOUT COMMUNITY ORGANIZING **248**

Using a Model of Client Empowerment **249**

BOX 8.5: INTERNATIONAL FOCUS: DISHA KENDRA **251**

CHAPTER 9   **Professional Concerns**   254

Ethical Considerations   255

    Codes of Ethics   257

    BOX 9.1: WEB SOURCES: FIND OUT MORE ABOUT CODES OF ETHICS   258

    Competence and Responsibility   261

    BOX 9.2: ETHICAL STANDARDS FOR PSYCHOLOGISTS: AMERICAN
            PSYCHOLOGICAL ASSOCIATION   263

    BOX 9.3: ETHICAL STANDARDS FOR SOCIAL WORKERS: NATIONAL
            ASSOCIATION FOR SOCIAL WORKERS   264

    Confidentiality   265

    Clients' Rights   268

    BOX 9.4: CODE OF PROFESSIONAL ETHICS FOR REHABILITATION COUNSELORS:
            CONFIDENTIALITY   270

    BOX 9.5: AMERICAN COUNSELING ASSOCIATION CODE OF ETHICS AND
            STANDARDS OF PRACTICE: CLIENT RIGHTS   271

    Ethical Standards of Human Service Professionals   272

    Ethical Decision Making   272

    BOX 9.6: ETHICAL STANDARDS OF HUMAN SERVICE PROFESSIONALS   273

GLOSSARY   283

INDEX   287

PREFACE

In writing the first five editions of this book, our goal was to offer instructors a textbook choice devoted entirely to human services—not psychology, sociology, or social work. We addressed the definition of the term *human services* in its broadest sense and described a variety of clients, the generalist human service professional, and the interaction between helper and client. We approached human services as a profession that continues to grow and develop. Our goals remain the same for this sixth edition of *An Introduction to Human Services*, but we have revised the book in ways that we believe improve it.

Our revisions are based upon the feedback we received from faculty and students during the review process. Many other revisions resulted from our own research and teaching; they document the changing face of the environment in which human services are delivered. And finally, we were guided by the changes that are occurring in our world, such as the shifting demographics, the increasing conservative influence, and developing technologies.

Part One describes human services. The focus of Chapter 1 continues to be the principles that define human services. The case of Almeada and baby Anne has been revised to better represent the human service delivery system and climate that exist today. The chapter has been condensed to provide a focused approach to defining human services. Chapter 2 combines a history of helping with an update on social welfare reform, a combination that allows thoughtful integration of human services into a long-standing historical context with developments to the present time. Chapter 3 offers a look at the current influences on human services: technology, managed care, the international dimension, and diversity. This chapter was revised to reflect the impact that these influences continue to have on human services. Chapter 4 concludes Part One by introducing three models that contribute to our understanding of human services. Updated case studies illustrate each model, and a final case study helps students integrate the three models. The human service model is expanded to include a strengths perspective.

Part Two continues to focus on the participants in the delivery of human services—the helper and the client—and includes new information about client populations. Chapter 5 adds a new discussion about environmental influences and defining strengths. Chapter 6 explores the identity of the human service professional.

Part Three focuses on human service delivery. Chapter 7 introduces the helping process. Revisions include crisis intervention and resolution-focused brief therapy to illustrate the helping strategies used by human service professionals. Chapter 8 reviews the environment in which human service delivery occurs. Revisions include an introduction to the agency setting and a description of the day-to-day challenges of human service work. Chapter 9 continues to focus on ethical issues.

FEATURES

Two unique features of the book remain. The first is that the book continues to be introductory rather than encyclopedic. It presents basic information that students need to know about the human service field and encourages the use of other books, electronic materials, media resources, and other sources to enrich students' knowledge of the introductory course content.

This knowledge will be more attractive to students when it is applied to case studies, books, current events, and audiovisual materials. In this book, you will find brief case studies, primary sources, and suggested additional readings for each chapter. A list and summary of relevant websites enhance the search for additional information. The instructor's manual that accompanies the text also identifies videotapes, movies, websites, and nonfictional accounts of clients. All these resources can enhance student understanding of human services. We encourage you to use these resources and to let us know of others that you discover on your own. Please note that by the very dynamic nature of the Web, URLs are subject to change. Therefore, while web links in this text were selected with care, some links that were active at the time of publication may no longer be functional.

A second unique feature of the book is the International Focus sections. As the cultural composition of the United States continues to shift, human service professionals must be prepared to work effectively with culturally diverse clients. At the introductory level, we continue our commitment to the expansion of the worldview of human service students. Each International Focus section is related to the content of the chapter and provides an opportunity for thought and discussion about the international dimension of human services and how it influences practice in the United States.

ACKNOWLEDGMENTS

Many friends and colleagues have contributed both to our growth as human service educators and to the writing of the sixth edition of this book. We are particularly grateful to our colleagues in the National Organization for Human Services and the Council for Standards in Human Service Education for their support, feedback, and contributions throughout the years. We would especially like to thank our students and the students in other programs throughout the country who use our book, for we have learned much from them about human services. Introductory students continue to be a favorite group for us to teach because of their enthusiasm and interest in the helping professions.

Our families have encouraged us during this endeavor, and we are grateful for their patience and support. The reviewers whose constructive comments helped us improve the manuscript include: Valerie Geaither, Metropolitan State University; Bud Lawrence, Corning Community College; John LeCapitaine, University of Wisconsin—River Falls; Tim Lindsay, Bethel College; Yvette Madison, Pennsylvania Highlands Community College; Terril Rector, University of Northern Colorado; and Lisa Turner, Clarion University.

We would also like to thank the staff at Brooks/Cole for all their work with this manuscript. This includes our editor extraordinaire, Marquita Flemming; Christina Ganim, Assistant Editor; Ashley Cronin, Editorial Assistant; and Karin Sandberg, Marketing Manager.

Marianne Woodside
Tricia McClam

ABOUT THE AUTHORS

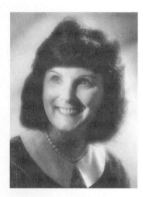

MARIANNE WOODSIDE

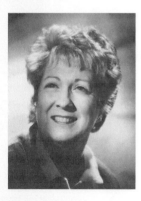

TRICIA McCLAM

As practitioners and instructors, we have been involved in human services for the past 35 years. As a result, we have experience both in delivering services and in preparing those who are learning to do so. From our years as practitioners in public schools and in rehabilitation settings, we have gained an understanding of helpers' commitment to their clients, their work, and their professions. In recent years, we have conducted in-depth interviews with practitioners and clients in an effort to better understand the methods of delivering services, the interaction between clients and human service professionals, and the changing context of service delivery.

In recognizing the complexity of clients' lives and the complicated problems they sometimes face, we have developed more effective communication skills, a realistic understanding of helping using the human service model, and an appreciation of the problem-solving process that is based on the strengths of clients and their environments. These were valuable skills and understandings for us as practitioners. As instructors, we have discovered the importance of developing them in our students if these new practitioners are to become effective human service professionals. Our work as educators has also contributed to our understanding of the evolving field of human services. As we develop curriculum with our colleagues, conduct research in human service education, participate in national and regional human service organizations, and travel and study internationally, we continue to be students ourselves. Concepts such as serving the whole person, using an interdisciplinary approach, training the generalists, and empowering clients have become basic to our work with beginning students.

Defining Human Services

Questions to Consider

- What are the perspectives for defining human services?
- How has human services evolved in the last 50 years? What factors influenced its development?
- How has society responded to the needs of people throughout history?
- What are the current trends in human service delivery? What is projected for the future?
- What model is most often used in human service delivery? How is it influenced by other models?

• • •

Human services may be a question mark to you as you begin this book. It is a difficult concept to define. Some think of it as the activities of workers who try to meet the needs of people. Others think of local and state agencies that used to be called departments of welfare or social services; today, many such agencies are departments of human services. Still others consider human services a **profession** for which a person receives special education and training.

Part One is titled "Defining Human Services." If you think of human services as a puzzle, the chapters in this part will provide you with the pieces necessary to understand this complex concept. Each piece will give you a different perspective from which to consider human services. Chapter 1 introduces Almeada, a client who needs help from the human service delivery system. Through Almeada's experience, this chapter examines both scholarly and professional definitions.

Chapter 2 provides an historical overview of helping, a 20th-century perspective on human services as a profession, and emerging 21st-century issues. Chapter 3 describes current influences on human service delivery and considers the future of such services. Chapter 4 describes three models of service delivery and includes a case study to illustrate each one.

An Introduction to Human Services

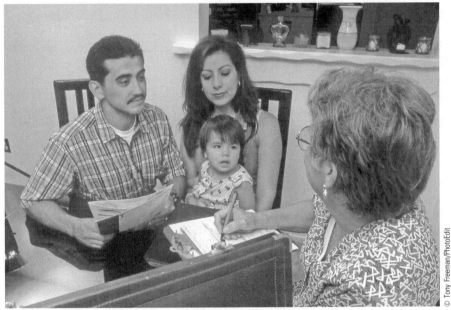

CHAPTER 1

© Tony Freeman/PhotoEdit

After reading this chapter, you will be able to:

- Identify the themes and purposes of human services.
- Define problems in living and provide an illustration of how individuals experience these problems.
- Compare the differences in the functions of social care, social control, and rehabilitation in terms of goals of care and treatment.
- Identify four tasks that human service professionals perform during the helping process.
- List abilities of human service professionals that enhance the helping relationship.
- Name three characteristics of human service teams.
- List the characteristics of the generalist human service worker used in today's delivery system.

Self-assessment

- What are the perspectives that provide definitions of human services?
- Explain how the human service delivery system provides Almeada with social care, social control, and rehabilitation.
- List the reasons problems in living occur.
- Why is it important to understand the client and the client's environment?
- How does networking help human service delivery?
- How does each of the principles of management enhance the effectiveness of service delivery?
- Describe the professional activities of the human service helper.

One of the first questions you will probably ask as you pick up this book is "What is human services?" This question has come up often in the last several decades as the field has changed and restructured. The purpose of this chapter is to help you gain an understanding of the term. The definition of *human services* is derived from six perspectives: (1) the themes and purposes of human services, (2) the interdisciplinary nature of human services, (3) the helping relationship, (4) management principles, (5) professional roles, and (6) professional activities. Understanding and integrating these diverse perspectives will help you formulate a definition of human services.

This chapter introduces the themes and purposes of human services as described by scholars and prominent leaders in the field. The six themes presented summarize the principles that guide the delivery of human services. A case study of Almeada, a young mother who is living in a large city with her baby daughter, Anne, illustrates these concepts. We also describe the interdisciplinary nature of human services and the relationship between client and helper. Important ideas to consider here are the nature of the client, the client's environment, and the interaction between the client and the helper.

Another important and defining characteristic of the human service delivery system is the management principles used by human service providers as they continually work to improve services to clients. The fifth perspective on human services introduces roles of professionals. Finally, a description of the professional activities of human service helpers illustrates their commitment to helping the client by providing needed services within a supportive environment.

Together, the six perspectives presented in this chapter will help clarify what human services is. They will also provide a basic understanding that will serve as a framework for the remainder of the book.

THEMES AND PURPOSES OF HUMAN SERVICES

The first perspective from which human services can be defined is a scholarly one. Scholars approach the definition of human services by describing the themes and purposes that guide human services; these themes and purposes have emerged over the past five decades. Those presented in this section represent the ideas of a range of scholars writing in the field today and include concerns with problems in living, the increase in problems in our modern world, the need for self-sufficiency, and the goals of social care, social control, and rehabilitation. A case study of Almeada and her daughter, Anne, illustrates these themes.

PROBLEMS IN LIVING

Human beings are not always able to meet their own needs. Human services has developed in response to the need of individuals, groups, or communities for assistance to live better lives. Examples of such people are often publicized in the media: the very young; the elderly; people with limited physical or mental capabilities; victims of crimes, disasters, or abuse; immigrants; people with acquired immune deficiency syndrome (AIDS); and many others. Assisting individuals is an example of the helping interaction. Families and groups also receive the attention of human service professionals, as do communities and larger geographic areas.

> Anne, a 1-year-old child, lives with her mother, Almeada, in a housing project in Chicago. Their home is a dirty, rat-infested, one-room apartment that offers little beyond protection from the weather. Almeada, 17 years old, works six days a week for a local clothing manufacturer for minimum wage. She spends day after day in a large, hot, noisy warehouse, sewing sleeves in dresses and shirts. Almeada feels lucky to have this job, since the plant has downsized twice. Most of her friends who work do so in the fast-food industry or in local supermarkets in the area.
>
> This summer, baby Anne is watched by a 10-year-old neighbor, Luis, from 7:30 A.M. until 5:30 P.M. Luis takes Anne to the playground each day and watches her while he plays with his friends. When she needs a nap, he puts her down to sleep on the only grassy spot. He changes her once a day at noon and feeds her a bottle of watered juice, a bottle of watered milk, and cut-up hot dogs. The playground is located in a rough neighborhood and is the hangout for one of the many street gangs in the area. Almeada leaves the house at 7:00 A.M. and does not return until 6:30 P.M. During the hours that Luis is not watching Anne, she is alone in her bed in the apartment. Almeada knows that she needs help for herself and Anne. Before she moved from her old neighborhood, Almeada had been seeing a child welfare worker, Barb LaRosa. She plans to call Ms. LaRosa tomorrow from work and hopes Ms. LaRosa will be able to give her some ideas about where to go for help in this new part of the city.

Baby Anne cannot take care of herself. She is one of the many individuals who require human services just to have the necessities of life. Anne lacks adequate food, housing, and developmental opportunities. She is in danger because she does not receive appropriate supervision during the day. There is also some question as to whether Almeada can take care of herself properly. She is only 17, works long hours for little pay, and has the major responsibility of raising a child, although she is little more than a child herself.

Human services recognizes problems such as Almeada's as **problems in living.** As part of this recognition, the focus is not on the past but rather on improving the present and changing the future. Doing so involves directing attention to the client, the environment, and the interaction between the two. Individuals grow and develop through the life cycle, encountering problems in living such as adolescent rebellion, parenthood, mid-life crises, caring for aging parents, and death and dying. Many difficulties in living arise in connection with families and communities; these may involve relating to children, spouses, and parents; maintaining progress in education; adapting to a new culture and language; sustaining performance at work; and assuming responsibility for the very young or the very old. An important aspect of problems in living is the difficulty individuals encounter in interacting with their environments. If unemployment is high, finding work is not easy; if friends and relatives abuse drugs and alcohol, abstaining is difficult; if parents and peers do not value education, choosing to stay in school is problematic; if the family is living in a new country and culture, adjustment is difficult. Human services addresses problems in living, with a focus on both the individual or group and the situation or event. These problems occur throughout the life span.

Anne's mother, Almeada Estrada, was 16 years old when Anne was born. Almeada received her early schooling in Chicago, but quit attending school regularly when she was in the fifth grade. She was held back in the first grade and again in the third grade because she had not mastered basic math and reading skills. Her parents, immigrants to the United States, did not think education was important; in fact, they spoke little English themselves and did not require that Almeada attend school at all. They were both alcoholics, continually unemployed and dependent on Almeada to structure their family life.

By the time Almeada was 10, she had discovered that life was more pleasant away from home. After school, she would spend long hours playing with her friends on the streets; nights, she would spend with girlfriends. She became sexually active at the age of 12 under pressure from her friends, who ridiculed her until she became "one of the gang." At the time she became sexually active, she knew about AIDS but did not understand it as a problem for her.

Between the ages of 12 and 16, Almeada was in constant turmoil, wondering how and where to live her life. She received advice as well as pressure from parents, friends, and teachers to do what they wanted. Occasionally, she was asked to join special programs at school, but her parents would not give their permission. No one was particularly interested in what she wanted to do. She was entangled in a troublesome adolescent rebellion in which she rejected parents and teachers and accepted peers as models. Relating to peers brought unwelcome pressure to go along with the gang.

In responding to the needs of clients, human service professionals are encountering an increasing number of problems to be solved, a rise that many experts attribute partly to a changing culture and lifestyle. This broad increase in problems is another theme in human services.

THE GROWING NUMBER OF PROBLEMS IN THE MODERN WORLD

Human services has emerged in response to the growth in human problems in our modern world. A growing number of people feel alienated and isolated from their neighborhoods and communities. No longer can they count on family and neighbors to share everyday joys and sorrows and assist in times of trouble and crisis. Households are in constant transition, as people leave family and friends to seek new job opportunities. Schools, religious organizations, and recreation centers still provide meeting places, but because of the constant turnover, newcomers are welcoming newcomers. Stress is a hallmark of today's world. We worry about how to feed, clothe, and shelter children, families, adults, and the elderly. Illiteracy, a lack of employable skills, and unemployment rates or low-wage employment add to people's feelings of helplessness and hopelessness, particularly in a technological age.

The lifestyles that were once assured with a good education are no longer guaranteed. People may be trained for jobs that are being phased out or no longer exist. New technology may also cause many to lose their jobs. The world appears smaller as we have increased our capability for global communication. As more information is available, more choices appear possible. At the same time, new sources of worry are the problems of overpopulation, malnutrition, urbanization, and the environment of the planet. There is also threat of nuclear war, terrorism, civil wars and genocide, and religious and social conflict. The media bring vivid pictures of all these problems into the home through television, radio, and the Internet.

> For the past two years, Almeada has felt the weight of daily problems in living. When she was 16, she discovered she was pregnant, and she received this information with mixed feelings. She was familiar with the problems of pregnancy because many of her friends had been pregnant. They often discussed choices, but to Almeada there was only one choice: to have the baby and take care of it. She tried to seek help from a reproductive health agency but was frightened when she had to walk through a picket line of abortion protesters to get there. Of course, she could not expect much support from her parents, who were the only family she had ever known. She could not expect help from the father of her unborn baby or any of the other males in her life; most were just passing through the neighborhood. She was not sure where she would live or how she would support herself, but she knew that she would make it.

Almeada lives in a complex world with little support. An effective human service delivery system will teach her to use the skills she needs to manage her own life and survive the difficult challenges that face her. This **self-sufficiency** is another theme of human services.

SELF-SUFFICIENCY

For many human service professionals, the key to successful service delivery is providing clients, or consumers of human services, with the opportunity and support to be self-sufficient. Economic self-sufficiency strengthens an individual's self-esteem.

BOX 1.1 | INTERNATIONAL FOCUS: *TEEN PREGNANCY*

Teen pregnancy rates in the United States were once the highest among developed countries. These rates have fallen steadily during the past decade for all racial and ethnic groups, including non-Hispanic white teens, black non-Hispanic teens, and Hispanic teens. Even so, of the one million teens who become pregnant each year, approximately 80% are unintended. Whether planned or unplanned, teen mothers are more disadvantaged than are other teens and have children who face negative health, cognitive, and behavior outcomes. *Healthy People 2010,* a federal initiative to improve health in the United States, includes a goal to reduce teen pregnancy among 15–17-year-old adolescent females.

In developed countries adolescent or teen pregnancy generally refers to girls younger than 18 years of age, most of whom are not married, and is considered a social issue. By contrast, teens in developing countries are often married, and the pregnancy may be accepted and welcomed. Unfortunately, in combination with malnutrition and poor health care, the pregnancy may lead to medical problems.

Sub-Saharan Africa has the highest incidence of teenage pregnancy in the world with 143 pregnancies per 1,000 girls aged 15–19 years. Generally speaking, women in Africa marry at much younger ages than women elsewhere and have earlier pregnancies. Of the 10 countries identified by Save the Children as places where motherhood carries the most risk for mother and baby, nine were in sub-Saharan Africa.

The situation in South Asia is similar: Early age at marriage means high adolescent pregnancy rates. This is truer in rural areas where knowledge and use of contraceptive methods is low. Some areas such as Indonesia and Malaysia are experiencing a decrease in the rate of early marriage and pregnancy, yet the rate remains high when compared with the rest of Asia.

In some areas of the world little information is available on sexual behavior. This is the case in the Pacific Islands although teen pregnancy is considered an emerging problem.

Regardless of location or society, there are some common outcomes of teenage pregnancy. One is the higher incidence of premature birth and low birthweight. For the baby, other problems may include developmental disabilities, behavioral issues, and poor academic performance. Daughters are more likely to become teen mothers, and sons are more likely to serve time in prison. Outcomes for the mother are lack of education, poverty, and a second child within 24 months.

When these individuals are able to contribute financially to meeting their own basic needs for food, clothing, and shelter, they gain a certain degree of independence, but they may still need some assistance. One important facet of moving clients to self-sufficiency is to empower them to make decisions and assume responsibility for their actions. Human services is committed to giving individuals and groups sufficient assistance to allow them to help themselves. Clients are encouraged to be independent and gain control of their lives as soon as they are able. They gain belief in themselves or the efficacy to make the changes needed to become self-sufficient.

It was difficult for Almeada to become economically self-sufficient when she was 16, barely educated, and pregnant. She had little parental guidance or support and few skills. She was forced to move back home to live with her parents and seek the little help they could give her. In fact, she began taking care of them again. She got a job as a cashier at the local grocery store. Almeada saved a few dollars a week and bought groceries for the family with the rest. Her parents tried to borrow money from her to buy alcohol; they took her money if she brought it home.

In the early days of her pregnancy, Almeada's life became routine. She worked from 8 A.M. to 5 P.M., walked home, prepared dinner, and visited with her friends later at night. Her advancing pregnancy changed her relationships with some of her friends because she did not have the stamina or the desire to share their evening activities. Even as her life changed, she was determined that no one would interfere with it; she did not want help. Almeada wanted to make her own decisions. Despite that fiercely independent attitude, she would soon need assistance.

Almeada was somewhat self-sufficient because she was working and her parents provided housing. As her pregnancy advanced, however, she had to quit work and rely on others. She also needed prenatal care, parenting skills, and an opportunity to assess her decision to keep the baby. Although economic self-sufficiency is a key for many clients, it would clearly be only a beginning for Almeada.

Social Care, Social Control, and Rehabilitation

Human services serves three distinct functions: social care, social control, and rehabilitation (Neugeboren, 1991). **Social care** is assisting clients in meeting their social needs, with the focus on those who cannot care for themselves. The elderly, children, people with mental disabilities or mental illness, and victims of crime, disasters, or crises are populations who might need social care.

Social control differs from social care in two fundamental ways: who receives the services and under what conditions they receive them. Social care is given to those who cannot provide for themselves (either temporarily or in the long term). In contrast, most recipients of social control are able to care for themselves but have either failed to do so or have done so in a manner that violates society's norms for appropriate behavior. Often society, rather than the individual, determines who receives services that represent social control. The purpose of such services is to restrict or monitor clients' independence for a time because the clients have violated laws of the community. Children, youth, and adults in the criminal justice system are examples of clients of social control.

Rehabilitation is the task of returning an individual to a prior level of functioning. What creates the need for rehabilitation? An individual who was once able to live independently becomes unable to function socially, physically, or psychologically. The inability to function can be caused by a crisis, a reversal of economic or social circumstances, an accident, or other circumstances. Rehabilitative services, which are designed to enable the individual to function near or at a prior level of independence, can have a short- or long-term focus. Veterans, people with physical disabilities, and victims of psychological trauma are among those who receive rehabilitative human services.

In actuality, separating these three functions of human services is often difficult. Many clients have multiple problems, so social care, social control, and rehabilitation may be occurring at the same time.

Almeada finally became involved in the human service system in mid-autumn, when she was seven months pregnant. She refused to go to school. Her parents let her continue to work at the neighborhood store—in fact, they encouraged her to. Life was easier for them when she was available to translate for them and help with their daily living needs. Her friends often missed school as well, so she saw them every day when they came to the grocery store to do their shopping. At evening, they all gathered at a shop in the neighborhood.

Two new programs were started at Almeada's school to provide more comprehensive support to many of its students. One program—Students, Parents Are Receiving

KARE (SPARK)—targeted students who had irregular attendance, low math and reading scores, no discipline record, and positive teacher reports. In the fall, the school officials noted that Almeada, who qualified for this new program, had not returned to school after the summer vacation. The second program—Students, Parents Each Are Special (SPEAS)—provided health care and other services to teen mothers. The case manager of SPARK, Barb LaRosa, visited the most recent address on the school records and found Almeada's father at home. He was in a drunken stupor and was unable to give Barb information about Almeada. When Ms. LaRosa talked to the neighbors, they suggested she try the grocery store where Almeada worked. Ms. LaRosa found Almeada in the middle of her daily shift and made an appointment to pick her up after work and take her home.

In the next few months, Barb LaRosa provided social care for Almeada and then for her baby, Anne. The school offered Almeada several options for continuing her education: She could receive homebound instruction until and after the baby was born; she could come back to school; or she could attend a special night school for potential dropouts who work during the day. Ms. LaRosa also referred Almeada to the SPEAS program. Almeada attended a prenatal care class taught by a local teacher one night a week at the school. Because of Almeada's youth and lack of parental support, Ms. LaRosa discussed with Almeada the options of keeping the baby or placing it for adoption. She also took Almeada to the health clinic located in the school to discuss these options further. Almeada remained sure that she wanted to keep her child. Ms. LaRosa introduced Almeada to the welfare worker who was available on school grounds one day a week. Almeada rejected welfare as an option.

Once the baby was born, Almeada needed rehabilitative assistance but, instead, returned to work immediately. She expected her parents to care for Anne while she was gone, but her parents refused to babysit. Almeada was afraid that one day they might harm Anne out of their own frustrations. Her parents could not stand to have the baby in the home because they had to compete with her for attention. Instead of receiving rehabilitative services, Almeada moved to a new neighborhood, rented a one-room apartment, and found a new job working in a garment factory six days a week. In her new neighborhood, Almeada again had neither human service support nor social support.

The story of Almeada's struggles and need for assistance is just one of many about individuals who cannot meet their own needs without assistance from others. A common element seen in all human services is that these services help individuals, families, and groups with their problems. There would be little need for these services if people did not need assistance and support from others. The term *human services* encompasses the variety of helping services that address the range of problems that people experience.

The themes and purposes of human services—problems in living, the growing number of problems, self-sufficiency, and social care, social control, and rehabilitation—contribute to a definition of human services. Examining the contributions of different disciplines also helps define human services.

THE INTERDISCIPLINARY NATURE OF HUMAN SERVICES

The study of human service delivery, an understanding of the professionals who deliver services, and familiarity with the clients who are recipients of services requires the integration of knowledge from a wide variety of academic disciplines. These disciplines include but are not limited to sociology, psychology, and anthropology.

TABLE 1.1	SUMMARY POINTS: ALMEADA'S CASE

- Both Almeada and baby Anne experience problems in living because their needs for adequate food, housing, and education are not met.

- Almeada's world is complex and she had little support during her pregnancy and after Anne's birth.

- Self-sufficiency was easier for Almeada when she was working, but her needs soon outgrew her resources.

- Social care provided Almeada with several choices to continue her education.

- Social control was not part of Almeada's case history because she maintained her independence throughout the pregnancy.

- Following Anne's birth, Almeada returned to work, moved, and found a new job rather than receive rehabilitative services.

Each discipline brings a unique perspective to the understanding of the nature of the individual, families, and groups of people. In addition, they focus upon the context of the environment in which "daily living" occurs and the interaction between the two.

> While Barb LaRosa was working with Almeada, she knew that it was important to understand as best as she could about Almeada and her environment. The program in which Ms. LaRosa received her training required her to take a large number of social science courses. According to her instructors, in order to understand the complexities of human behavior within the social environment, the study of sociology, psychology, and anthropology is helpful.

Sociology, as a discipline, examines the ways in which human societies influence the people who live in these societies. In other words, sociology assesses the individual and the broader culture, and tries to account for and understand the differences within human culture. Some of these differences are described very simply: "The Chinese wear white to funerals, whereas people in the United States prefer black. People in England and the United States say a watch 'runs' whereas the Spanish say it 'walks' and the Germans say it 'functions'" ("What is sociology," n.d.). Sociology helps human service professionals understand elements of life that affect living, such as family structure, family roles, gender, race, and poverty.

According to the American Psychological Association, "Psychology is the study of the mind and behavior. The discipline embraces all aspects of the human experience—from the functions of the brain to the actions of nations, from child development to care for the aged. In every conceivable setting from scientific research centers to mental health care services, 'the understanding of behavior' is the enterprise of psychologists" (American Psychological Association, 2006). Many individuals believe that psychology helps explain "what makes people tick." Numerous theories examine how people think, feel, and behave and explores why they think, feel, and behave in the ways in which they do. These theories analyze behavior and mental processes from the physiological, behavioral, cognitive, and psychodynamic perspectives. As they study psychology, students use these theories to develop a better understanding of people.

BOX 1.2 | WEB SOURCES: *FIND OUT MORE ABOUT MEETING ALMEADA'S NEEDS*

http://www.kidscount.org

The Annie E. Casey Foundation website has an online database about children that allows the reader to create custom maps, profiles, graphs, and rankings nationally and state-by-state.

http://www.jstor.org

This website is for a research journal, *Family Planning Perspectives*. Family planning is broadly defined to include contraceptive practices, adolescent pregnancy, abortion, and public policies.

http://www.acf.dhhs.gov

This website is for the Department of Health and Human Services. This department administers the major federal programs that provide services for children and families, such as Head Start and Temporary Assistance to Needy Families

(TANF). This site has information about these programs as well as fact sheets and statistical information relating to children and families.

http://www.childrennow.org

Children Now disseminates information on children's issues, especially children and the media. This site has statistics on the status of children, polls on children's attitudes, research on television and the media, the *Media Now* newsletter, action alerts, and many links to sources of statistics and to education, safety, parenting, and governmental information.

http://www.futureofchildren.org

The goal of the Future of Children website is to provide the research and analysis to promote effective policies and programs for children.

Anthropology studies the cultural, physical, and social development of humans and the variation in their customs and beliefs. A critical component of the study of anthropology is fieldwork. Anthropologists often live at the site they are studying as they try to learn about human groups and the role of culture in the lives of the individuals within these groups.

Today anthropologists study culture in its broadest sense. Not only are they studying about such groups who live in remote areas of the globe, but also they are studying individuals in mainstream culture in diverse settings. Similar to the tasks of the organizational psychologist, anthropologists are working in the business environment and studying topics such as the culture of work, employee relations, and human resources. In other words, they are learning about employee problems on the job by learning about employee perceptions and behavior. Directly related to human services are projects that help bring more clarity about the clients served. For example, one project may focus on individuals with AIDS. Another may explore the life and problems of the homeless in contemporary society.

As Barb LaRosa tried to think about Almeada and her new life with baby Anne, she realized that the young woman's life would change as she moved away from her neighborhood, her friends, and her parents—and Barb LaRosa was worried about her. For many years Barb has been able to use the information she learned in school to understand her clients and the situations they face. Almeada would be struggling to care for baby Anne and herself without a social support network or formal human services. In fact, Almeada would not even speak Spanish, the primary language spoken in the neighborhood. Even though Almeada was strong and determined, the difficult environment within which she was living would present challenges that would be difficult to meet without help.

The work of human service delivery is an interdisciplinary endeavor that requires knowledge of individuals, an understanding of society and its relationship to individual and family life, and a view of the culture in which people live. Helpers like Barb LaRosa often work with clients who are very different from themselves. By integrating disciplines such as sociology, psychology, and anthropology, human service professionals can better understand the nature of their clients and their environments. This allows them to understand and relate to their clients more effectively.

THE RELATIONSHIP BETWEEN CLIENT AND HELPER

The delivery of human services involves both the client and the helper. The process of helping is client oriented as the helper focuses on assisting clients to meet their needs. To do this, the helper performs many roles and assumes a wide variety of responsibilities. Let us look at Almeada and her human service worker, Barb LaRosa, to see the helping relationship in action.

> When Barb LaRosa first approached Almeada, she talked at length with Almeada about her situation. Barb had contacted Almeada to learn whether she would come back to school and to help her with problems that were barriers to her school attendance. After they talked, it was obvious that Almeada faced many problems. Barb planned to work with Almeada, baby Anne, and Almeada's parents if they would accept the help. First, Barb wanted to introduce Almeada to services available at school, because Almeada and her parents were familiar with the school context.

At one time, a worker in Barb LaRosa's position would have focused on school-related issues; she would not have assessed Almeada's needs in other areas or referred her to other services. She might have told Almeada about other human service agencies, but Almeada would have had to contact them on her own. Today, human service professionals assist the whole person and empower clients to help themselves. Barb LaRosa was not able to meet all Almeada's needs, but she did work actively to connect her with other human service agencies in and outside of the school setting. In fact, multiple services at school reflect a current trend in human services to integrate client services. Barb LaRosa was providing assistance to Almeada and Anne, who need help with their social, psychological, and economic problems. She also was coordinating the care that Almeada and Anne received.

As a human service professional, Barb LaRosa has the skills to develop a relationship with Almeada. In this situation, much of Ms. LaRosa's success is dependent on her personal interaction with Almeada and her ability to use professional skills such as active listening, observation, and assessment to establish a relationship. She is also able to apply her problem-solving skills to address the needs of Almeada and Anne. Using the problem-solving process, she initiates human service delivery by considering the relationship of her client with the environment and other professionals in the human service delivery system.

> Barb LaRosa, the human service professional who helped Almeada, was a very effective helper. First, although she was employed by the school system, she was able to work with other professionals to develop a plan of assistance for Almeada and Anne, using the existing human service organizations for their benefit. Second, she established a helping relationship with Almeada and worked to understand Almeada's perspective. Third, Barb had the ability to engage in problem solving with Almeada and to recommend alternatives. She took a special interest in Almeada, provided a structure for Almeada's service plan, and linked Almeada with other organizations. For Barb LaRosa, Almeada was an important person, and one to be treated with respect and dignity.

The Client and the Client's Environment

Individuals who receive help do not exist in a vacuum; they are active participants in many different systems that influence their circumstances. Services to the client must be delivered with an understanding of the client's culture and with the client's participation. To be effective, the human service professional must ask the client questions about present conditions, current stresses and relationships, and everyday events. The helper listens to the client, always attempting to see a situation through the client's eyes. Questioning and listening should help the human service professional understand the client's world. The helper must show both a strong commitment to the client and concern for the client's well-being. The helper also assists the client in identifying personal strengths and limitations and developing new skills and abilities to enhance personal development.

Human service professionals also function as educators. As educators, these professionals help clients develop certain skills to increase their intellectual, emotional, and behavioral options. The client is a complex individual with many intellectual, emotional, and behavioral possibilities. Clients feel better about themselves when human service professionals treat them as thinking, feeling, and acting human beings who are capable of change. If the human service professional believes in and promotes change, then change will be easier for the client.

In many situations the human service professional helps the client learn how to use the problem-solving process. The purpose of performing the teaching role is to empower the client to solve future problems independently of the human service professional or agency. This leads to clients who begin to operate with increasing independence and self-esteem.

> Almeada now lives in her new neighborhood with her daughter, Anne, and works six days a week in a garment factory. She knows she needs help. Because her major contact has been with human service professionals in another neighborhood, she does not really know who to call, so she calls her previous worker, Barb LaRosa.
>
> Ms. LaRosa is delighted to hear from Almeada again and is alarmed at her plight. Almeada talks of her current work and child-care situation in depressed and hopeless terms. Almeada seems to feel that she has limited options, especially since most of her neighbors speak little English, and Barb wants to refer Almeada to a source that can help increase those options. She tells Almeada that she will make a few phone calls and then call her back. Barb also wants to bolster Almeada's confidence in herself. As she gathers information about Almeada's move, her new employment, and her care of Anne, she praises Almeada's responsibility and maturity. She helps Almeada see how she has been a successful problem solver, reinforcing her strengths. She also praises Almeada's calling her and reaching out for help. Ms. LaRosa knows that any positive change Almeada can make will help solve the rest of her problems.

A function of the human service professional is to help clients develop their ability to assess fundamental needs and to focus on the problems early in the helping process. Abraham Maslow, a psychologist, described a hierarchy of human needs that begins with basic physical needs and rises through higher levels to address safety and security needs, social belonging needs, self needs, and finally, self-actualization needs at the highest level. He stressed that addressing higher-level needs is difficult unless an individual's basic needs have been met (Maslow, 1971). In other words, if a child is

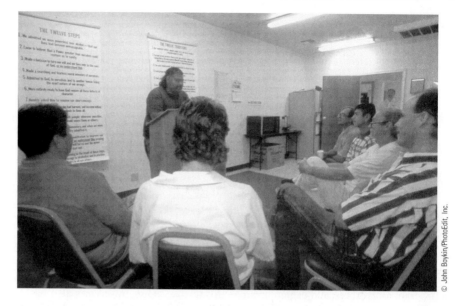

© John Boykin/PhotoEdit, Inc.

hungry or very tired, or an adult is very scared, that child or that adult will have difficulty focusing on needs related to belonging or self-actualization. Clients are often so overwhelmed by their situations that they do not know how to identify what they need or where to begin to look for help or solutions. A good place to start is with the most basic needs, which are often the simplest to address and give the client satisfaction early in the helping process.

As an educator, the helper also teaches clients to recognize how their physical and interpersonal environments affect them. Clients are responsible for their own thoughts and behavior. Sometimes, however, clients are unable to make changes because their environments do not support such changes. Clients must be taught to determine the influence their environments have on their lives and to assess when and how their environments can be changed. Sometimes, such changes are very difficult or impossible.

In summary, an important conception of human services is the relationship between the helper and the client. The helper is committed to developing a relationship with the client that facilitates problem solving within the client's own environment. Many times the human service professional is also an educator who is teaching the client important skills that can be used long after the helping relationship has ended.

MANAGEMENT PRINCIPLES IN HUMAN SERVICE DELIVERY

Understanding how services are delivered is an important part of defining human services. Three principles of management related to the delivery of services characterize the profession today: networking to develop a human service umbrella, forming teams and partnerships to provide service, and using case management to facilitate client growth. These management strategies help professionals provide more effective and efficient assistance to clients as well as enhance their own work environment.

BOX 1.3 | A PIONEER IN HUMAN SERVICES

Dr. Harold McPheeters, a psychiatrist by training, is considered a key figure in the development of human service education. After serving as an administrator in the department of mental health in two states, he joined the Southern Regional Education Board (SREB) in 1965 as director for the Commission on Mental Health and Human Services and director of health programs.

His work began with a planning grant to bring together mental health professionals and community college officials to explore the feasibility of educating mental health practitioners in two-year colleges. That grant provided the groundwork for 20 years of research and training in the mental health and human service field. Defining the concept of the generalist worker, providing support for training mental health/human service professionals, developing a certification program for workers, and beginning an approval process for training programs were efforts completed under Dr. McPheeters's leadership and with his support. Before his retirement from the SREB in September 1987, Dr. McPheeters wrote (at our request) the following definition of human services, based on his 30 years of experience in the field. His definition integrates many of the ideas that have been presented.

I never came up with an absolute definition of human services. Originally, our work began with the associate degree programs that were training people to work in some aspect of mental health. However, it soon became apparent that the graduates of those programs and the graduates of other programs that were titled according to other human service fields, such as child care workers, youth service workers, and aging program workers, were all finding employment in a variety of human service fields—not just in the narrow subspecialty areas of mental health, addiction, aging, and so on. So the terminology began to change to "human services" although no very precise definitions were applied.... Human services works with those same problems and people, but with a blend of primarily psychological and sociological theories and principles. Human services also has an eclectic approach to collaborating with whatever approaches (for example, medical) are needed to help people solve their problems. I suppose my definition would be something like this: Human services is the occupation/profession that uses a blend of primarily psychological and sociological theories and skills in preventing, detecting, and ameliorating psychosocially dysfunctioning people and in helping them attain the highest level of psychosocial functioning of which they are capable.

NETWORKING TO DEVELOP A HUMAN SERVICE UMBRELLA

Human services is not a single service delivery system but a complex web of helping agencies and organizations whose primary goal is to assist people in need. It encompasses a variety of services that include but are not limited to child, youth, and family services; corrections; mental health; public health; crisis intervention; and education (see Figure 1.1).

Karin Eriksen (1981), a founding scholar in human service education, notes that "human services is often called the umbrella for our society's professions which are involved either directly or indirectly in promoting and reinforcing satisfying, healthy living and community cohesiveness" (p. 8). Going beyond the metaphor of the umbrella, Eriksen describes human services as a "bridge" between people and systems. One function of bridging is to narrow the gap between the services being offered and the needs of the individuals who are receiving those services.

Another bridging responsibility is to link human service agencies. Agencies and organizations share the common goal of assisting people in need. In the past,

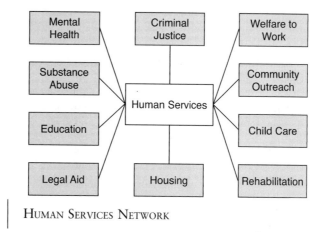

FIGURE 1.1 | HUMAN SERVICES NETWORK

there has been little coordination, and the result has been overlapping professional responsibilities and competition for resources. Today, as service delivery philosophy changes and resources become scarce, agencies are limiting services, tightening eligibility criteria, and focusing on short-term interventions. Only increased communication, cooperation, and collaboration among helpers and agencies can promote effective service delivery. **Networking** is one way that service providers work together to serve clients.

> Barb LaRosa wants to help Almeada in her new neighborhood, and she knows that finding a good entry into the system is critical. Ms. LaRosa worries that, without the right help, Almeada will be lost in the human service delivery system. She needs to find another professional who is familiar with Almeada's neighborhood human service system and knows the formal and informal linkages that need to be made to deliver multiple services. She is looking for a worker who will help Almeada move between the many agencies whose services she will require.
>
> Almeada needs the support of those who provide child care and teach parenting skills. In addition, she needs assistance in improving her work skills and health. Vocational development and public health services are rarely offered together. Coordination, monitoring, and evaluation are key services that are needed. Where will Barb LaRosa locate such a professional?

For Almeada or any other client to assume the responsibility of negotiating, the networking would be difficult; human service professionals must build the bridges between agencies, organizations, and services. Working together to provide services for the good of the client is often called **teaming** and is another management tool used for delivering good quality services to the client.

FORMING TEAMS AND PARTNERSHIPS TO PROVIDE SERVICES

Working as a team to provide services is part of the history of human services. Developers of the human service movement from early in its history stressed the importance of working with other professionals to assist the client in receiving services. More recently, the concept of working as a team has expanded, and "teaming" has become a common approach to organizing the work of an agency or organization.

> After talking to several child and youth services offices, Barb LaRosa contacted Hernando Alvarez, a case manager in the child services division of the state department of human services. He recommended that Almeada call his office and schedule a meeting with an intake worker. His office, just recently reorganized to be more customer oriented, was open for intake and service from 7 A.M. to 10 P.M. Mondays through Thursdays and on Saturdays from 8 A.M. until noon. Almeada would be assigned to a case manager who would not provide services but would coordinate them. In addition, four other workers would help plan, implement, and evaluate work with Almeada. A backup case manager would also know Almeada's case in detail and be available to support her if her primary case manager was absent.
>
> This particular team treats the entire human service delivery system as a larger team. They cooperate with each organization, sharing problems and finding creative solutions that benefit clients. One warning that Mr. Alvarez gave was the uncertainty of the agency's funding because of the evaluation of welfare return efforts. He hoped that Almeada would not get lost in the possible changes. At the conclusion of her conversation with Mr. Alvarez, Barb LaRosa felt she could make a good referral for Almeada, and she made a promise to herself to contact Hernando Alvarez in two months to check on her client's progress.

The primary beneficiary of teaming in a human service setting is the client. The team approach yields more efficient and more effective service. As suggested in the case of Almeada, many professionals, functioning as a group, are working together to provide creative, coordinated services. Such teams are able to evaluate their own performance and make changes to improve their service delivery. The bottom line is improving the delivery of services to clients.

Partnerships are also emerging as a way that organizations in the human service delivery system can work together to serve their clients more completely. These partnerships are formed when two or more human service organizations agree to work together toward common goals. In addition, partnerships form with corporations, businesses, and government entities as those organizations outside the human service delivery system see benefits in supporting the social service sector. Partnering requires many of the same qualities as teaming: a high degree of cooperation, a commitment of time, and a high level of trust. When partnering is successful, there is mutual gain for each of the parties involved.

The concept of partnership has emerged as a way for human service organizations to relate to each other for several reasons. Many of them are financial. As the cost of service provision increases and available financial resources decrease, many organizations are finding that they can provide services more cost effectively when they work with other agencies. Partnerships have also been encouraged by the increasing pressure to be accountable for resources expended. Agencies find that combining their resources and expertise enables them to provide better services to their clients.

> Hernando Alvarez contacted Almeada the day after he talked with Barb LaRosa. Rather than place the burden of contacting the state department of human services (DHS) on Almeada, he went to see her at her workplace. He explained that Ms. LaRosa had called him and that he was interested in working with Almeada

TABLE 1.2	SUMMARY POINTS: ALMEADA'S CASE

- Integrating different social science perspectives helps human service professionals understand clients and their environments.

- Barbara LaRosa illustrates the importance of integrating and coordinating services as she teaches Almeada about problem solving and the influence of her environment on her life.

- Barbara LaRosa's networking skills are useful in locating a human service professional who is knowledgeable about services in Almeada's new neighborhood.

- Almeada benefits from the creative, coordinated services provided by Hernando Alvarez and his team.

- A case management approach to Almeada's situation involves both providing and co-ordinating services.

to decide what services she needed and to help her find a way to access those services.

Because the department had partnerships with many businesses and industries, he was able to schedule a time when he could meet with Almeada at her business site. Her employer had a small office for DHS workers and encouraged his employees to use the services the agency made available. Hernando knew that some services could be provided very quickly; others would evolve more slowly.

Hernando Alvarez and other DHS workers increased their ability to work effectively with clients through their partnership agreements with many local corporations and businesses. For DHS and other agencies, partnerships are usually established at the organizational level and are marked by a general statement of agreement that two or more organizations will work together. The text of the agreement contains language similar to the following: "This statement represents an acknowledgment by Organization A and Organization B of their mutual interest in forming a joint, long-term cooperative relationship whose purpose would be to encourage interaction between the two organizations." Later, the organizations work together to find specific projects and activities that would invite mutual support, and in Almeada's case, her employer encourages DHS to support his employees.

Just as teaming and partnerships have emerged as powerful tools to improve the delivery of human services, another tool, the role and responsibility of case management, is emerging as a way to expand services available to meet the needs of the multiproblem or long-term client.

CASE MANAGEMENT

Several factors make **case management** a viable alternative for service delivery today. One is the shift from large, state-operated institutions to smaller, community-based facilities. This shift gives special importance to interorganizational coordination, a team approach, and helping professionals with a concern for the whole person because services are not being assessed or delivered in one comprehensive system.

A second factor is the categorical public funding of the past, which resulted in highly complex, redundant, fragmented, and uncoordinated services. The resulting system is burdensome for people with complex problems who are least able to act as advocates for themselves. In many cases, multiproblem clients are assigned a different worker within a given agency for each service and different workers in different agencies. Often there is no central worker who knows and understands the client's total situation or who is responsible for planning and coordinating treatment strategies.

A third factor is the very nature of human service work today. Service providers increasingly find themselves with a dual role: providing direct services and coordinating services from other agencies and/or professionals. Thom Prassa likens having a caseload to being an air traffic controller, coordinating and sometimes juggling many different cases. On a case-by-case basis, he often feels like he is "parachuting into a fire. We put out fires all the time: suicide attempts, arranging placements, paperwork, talking with parents, and so forth" (personal communication). This dual role can create problems in terms of time management, effective and efficient service delivery, and quality assurance.

The goal of case managers is to teach those who need assistance to manage their own lives but to support them when expertise is needed or a crisis occurs. In reality, the use of case management is expanding rapidly into areas unheard of five years ago. Long-term care involving work with individuals encountering problems associated with aging, mental illness, disability, and mental retardation uses case management as a method of coordinating and delivering services. A new use of case management is to link it with outreach functions to service targeted populations, such as prenatal care for low-income, inner-city women; grandparents raising grandchildren; and substance abusers.

What exactly do case managers do? They gather information, make assessments, and monitor services. In addition, they arrange services from other agencies, provide advocacy service, and assume responsibility for allocating scarce resources and providing quality assurance. They also provide direct services. Many human service professionals believe that being a case manager means they will do whatever they must to help their clients.

The case management structure affects both coordination of services and client access to services. Given the fragmented state of service delivery and claims of coordination that are not borne out in practice, what is needed is interorganizational and interagency coordination that does not shuffle clients from one office to another. Exchanging resources rather than clients would ensure that clients do not get lost in the system or become frustrated with service delivery. Another necessary structural change is the establishment of a single point of access rather than entry points at each agency. Another approach is to introduce clients to an array of community services. True coordination and integration allow clients to proceed through central intake, have their needs assessed, and be assigned to providers.

Part of preparing for case management is learning to be proactive. Problems today call for professionals who understand the need for case management and have the skills to perform effectively in that role. As case manager positions increase, human service professionals will be ready to assume that responsibility; but equally important, those trained as case managers will help develop organizational structures in which case management can work. We need professionals within the **human service system** who are able to promote these changes. The management principles described in the preceding paragraphs define the emerging context in which human services are being delivered. Equally important to understanding human services is knowing the broad range of agencies and organizations that provide these services.

ROLES AND ACTIVITIES OF THE HUMAN SERVICE PROFESSIONAL

The human service professional provides services in a variety of settings. To respond to the many settings and the diversity of clients these settings represent, the helper needs a broad-based education and a willingness to adapt to changing roles and circumstances.

THE GENERALIST

The concept of the **generalist** is fundamental to human services. It describes the kinds of skills the professional has and the types of functions the professional performs. The term *generalist* has not always been associated with human services; the concept has evolved over the last few decades. Early in the history of human services, the term referred to a person who worked within a specific discipline, such as psychology or psychiatry. Professionals in these disciplines performed many functions: interviewing, diagnosis, therapy, and follow-up. As a generalist, the professional performed all the duties expected of a member of that particular profession.

As the role expanded, the term took on a new meaning, connected to a specific client group. Generalists performed duties and had the skills to work with only one group. For example, youth mental health workers specialized in working with children. This would include working with individuals and with groups in educational, recreational, and counseling situations. Such workers would also be familiar with social, biological, and developmental problems of children and adolescents; they would also understand the importance of working with the family.

A third emerging concept of the generalist is most representative of human services today. The human service generalist has the knowledge, values, and skills to perform several job functions in most human service settings. The generalist also understands how these functions fit with client and agency goals. For example, a helper trained to conduct interviews, write social histories, and define a treatment plan should be able to perform those responsibilities with the elderly, young children, or people with mental retardation.

The human service generalist works with the client using both micro and macro perspectives. The micro system is represented by the individuals in the client's environment and might include family, friends, teachers, coworkers, and individuals within the human service delivery system. The macro system is represented by the organizations, agencies, communities, and neighborhood locales with which the client interacts. For example, if the human service professional is working with the individual client using the micro perspective, then the professional is interviewing the client, establishing rapport, and engaging in planning and problem solving. Using the macro perspective, the same professional works with the client to understand his or her larger environment. This might include learning how to use the human service bureaucracy to convert needs into political action or to understand how school relates to the neighborhood. It is interesting to examine follow-up studies of graduates of human service programs to see the development of the generalist concept as well as the broadening definition of human services.

Early studies compiled by the Southern Regional Education Board indicated that graduates of human service programs were getting jobs in state hospitals, educational settings, mental health centers, children's agencies, and general hospitals. Three-fourths of the jobs were in mental health agencies. Although these graduates were performing a wide range of services, most were indirect services dealing with patients and other staff members. Their job functions were client advocacy, community consultation, and collecting basic research data—in other words, working from the macro perspective (Southern Regional Education Board, 1979).

Studies of graduates of human service programs since 1972 differ significantly from the earlier surveys. The results reflect a diversity of employment settings for graduates, including state hospitals, mental health centers, centers for the developmentally disabled, schools, child and family services centers, correctional facilities, nursing homes and other service facilities for the aging, abuse prevention and treatment centers, recreation centers, centers for people with physical disabilities, crisis intervention units, child- and elder-abuse prevention and treatment centers, group homes, and specialized fund-raising organizations. The job functions of these graduates include direct service activities, group and individual counseling, patient advocacy, interviewing, referral, gathering and recording information, treatment planning, discharge, follow-up, grant writing, fund-raising, and administration. These responsibilities reflect work within both the micro and the macro perspectives.

Future job opportunities for human service graduates are expected to be excellent and will continue to reflect the generic nature of helping. The expanding elderly population, which will be discussed in Chapter 3, will require many more human services. Other diverse employment settings for human service graduates include employee assistance programs, funeral homes, and shopping malls.

ACTIVITIES OF THE HUMAN SERVICE PROFESSIONAL

The professional activities of the human service helper are often discussed in the professional literature and are defined by the helper's relationship with clients and other professionals, academic training, ethical standards, continuing education, and measured competence. Human service professionals often work with individuals who have few material possessions and little emotional support and who need many professional services and much professional care. The human service professional is often the first to provide support when the client enters the system. Clients become involved with helpers because they hope for a better existence. They view human service professionals as important people with special information and skills to help them identify and work toward their goals.

A human service professional's activities include academic training founded on a systematic body of knowledge. Academic preparation for human services takes either two or four years, depending on the training program. This intense training, academically and experientially based, focuses on the acquisition of knowledge and skills pertinent to human service systems, professionals, and clients. The training is also systematic. It begins with the study of introductory concepts of human services, then explores types of clients, problems, and methods of addressing those problems, and culminates in supervised field experiences. The body of knowledge on which the training is based is interdisciplinary, drawn from other helping fields including psychology, criminology, rehabilitation, counseling, and social work. Human service field practice is unique in its diversity of settings and populations; however, the basic helping skills and methods of addressing client needs are both unique to human services and borrowed from other helping professions. Trained as generalists, human service professionals are thus taught knowledge and skills that can be transferred to diverse settings and populations. Even the guiding theories and principles include knowledge and values from disciplines such as psychology, sociology, biology, and anthropology. Practitioners need such a multidimensional approach to deal with the complex individuals and environments they encounter.

The good relationship the human service professional has with other social service professionals is a measure of the status of human services. Other helpers work with human service professionals side by side in a professional setting. For some, this professional is the one individual who is specifically designated to focus on the client's mental health and to coordinate social care.

In a nursing home, for example, the human service professional admits the client, takes a social history, monitors and facilitates the client's adjustment, coordinates services with family needs, counsels the client during troubled times, and attends treatment team meetings with the staff to discuss the client's admission, progress, and discharge. Other professionals, including physical therapists, physicians, nurses, and pharmacists, focus on the client's physical health. These professionals look to the human service worker to address the client's mental health needs, which may involve support or referral to a specialist. In other settings, the human service worker is one of many mental health professionals. In a mental health institution, for example, psychiatrists, psychiatric nurses, psychiatric social workers, psychologists, human service workers, and psychiatric technicians all focus on the mental health of the client. Each of these professionals has a particular function within this setting, and each relies on the others to perform their appropriate tasks effectively. For clients and other social service providers, the work of human service professionals is essential.

Ethical standards also define professional human service activities. Human service professionals are committed to the ethical treatment of clients and the development of

TABLE 1.3 | SUMMARY POINTS: PROFESSIONAL ACTIVITIES

- Acquire the knowledge and skills that can be transferred across settings and populations.
- Establish good working relationships with other professionals.
- Abide by the ethical standards that guide professional behavior.
- Pursue continuing education opportunities to learn and develop as a professional.

---

ethical relationships with coworkers, other professionals, and the system. Ethical standards guide this behavior. Because clients are the central focus in human services, their treatment and rights are of great concern, including issues of confidentiality and respect for the client's values, heritage, beliefs, and self-determination. Human service professionals are usually bound by two sets of ethical standards: those developed by human service professionals and educators, and those developed specifically for the populations they serve. See Chapter 9 for the Ethical Standards of Human Service Professionals.

Another important professional activity of human service professionals is continuing education. A commitment to continued learning and development while working in the field is essential for such professionals. This continuing education takes many forms. According to follow-up studies of human service program graduates, many seek advanced degrees. More than half the graduates of two-year programs seek a bachelor's degree—most often in human services, psychology, sociology, criminal justice, or related fields. Graduates of four-year human service programs seek master's degrees in social work, public health administration, nursing, counseling, educational psychology, rehabilitation, and related fields. Human service professionals also continue their education by belonging to professional organizations. Many of these organizations are related to the specific fields in which their members work or the specific population they serve. A final way human service professionals grow and develop is through in-service training. Many agencies sponsor seminars on current social or policy issues, on skill development, or on professional issues. Agencies that do not offer such seminars often encourage their workers to attend seminars sponsored by others.

In the mid-1990s, the federal government took on a project to establish standards for a number of emerging professions. The Human Service Research Institute (HSRI) was given the responsibility for researching the current status of human service occupations and describing the contemporary workplace within the human service delivery system. This project developed for human service practitioners skill standards, activities the professional assumes, and practical outcomes of the work. The result of this study is the document *The Community Support Skill Standards: Tools for Managing Change and Achieving Outcomes,* which more clearly defines the work of human service professionals (Human Services Research Institute, 2006).

In summary, human service professionals are concerned about and participate actively in training, ethical commitment, continuing education, and registration and certification. It is a relatively new occupation involved in professional activities of value to those who receive its service.

KEY TERMS

case management	networking	profession	social care
ethical standards	partnerships	rehabilitation	social control
generalist	problems in living	self-sufficiency	teaming
human service system			

THINGS TO REMEMBER

1. Human services has developed in response to the need of individuals or groups for assistance to live better lives.

2. Because human services recognizes client needs as problems in living, it does not focus on the past but seeks to improve the present and change the future.

3. Human services has emerged as a response to the increase in human problems in our modern world.

4. Human services provides three distinct functions: social care, social control, and rehabilitation.

5. Human services uses an interdisciplinary approach to understanding clients, helpers, and the context.

6. Human services consists of those services that help people with their problems.

7. The relationship between client and helper is the foundation for human service delivery.

8. Certain management principles influence delivery and reflect the value of focusing on the client.

9. The interaction between the client and the human service system also defines human services.

10. The services provided are designed to improve an individual's well-being.

11. In the successful delivery of services, the client develops new insights, skills, and competencies.

12. The field of human services is respected by its clients and other helping professions.

13. Human service work is a profession committed to ethical standards and continuing education.

ADDITIONAL READINGS: FOCUS ON POVERTY

Ehrenreich, B. (2002). *Nickel and dimed: On (not) getting by in America.* NY: Owl Books.
    Essayist Barbara Ehrenreich explores how women in the labor market survive as low wage earners by looking for a job and a place to live, working, and trying to make ends meet. She tries waitressing in the Florida Keys, working as both a cleaning woman and a nursing home assistant in Maine, and clerking at Wal-Mart in Minnesota.

Hays, S. (2003). *Flat broke with children: Women in the age of welfare reform.* New York: Oxford University Press.
    Welfare reform resulted in a dramatic decline in the welfare rolls. This author "puts a face" on welfare reform with her research in two towns. She addresses the challenges from inside the welfare office and from welfare mothers.

New York Times. (2005). *Class matters.* New York: Times Books.
    Fourteen *New York Times* reporters use storytelling to examine class as an important facet of contemporary American culture. Heart attack victims, immigrants, interclass marriage partners, a foster child, and the wife of a corporate executive show the ways class is defined today.

Rank, M. R. (2005). *One nation, underprivileged: Why American poverty affects us all.* New York: Oxford University Press.

The author suggests that poverty results from economic and political policy failures rather than individual inadequacies or attitudes and suggests a new paradigm for understanding poverty and strategies to reduce it.

Smith, S. C. (2005). *Ending global poverty: A guide to what works*. New York: Palgrave Macmillan.

Grass-roots programs and organizations help people in urban slums and rural areas break free of poverty. The author examines innovative and effective programs, describes how companies and foreign investors can help, and offers tools, guidelines, and suggestions.

REFERENCES

Action evaluation. (2006) *An overview*. Retrieved September 9, 2006, from http://www.uwstout.edu/bpa/ir/laptop/monitor.pdf#search=%22action%20evaluation%22.

American Psychological Association. (2006). *About APA*. Retrieved September 15, 2006, from http://www.apa.org/about/.

Eriksen, K. (1981). *Human services today*. Reston, VA: Reston Publishing.

Human Service Research Institute. (2006). *Community support skill standards project*. Retrieved September 7, 2006, from http://www.hsri.org/ddworkforce/csss/aboutcsss.html.

Maslow, A. (1971). *The further reaches of human nature*. New York: Viking Press.

Neugeboren, B. (1991). *Organization, policy, and practice in the human services*. New York: Longman.

Southern Regional Education Board. (1979). *Staff roles for mental health personnel: A history and a rationale*. Atlanta, GA: Author.

What is sociology?: The sociology page. (n.d.). Retrieved September 15, 2006, from http://www.macionis.com/.

A History of Helping

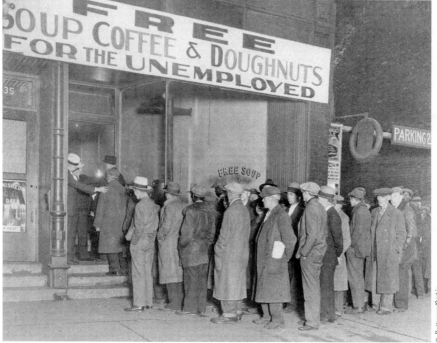

CHAPTER 2

© Bettmann/Corbis

After reading this chapter, you will be able to:

- Trace the historical development of helping.
- Describe the evolution of human needs since the Middle Ages.
- Illustrate three 19th-century philosophies about human needs and how those beliefs shaped human services.
- Identify the significant legislation that supported the development of human services in the 20th century.
- Trace U.S. government involvement in human services in the 20th century.
- Summarize the conditions that led to the decline of government involvement in the last 30 years.

Self-assessment

- Describe the major characteristics of helping those in need prior to the Middle Ages, during the Middle Ages, and immediately following the Middle Ages.
- Explain how the Elizabethan Poor Laws influenced colonial America's approach to helping the poor and needy.
- Trace the development of care for the mentally ill and children from the 1850s to the 1930s.
- How was the federal government involved in human services from the 1930s to the present?
- In what ways has major legislation influenced the development of human services?

Chapter 2 presents an overview of the history of helping to provide insight into the emergence and growth of services to people in need. History in this chapter traces how beliefs change over time. It describes who is "less fortunate" and examines the different categorizations of less fortunate people throughout history. The categories familiar to us today—the poor, people with mental impairments, and criminals—have not always been used. What is central to a definition of *less fortunate*, both then and now, is consideration of the "have-nots" in society, who meets their needs, and how those needs are met. In addition, we examine the emergence and growth of the human services. This chapter assists us further in defining human services.

EARLY HISTORY: A SUMMARY

Until the Middle Ages, people believed that mental illness was caused by evil spirits, and early forms of treatment focused on ridding the body of these demons. One treatment used was trephining the skull (using a crude saw to remove circular disks of bone). This hole in the head allowed evil spirits to escape. Another popular method of treatment was exorcizing evil spirits through religious rites. People with mental illness were feared because their supposed possession by spirits was perceived as a link with the supernatural. Other attempts to control the demons included chaining, beating, starving, and bleeding the unfortunate human host (National Institute for Mental Health, 1971).

Hippocrates, a physician in the third century BC, was one of the few professionals who used the scientific approach to explain and treat problem behavior and mental illness. He believed that problem behavior was a function of natural illness and that

Early History: A Summary Timeline

Early History	Mental illness, evil spirits
200 BC	Hippocrates defines mental illness
1500s AD	St. Thomas, St. Francis—First human service workers
1500–1600s	England protects mentally impaired
1601	First Elizabethan Poor Law
1700s	Almshouses established
1792	Pinel's humane treatment of the mentally ill

mental disorders had natural causes such as brain disease, heredity, or head injuries. In other words, evil spirits were not probable causes of mental illness. Hippocrates was also able to distinguish between different types of mental problems; among his most significant contributions were labels for illnesses, such as *melancholia* and *epilepsy,* which are still used in mental health today. His work marks the beginning of the medical model of service delivery.

Until the 1500s, the Catholic Church was chiefly responsible for providing human services. Religious figures such as St. Thomas Aquinas and St. Francis of Assisi are considered by some to be the first human service professionals. Under the Church's guidance, many institutions were founded for the poor, orphans, the elderly, and people with disabilities. At this time, deviant behavior was perceived as a sickness, and **asylums** were established to house those who were so labeled. After AD 1500, the power of the Church declined and that of government increased, producing conflict between church and state.

In addition to services provided by the Church, the needy in England also received attention from the government. In fact, the English Crown's right and duty to protect people with mental impairments had existed from the 13th century. For people with mental impairments, two categories were established: (1) natural fools or idiots and (2) those who were *non compos mentis. Idiots* became the preferred term for the first category, which included people with retarded intellectual development whose condition was permanent, present at birth, or both. The second category, *non compos mentis,* was the umbrella term for all other mental disabilities. By the 15th century, the term *lunatic* had replaced *non compos mentis.*

Diagnoses of mental illness were determined by inquisitions (unrelated to those established by the Catholic Church), which were conducted by a government official and a jury of at least 12 men (Neugebauer, 1979). The following questions were asked in the investigation:

- Was the person an idiot or a lunatic?
- When, how, and in what manner was the individual lucid?
- What lands and other property did the individual own?

The Crown's rights and duties were determined by these diagnoses. It was the king's duty to protect an idiot's lands and property and to provide the individual with the necessities of life; and the king was entitled to all the revenues from those lands.

Before the Middle Ages, feudal lords had assumed responsibility for much of the care of poor and sick people who lived on their lands. During the Middle Ages, needy people received aid from human service institutions such as orphanages, the Church, and late in this period, the government. Several types of institutions provided services during the Middle Ages.

One important source of aid to the needy was hospitals. Not only did they provide medical assistance to the ill, but they also fed and housed tired travelers, orphans, the elderly, and the poor. A second type of institution, the insane asylum, was established in Europe during the 15th and 16th centuries. These institutions represented some concern for the care and housing of people with mental illness, but the patients did not receive effective treatment, and their living conditions were poor. The following excerpt describes the conditions at London's Bethlehem Hospital, an institution typical of the asylums established during that time:

> London's Bethlehem Hospital, better known as Bedlam, founded in the thirteenth century as a priory, converted in the fourteenth century into a hospital, given by Henry VIII to the City of London in 1547 as Britain's first insane asylum, became, within a few decades, little more than a dungeon. Women were chained by the ankles to one long wall. Men were liable to be attached by the neck to a vertical bar. One man was kept that way, even in the eighteenth century, for twelve years. (Friedrich, 1976, p. 49).

Relief for the poor was the responsibility of the Church during the Middle Ages. Church authorities at the diocese or parish level administered relief to feed and protect the poor within their districts. The money available for their care was sufficient to meet the needs in these local districts (Trattner, 1999). In ministering to the poor, the Church served in the capacity of a public institution, and the tithe was considered a public tax. The care of the poor by the Church altered as the nature and incidence of poverty changed with the socioeconomic conditions. Specifically, the decline of feudalism, the growth of commerce, and the beginning of industrialization made it necessary to find new ways of assisting those in need. The poor, the unemployed, the disabled, widows, dependent children, the elderly, people with mental retardation, and people with mental illness who were previously cared for on the feudal estates by the feudal lords now had no place to go. Most wandered around, often settling in cities that were ill equipped to handle them.

TABLE 2.1 | SUMMARY POINTS: EARLY METHODS OF TREATMENT

- Trephining the skull involved using a crude saw to remove circular disks of bone.
- Exorcizing evil spirits was a religious rite to rid the body of their presence.
- Hippocrates believed that mental illness was a disease.
- Institutions were founded for the poor, orphans, the elderly, and people with disabilities.
- Asylums housed those with deviant behavior.
- Inquisitions determined diagnosis of mental illness as *non compos mentis* or idiots.
- Poor relief was the responsibility of the Catholic Church during the Middle Ages.
- The Elizabethan Poor Law was passed to mount a large-scale attack on poverty.

BOX 2.1	ELIZABETHAN POOR LAWS

The Elizabethan Poor Laws were passed as a response to the increasing number of poor in Great Britain. Few of the poor had the skills to earn a living wage, and as their numbers increased, pauperism became a national problem. The Poor Law of 1601 provided a clear definition of the "poor" and articulated services that they were to receive. It also defined what punishment those who returned to work would receive. This legislation is the foundation for the current social welfare system existing today in Great Britain. The following describes the law:

Poor Law of 1601

By this act two or more "substantial householders" were to be yearly nominated by the justices of the peace to serve as overseers of the poor in each parish. The overseers were to raise

> weekly or otherwise, by taxation of every inhabitant, such competent sums of money as they shall think fit, (a) for setting to work the children of all such whose parents shall not be thought able to keep and maintain them; (b) for setting to work all such persons, married and unmarried, having no means to maintain them, and who use no ordinary and daily trade of life to get their living by; (c) for providing a convenient stock of flax, hemp, wool,

thread, iron, and other ware and stuff to set the poor on work; (d) for the necessary relief of the lame, old, impotent, blind, and such other among them being poor and not able to work.

> Children whose parents cannot maintain them are to be apprenticed till the age of four-and-twenty years in the case of boys and twenty-one years or the time of marriage in the case of girls. The overseers may, with the leave of the Lord of the Manor, erect houses for the impotent poor on any waste or common ... in many parishes of this land, especially in country towns; but many of those parishes turneth forth their poor, yea and their lusty laborers that will not work, or for any misdemeanor want work, to beg, filch, and steal for their maintenance, so that the country is pitifully pestered with them; yea, and the maimed soldiers that have ventured their lives and lost their limbs on our behalf are also thus requited ... So they are turned forth to travel in idleness (the highway to hell) ... until the law bring them unto the fearful end of hanging.

Source: Excerpt from *The New Encyclopedia of Social Reform*, by W. Bliss, pp. 918–920. Copyright © 1908 Funk and Wagnalls.

A new type of economy and the employment needs of the industrial revolution also affected a number of poor people. The growth of commerce encouraged the development of a money economy, based on capital investments, credit, interest, rent, and wages. This system was very different from the rural economy, which depended on the bartering of goods and services. As the poor could no longer survive by bartering and had little money, they often could not afford food, housing, and clothing. In England, the pressures of the poor in the cities created the need for a large-scale attack on poverty and prompted the passage of the Elizabethan Poor Law of 1601. This legislation was critical in the history of human services. It guided social welfare practices in England and the United States for the next 350 years by specifying who was to provide what services to those in need. For example, parents were legally responsible for their children and grandchildren, and children were responsible for the support of parents and grandparents. More significant, however, was the acknowledgment in the legislation that the state had a responsibility to relieve need and suffering and that the disadvantaged not only deserved assistance but also had a legal right to it.

The law included three main features. The first was compulsory taxation to raise funds to help the needy. The administration of this money resembled the Church's

TABLE 2.2	SUMMARY POINTS: ELIZABETHAN POOR LAW OF 1601

- Law passed as the number of poor increased
- Compulsory taxation to raise funds to help the needy
- Classification of dependents according to ability to work: children, the able bodied, and the "impotent poor"
- Responsibility for those in need was first with the family and then with the government

system developed during feudal times. Second, dependents were classified according to their ability to work: children, the able-bodied, and the "impotent poor" (adults unable to work). Relief was provided to each group: Dependent children were apprenticed or indentured; the able-bodied worked or were punished; and the lame, the blind, and other poor people unable to work received home or institutional relief. Third, the responsibility for the sick, the poor, and others in need rested first with the family. If the family could not provide assistance, the government was responsible for doing so.

By the end of the 18th century, a dramatic change in the care of people with mental illness occurred. A move toward more humane treatment of those in mental institutions began in 1792 when Philippe Pinel unchained 50 maniacs at Bicetre Hospital in Paris (see Chapter 4). This period is often called the first revolution in mental health. For those in mental institutions, this period meant improved diets, regular exercise, religious observance, and the development of the mind. As you will read later in this chapter, in the United States these efforts were led by Benjamin Rush. Unfortunately, the rise in moral treatment lasted only until the mid-19th century because of limited resources, overcrowding, and the passage of time (Macht, 1990).

HUMAN SERVICES IN THE UNITED STATES: COLONIAL AMERICA

As we examine the history of human services in the United States, we see the influence of the English approach to human services discussed in the preceding section. During the years of colonization, public relief was supported by individuals and groups, who donated resources and labor to institutions such as schools and hospitals or directly to needy people. Much assistance took the form of neighborly kindness or mutual aid. As the populations of the cities in the colonies grew, so did the number of indigents, idlers, criminals, orphans, and others who needed assistance. The colonists used the Elizabethan Poor Law as a model of how to meet the needs of those individuals.

The four principles that formed the basis of the local practice of poor relief in the colonies can be traced directly to the Elizabethan Poor Law of 1601. The first principle defined **poor relief** as a public responsibility. The second principle, the question of legal residence, therefore became a practical one, as services were provided at the local or parish level. The third principle spelled out the responsibility family members had to needy individuals; public aid was denied those who had parents, grandparents, adult children, or grandchildren. Finally, legislation combined concerns about children and

1600s	Recognition of the needs of the poor
1600–1700s	Almshouses established
1773	State hospital opens in Williamsburg, Virginia
1792	Philippe Pinel advocates more humane treatment
1800s	District workhouses established

work by declaring that the children of paupers were to be apprenticed to farmers and artisans, who agreed to care for them.

Like England, the colonies responded to the needy by developing institutions. The first almshouse was built in Massachusetts in 1662 for dependents such as people with mental illness, the elderly, children, the able-bodied poor, those with physical disabilities, and criminals. **Almshouses** were not developed systematically, but over the next 150 years they were established throughout the colonies as the need arose. The numbers of these houses made it increasingly obvious that there were large groups of needy individuals the towns could not support. With this realization began the trend for larger governmental units to accept the responsibility for the "state poor." By the early 1800s, a system of district workhouses had been developed. Besides the almshouses, there were very few specialized formal institutions. Criminals were held in jail until trial and, if found guilty, were fined, whipped, or executed. Poor strangers or vagrants were simply told to leave town. People with mental illness had no special facilities before the American Revolution; their care was the responsibility of their families. Those without relatives to care for them were placed in almshouses. Those with mental illness were often locked up by their families in an attic or cellar or left to wander about the countryside.

Benjamin Franklin was instrumental in establishing one of the few formal institutions for people with mental disturbances, a section of the Pennsylvania Hospital. Another facility devoted exclusively to those with mental disturbances was a state hospital at Williamsburg, Virginia, which opened in 1773. Little attention was given to the treatment of mental disease because it was viewed as an economic and social problem rather than a medical one. Determining insanity was the responsibility of officials, such as governors and church wardens, not members of the medical profession.

Providing services for those in need continued to be a concern for reformers and federal and state leaders. Widespread change in the 19th century required a different approach to providing services.

THE 19TH CENTURY: A TIME OF CHANGE

Large-scale immigration, rapid industrialization, and widespread urbanization led to many societal changes during the colonial years. These changes brought more poverty and more outlays for relief of the poor. During the Middle Ages, need was believed to arise from misfortune, for which society should assume responsibility. Belief in the right to public assistance was established and endorsed by the Elizabethan Poor Law, which placed the responsibility on the government. In the early years in the United States, colonists used the English system as a model for their philosophy

THE 19TH CENTURY: A TIME OF CHANGE TIMELINE

1800s	Rapid industrialization
1813	Practice of probation begins
1810s	Benjamin Rush influences mental health care
1820s	Rise of the philosophy of individualism
1840s	Dorothea Dix teaches prisoners
1850s	Rise of the philosophy of Social Darwinism
1854	Care of mentally ill becomes state responsibility
1880s	Philanthropy emerges
1889	Opening of Hull House

toward and services for the poor and needy. By the early 1800s, however, the philosophy in the United States had changed.

Destitution was viewed as the fault of the individual, and public aid was thought to cause and encourage poverty. This punitive attitude toward the poor—the belief that to be poor was a crime—was manifested in the Poor Law Reform Bill of 1834. Its purpose was to limit the expansion of services provided to the poor or the have-nots. This bill introduced the concept of "less eligibility," stating that assistance to any person in need must be lower than the lowest working wage paid. The social philosophies of individualism, the work ethic, economic laissez-faire, and Social Darwinism promoted further changes in attitudes toward the poor and the needy.

SOCIAL PHILOSOPHIES

During the 19th century, those espousing the philosophy of **individualism** viewed America as the land of opportunity. Hard work was the road to success, and that road could be traveled by anyone. The individual was held solely responsible for any failure. Similarly, proponents of the work ethic emphasized the importance of hard work and thrift for financial success and viewed poverty as a sign of spiritual weakness. Wealth was virtuous, and hard work represented the road to salvation.

Laissez-faire was an economic concept that focused on societal rather than individual responsibility. The original French phrase means "leave alone," and this concept encouraged a social attitude of "live and let live." The most desirable government, then, was the one that governed least—negating society's responsibility to help its less fortunate citizens. Those adhering to this philosophy opposed the provision of any human services as a right of the individual.

Social Darwinism, in combination with laissez-faire and the work ethic, created a climate for the reform that was to follow. An outgrowth of Charles Darwin's theory of evolution, it was used to explain social and economic phenomena. According to those who interpreted Darwin in social terms, the natural order of life was that the fittest would survive, creating a society of perfect people. Those who were unfit would not be able to meet their own needs and would not survive.

Supporters of Social Darwinism called for the repeal of poor laws and state-supported human services that facilitated the survival of the "unfit," as they believed that all change must be natural. Any attempt to help the less fortunate would be against progress, which depended on "natural selection." This belief was especially popular between 1870 and 1880. In reality, it often served as a rationalization for unscrupulous business practices. Furthermore, it encouraged the belief that nothing could be done about the situation of the working class and the poor, who faced long work hours, low wages, child labor, and unhealthy working conditions.

These prevailing philosophies discouraged the provision of human services and limited services to those who desperately needed assistance. The private sector became very important in filling the need. Wealthy individuals were instrumental in organizing and reforming institutions. Mental hospitals, almshouses, workhouses, penitentiaries, and institutions for unwed mothers and delinquent youths appeared. Philanthropic societies were formed to support these institutions. By the middle of the 19th century, public and private sectors were working side by side. As welfare problems grew, the private sector was unable to meet increasing needs. In spite of the prevailing philosophies, there was growing demand for public agencies to assume more responsibility for the poor and needy.

By the 1850s, specialized institutions had been established for persons with mental illness, juvenile delinquents, the deaf and blind, and criminals. These institutions were established primarily in the belief that reform, rehabilitation, and education were possible. Institutions could improve society by protecting individuals from negative environmental influences.

In summary, the 19th century was a time of dramatic change in the way society viewed its responsibilities toward the poor and needy. Government relinquished some of its role in providing services, and the private sector assumed more responsibility. Unfortunately, the problems of those in need multiplied, and gradually the government began to increase its assistance again. Institutions also developed in response to the needs of specific populations. Probation, mental health, and child welfare provide examples of how 19th-century attitudes affected the delivery of human services to specific populations.

PROBATION

In the United States, the earliest practice similar to **probation** as we know it today occurred in 1813, when Judge Peter O. Thatcher of Boston began placing youthful offenders under the supervision of officials such as sheriffs and constables. In 1841, the concept of "friendly supervision" was introduced by John Augustus, a shoemaker. He helped drunks and other unfortunates by bailing them out, sometimes paying their fines, and then providing "friendly supervision" as they adjusted to a new life. The most well-known organization to provide assistance to ex-convicts was the Salvation Army, created in England in the late 19th century by William Booth. Its members believed in taking a more sympathetic approach to the problems and circumstances of those in need. For example, members of its Prison Gate Brigade met prisoners upon their release and provided whatever assistance they could, including a home, food, and employment (Irvine, 2002).

TABLE 2.3 | SUMMARY POINTS: SOCIAL PHILOSOPHIES OF THE 19TH CENTURY

- **Individualism**—hard work was the road to success and poverty was a sign of spiritual weakness.

- **Laissez-faire**—an economic concept that focused on societal rather than individual responsibility.

- **Social Darwinism**—any attempts to help the less fortunate would impede progress and facilitate the survival of the "unfit."

TREATMENT OF PEOPLE WITH MENTAL ILLNESS

Patients in the early asylums were mostly psychotic or severely retarded. Treatment was medically oriented, and many patients were treated as if they had a physical illness. The beginnings of reform in the late 1700s can be attributed to Dr. Benjamin Rush at the Pennsylvania Hospital in Philadelphia. Dr. Rush, who is considered the father of American psychiatry, fought the superstition and ignorance surrounding mental illness and elevated the study of mental illness to a scientific level. Before his study, mental patients lived in atrocious conditions and were treated with brutality and cruelty; customary treatment methods were bleeding, restraint, and cold showers. Dr. Rush introduced occupational therapy, amusements, and exercise for patients.

Dorothea Dix was another pioneer who fought to improve conditions and services for people with mental illness during the 19th century. She became involved in social reform when, in 1841, she accepted an offer to teach a Sunday school class of 20 female prisoners in the jail at East Cambridge, Massachusetts. She was appalled at the conditions she found in the jail: overcrowding, filthy quarters, and little or no heat. What alarmed her most was the crowding together of criminals and the insane. She began a personal investigation of all the jails and almshouses in Massachusetts and made careful, systematic records of what she saw. Backed by a group of broad-minded, public-spirited citizens, Dix launched a whole new career as a moral reformer, calling for more enlightened treatment of those with mental illness. Controversy and outrage engulfed her, but those who checked her accounts found them to be factual (Marshall, 1937).

She encouraged the national government to assume additional responsibility for the care and treatment of people with mental illness. Using such methods as fact gathering, preparing memoranda and bills, and rallying public opinion, she began her campaign in Massachusetts, where the number of dependent insane was twice the total capacity of the state's three mental institutions (Trattner, 1999). The years between 1843 and 1853 are sometimes called her "decade of victory," because she was personally responsible for founding state hospitals in nine states.

By 1854, the U.S. Congress had declared the financial care of people with mental illness the responsibility of the states. This responsibility included paying for construction of proper facilities and needed treatment. In reality, however, the state systems were custodial warehouses, characterized by inadequate doctor–patient ratio, untrained personnel, overcrowding, and lack of public interest.

By the late 19th century, states began to separate people with mental illness and those with developmental disabilities. There was an attempt to upgrade research, treatment, and physical facilities, and the hospitals eventually provided aftercare and outpatient clinics. The medically oriented approach continued to prevail in institutions, and mental disorders were defined and classified into two groups: those caused by organic brain disturbance and those with no apparent physical cause (psychogenetic).

CHILD WELFARE

The first juvenile reformatory in America, the House of Refuge for Juvenile Delinquents in New York City, was supported by state funds. Massachusetts and Ohio quickly followed by establishing juvenile facilities. After the 1830s, the number of such institutions multiplied, as the public demanded the removal of children from alms-houses. Unfortunately, juvenile institutions were not always an improvement, and overcrowded conditions and poor care prompted the establishment of a system that placed children in private homes.

Other forms of child welfare were the provision of mothers' or widows' pensions, the creation of juvenile courts and probation systems, the passage of compulsory school attendance laws, and crusades against child labor. There were several reasons for these actions. Many people believed that children were the most vulnerable and deserving group in society, and it was difficult to argue that the children were responsible for their own conditions. Children also constituted one of the largest groups of neglected and needy.

REFORM MOVEMENTS

By the latter half of the 19th century, two population shifts were affecting the provision of services to people in need: immigration from abroad and migration from rural to urban areas. In 1860, one-sixth of Americans lived in the cities; by 1900, this figure was one-third; and by 1920, one-half (Trattner, 1999). Between 1860 and 1900, approximately 14 million immigrants from abroad settled in cities, creating an urban population that consisted primarily of former farmers and immigrants. Most were unskilled or semiskilled workers in search of employment. This population explosion in the urban areas created many problems for the urban governments. Two responses to these problems were the organized charity movement and the settlement house movement.

THE ORGANIZED CHARITY MOVEMENT   The goal of the organized charity movement was to eliminate difficulties such as fraud or duplication in the provision of services (Trattner, 1999). According to the movement, the best way to deal with poverty was through personal contact or "friendly visiting" between the rich and the poor. Influenced by laissez-faire, individualism, and Puritanism, the movement soon shifted to reform, seeking better conditions in institutions, promoting better sanitation and health regulations, developing parks and recreation areas, and writing and enforcing housing codes.

The Charity Organization Society, a forerunner of the Community Chest and the United Way, is an example of society's response to the expanding urban

INTERNATIONAL FOCUS
Mental Health in Developing Countries

All countries have systems of economics, religion, education, and law that have developed over time. Colonization by Western European countries interrupted the evolution of these systems in many developing countries, as Western traditions supplanted earlier systems, including mental health care systems.

Examples of developing countries using European systems of institutionalization or custodial care can be found in Southeast Asia in the early 1800s. In Singapore and Penang, lunatic asylums and hospitals for the insane were modeled after European facilities. No better than warehouses for people with mental illness, these institutions also housed criminals, vagrants, and other social undesirables. With little hope of better care, many stayed for the remainder of their lives. By the end of the 19th century, the practice of institutionalization had expanded into India and Indonesia. Because such custodial care facilities did little to better the lives of people with mental illness, a negative perception of institutionalization still influences the attitudes of people in Southeast Asia today.

Based on studies in several parts of the world, the World Health Organization (1975) concluded that there are no fundamental differences among nations with regard to the range or prevalence of mental disorders. In the predominantly rural populations and rapidly growing cities of developing countries, however, a combination of overcrowding, unemployment, limited and outdated health facilities, and rapid social change makes mental disorders take the form of physical complaints or criminal activity.

Mental disorders may be a source of fear, not only to family members and friends but also to administrators, health workers, and politicians. The belief that these conditions are caused by the supernatural continues to be widespread; it can lead to a person's rejection by or isolation from family members and community, skepticism among the public about treatment programs, and regressive attitudes regarding the development of mental health services. Institutionalization remains a dominant form of treatment.

population. Members of the Charity Organization Society believed that giving handouts of money and food actually encouraged people to remain poor and to beg for services. They supported the systematic distribution of alms only to the poor who needed them, thus helping the deserving poor while discouraging begging. They hoped to encourage thrift and independence among the poor. Eventually, this group evolved into a clearinghouse for all the city's charitable organizations, similar to the United Way of today.

THE SETTLEMENT HOUSE MOVEMENT   The development of the **settlement house** movement was in large part a reaction to the inability of the organized charity movement to improve the living and working conditions of the poor. The leaders of the settlement house movement, unlike the leaders of the organized charity movement, did not support the laissez-faire philosophy. They wanted reform that included adequate housing, better schools, the abolition of child labor, and an end to the sweatshops. They thought that the best way to achieve this reform was not through alms or "friendly visiting" but through "social engineering." Human service workers and reformers were "engineers"; they must participate in the system all the time, not only when something was wrong. Individual workers and reformers were perceived as members of an active and attentive movement that intervened at the neighborhood level. The settlement house is an example of social engineering in practice.

Typically, a settlement house was a large house in a slum area. It served as a community center, sponsoring such activities as recreation; classes in English, cooking, and citizenship; vocational training; and child care. Key elements to the success of a settlement house were the commitment of the workers and the location of the house. Social engineering could not be accomplished from afar; workers lived in the house or in the community in which they served. The house was part of the community.

Perhaps the best example of a settlement house is Hull House in Chicago, founded by Jane Addams in 1889. Addams was inspired by Toynbee Hall, a pioneer English settlement house she visited while in England in the 1880s. Upon returning from Europe, she and her college friend, Ellen Starr, moved to the poor section of Chicago and began raising money to support what was to become Hull House, located in the middle of the immigrant section in Chicago. Addams and Starr moved in and invited their immigrant neighbors to read Italian novels and see slides of Italian art. The women came and brought their children; the presence of children necessitated a nursery. Soon a boys' club was established, and then a men's club. Over the years, more than 50 services were available at Hull House.

These movements are important because they illustrate the continual struggle during the 19th century to assist those in need. Generally, the assistance took two forms: provision of services and advocacy of reform. It was difficult to blame all the problems of urban poverty on the individual. The settlement house movement, in particular, introduced a new philosophy of helping that recognized the impact of societal forces on the lives of individuals. This new philosophy continued to develop in the 20th century.

EARLY 20TH CENTURY: NEW DIRECTIONS

The beginning of the 20th century marked a change in the country's response to individuals in need. During this period of social reform, the first seeds of the mental health movement were formed, and federal legislation provided broad government support for many Americans.

The early 1900s, sometimes called the *sociological era,* continued the period of social reform. During this time, two significant events or changes affected the history of helping and human services. The first was the development of a new profession. Settlement house and Charity Organization Society workers became known as **social workers.** The basis for the new profession was the belief that such people needed specific skills, knowledge, and understanding to work effectively with the poor. Good intentions were admirable but not sufficient to provide assistance. During this time, social diagnosis, or casework, evolved as the method of practice. Mary Richmond, the author of *Social Diagnosis* (1917), identified this process as one of investigation, diagnosis, prognosis, and treatment. Her book is regarded as the first treatise on social casework theory and method (Zimbalist, 1977). The development of the social work profession is significant; it represents the beginning of the professionalization of human services. Later in this century, the fields of welfare, mental health, child guidance, and probation also became professionalized.

Also during the early 20th century, a reexamination of the causes of poverty took place. A group of writers called "muckrakers" actively criticized the wealthy, accusing

EARLY 20TH CENTURY: NEW DIRECTIONS TIMELINE

Early 1900s	Beginning of Social Work Profession
1909	National Committee for Mental Hygiene founded
1910s	Muckrakers publicized social ills
1920–1930s	Free clinics for mentally ill opened
1935	Social Security Act passed
1945	Beers published *A Mind That Found Itself*
1955	Joint Commission on Mental Illness and Health met

them of moral decay, cheating, and bribery. (The term was first used by President Theodore Roosevelt in criticizing sensationalist, untruthful writers.) Muckrakers such as Lincoln Steffens and Upton Sinclair exposed unfair business, government, and labor practices. They supported the idea that poverty was caused by social and economic conditions, not by the individual, and proposed that poverty was a condition that prevented people from reaching their potential. They claimed that because poverty and need resulted from societal shortcomings, improvements in housing and working conditions could help eliminate poverty.

SEEDS OF THE MENTAL HEALTH MOVEMENT

Clifford Beers, a victim of mental illness, was confined for three years in public and private mental institutions, where he experienced deprivation and cruelty. To publicize the plight of those with mental illness, he wrote about his collapse and treatment in *A Mind That Found Itself* (1945). In 1908, he founded the Connecticut Society for Mental Hygiene, considered by many to be the beginning of the organized mental health movement in America. By the following year, this pioneer state society had written a prospectus that included the following guidelines (Beers, 1945, p. 395):

> I "After all, what the insane most need is a friend!" By coordinating the friendly impulses of those who, if they but knew how, would gladly help the insane, the Society for Mental Hygiene can prove itself that friend.
> II It is the aim of the Society for Mental Hygiene to become a permanent agency for education and reform in the field of nervous and mental diseases; an agency for education always, for reform as long as radical changes may be needed.
> III The chief object of the Society for Mental Hygiene shall be the improvement of conditions among those actually insane and confined, and the protection of the mental health of the public at large.

Beers also proposed a national society, the National Committee for Mental Hygiene, which was formed in 1909. This group later changed its name to the National Association for Mental Health and is known today as the Mental Health Association. Its aim is to improve mental hospitals, arouse public concern, and prevent disease. By providing education on causes, diagnosis, prevention, and treatment, this organization furthered the development of the mental health movement.

| BOX 2.3 | AN ASYLUM IN 1902 |

After fifteen interminable hours the straitjacket was removed. Whereas just prior to its putting on I had been in a vigorous enough condition to offer stout resistance when wantonly assaulted, now, on coming out of it, I was helpless. When my arms were released from their constricted position, the pain was intense. Every joint had been racked. I had no control over the fingers of either hand, and could not have dressed myself had I been promised my freedom for doing so.

For more than the following week I suffered as already described, though of course with gradually decreasing intensity as my racked body became accustomed to the unnatural positions it was forced to take. This first experience occurred on the night of October 18th, 1902. I was subjected to the same unfair, unnecessary, and unscientific ordeal for twenty-one consecutive nights and parts of each of the corresponding twenty-one days. On more than one occasion, indeed, the attendant placed me in the straitjacket during the day for refusing to obey some trivial command. This, too, without an explicit order from the doctor in charge, through perhaps he acted under a general order.

During most of this time I was held also in seclusion in a padded cell. A padded cell is a vile hole. The side walls are padded as high as a man can reach, as is also the inside of the door. One of the worst features of such cells is the lack of ventilation, which deficiency of

course aggravates their general unsanitary condition. The cell which I was forced to occupy was practically without heat, and as winter was coming on, I suffered intensely from the cold. Frequently it was so cold I could see my breath. Though my canvas jacket served to protect part of that body which it was at the same time racking, I was seldom comfortably warm; for, once uncovered, my arms being pinioned, I had no way of rearranging the blankets. What little sleep I managed to get I took lying on a hard mattress placed on the bare floor. The condition of the mattress I found in the cell was such that I objected to its further use, and the fact that another was supplied, at a time when few of my requests were being granted, proves its disgusting condition.

For this period of three weeks—from October 18th until November 8th, 1902, when I left this institution and was transferred to a state hospital—I was continuously either under lock and key (in the padded cell or some other room) or under the eye of an attendant. Over half the time I was in the snug, but cruel embrace of a straitjacket—about three hundred hours in all.

Source: Excerpt from *A Mind that Found Itself,* by Clifford W. Beers, pp. 133–134, 395. Copyright © 1907, renewed 1953 by the American Foundation of Mental Hygiene, Inc.

Services for people with mental illness continued to improve and expand. By the 1920s and 1930s, most large cities had free clinics for mental patients, where treatment and social services were provided. In fact, human services as we know it today began with the impact of World Wars I and II on the mental health field. By the end of World War II, the profession of clinical psychology was created, in part because the number of veterans who were hospitalized in Veterans Administration (VA) facilities for psychiatric evaluation had reached more than 40,000 (Cranston, 1986).

Until the 1930s, individual leaders such as Jane Addams, Clifford Beers, and the muckrakers spearheaded the development of services and the reform of conditions for the impoverished. As described previously, the development of professions that trained workers in social services also began. As important as these contributions were, they had little impact on poverty, mental illness, or other human service concerns on a large scale or at a national level. As a result, the federal government increased its financial commitment to those in need. Presidents of the United States assumed a leadership role in providing services.

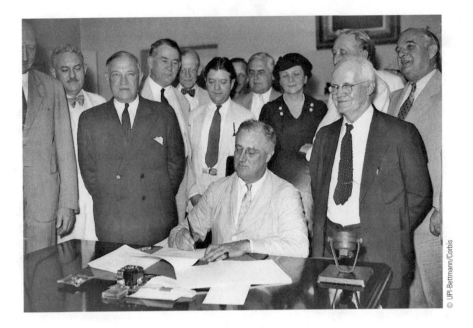

© UPI-Bettmann/Corbis

INCREASED FEDERAL INVOLVEMENT

The Great Depression was marked by vast unemployment, failing business ventures, and the collapse of banks. The economic situation created a wave of panic and long-term psychological and economic depression for individuals who could see no end to financial hardship. President Franklin D. Roosevelt introduced New Deal legislation that fundamentally changed the federal government's role in providing human services, focusing on two goals. The first was to provide short-term aid to those who were unemployed. The Works Progress Administration (WPA) and the Civilian Conservation Corps (CCC) were but two of the work relief programs he initiated. The second focus was the enactment of the Social Security Act of 1935 as protection against future economic hardships.

The **Social Security** Act of 1935, the cornerstone of the present American social welfare system, was passed in response to the need for human services. This landmark piece of legislation was significant for several reasons. First, it translated into action the belief that Americans had the right to protection from economic instability. The federal government assumed responsibility for the economic security of all citizens, and thus began the American welfare state. Second, it expanded welfare activities and improved their standards by establishing a new alignment of responsibility in public welfare. The policy of federal aid or grants to states began, thus closing the door on three centuries of the "poor law" principle of local responsibility.

What the act actually did was to provide assistance in three areas: social insurance, public assistance, and health and welfare services. Social insurance programs included old-age, survivors, disability, and unemployment insurance, all of which supported an individual's right to benefits regardless of need. Public assistance provided federal funds to states to establish programs such as Aid

TABLE 2.4	SUMMARY POINTS: SOCIAL SECURITY ACT (1935)

- Social insurance programs (old-age, survivors, disability, and unemployment insurance) supported an individual's rights to benefits regardless of need.
- Public assistance helped states establish programs for the needy (e.g., Aid to Families with Dependent Children, Old Age Assistance, and Aid to the Blind).
- Health and welfare services provided programs for public health, vocational rehabilitation, and child welfare among others.

to the Permanently and Totally Disabled (APTD), Aid to Families with Dependent Children (**AFDC**), Aid to the Blind, and Old Age Assistance (OAA). Also available under this category were programs of general assistance to needy people who were not eligible under any other program. The third area, health and welfare services, focused on child welfare, vocational rehabilitation, public health, children with disabilities, and maternal and child health.

Of course, some pieces were missing from these new social welfare efforts. The Social Security Act did not provide for long-term hardships. Unemployment benefits were available for only a limited amount of time, and neither health insurance nor permanent physical disability insurance was provided. In spite of these limitations, the initiatives of the Social Security Act became well-established components of the social welfare system.

MID-20TH CENTURY: FOCUS ON MENTAL HEALTH

Forerunners of the mental health movement, such as Phillipe Pinel, Benjamin Rush, and Clifford Beers, all spoke eloquently about the needs of the mentally ill. The growth of mental health and human services continued during the middle years of the 20th century as the commitment to helping others increased. The social welfare system expanded to provide better service to the mentally ill, children, and the poor, to name a few.

An important step in the provision of services to those with mental illness was the passage of the National Mental Health Act of 1946 (Public Law 79–487).

MID-20TH CENTURY: FOCUS ON MENTAL HEALTH

1946	National Mental Health Act of 1946 created a Mental Hygiene Division to address preventive measures
1955	Mental Health Study Act acknowledged personnel shortage in mental health
1963	Community Mental Health Centers Act passed establishing National Health Institute for Mental Health
1965	President Lyndon Johnson declared "war on poverty"
1970s	National Organization for Human Service Educators and Council for Standards in Human Service Education established formal preparation of human service workers

This act created a Mental Hygiene Division within the U.S. Public Health Service and a center for information and research, which later became the **National Institute for Mental Health** (NIMH). The Mental Hygiene Division emphasized preventive health measures. Its functions were to assist in the development of state and community health services; to study the causes, prevention, and treatment of mental illness; and to support training of psychiatrists, psychologists, social workers, and nurses. This agency played a critical role in the developing human service movement.

A second piece of legislation that helped set the stage for the emergence of human services was the Mental Health Study Act of 1955 (Public Law 84-82), which provided funding for a Joint Commission on Mental Illness and Health. The charge to the commission was "to analyze and evaluate the needs and resources of the mentally ill in the United States and make recommendations for a national mental health program" (Albee, 1961, p. x). The commission made recommendations for training, research, facilities, and programs.

Two of the commission's recommendations directly affected the human service movement. First, the commission concluded that the professional sector alone could not meet the health care needs of the majority of people if only traditional mental health professionals were used. According to the commission,

> [a]ll mental health professions should recognize that nonmedical mental health work-ers with aptitude, sound training, practical experience, and demonstrable competence should be permitted to do general, short-term psychotherapy—namely, treating per-sons by objective, permissive, nondirective techniques of listening to their troubles and helping them resolve these troubles in an individually insightful and socially useful way. Such therapy, combining some elements of psychiatric treatment, client counsel-ing, "someone to tell one's troubles to," and love for one's fellow man, obviously can be carried out in a variety of settings by institutions, groups, and individuals, but in all cases should be undertaken under the auspices of recognized mental health agencies. (Albee, 1961, p. x)

The commission also recommended that "a national mental health program should set as an objective one fully staffed, full-time mental health clinic available to each 50,000 of population" (Albee, 1961, p. xiv). A major impact of the Mental Health Study Act on the human service movement was that it acknowledged the personnel shortage that existed, suggested a new type of mental health worker who could be trained in less time, and recommended a setting in which such new workers could be utilized effectively.

The commission's recommendations were well received and quickly became law. The conditions that encouraged this immediate action were an awareness of the increasing numbers of people with mental health problems, the rising costs of institutional care, and the need for more effective use of personnel, treatment facilities, and treatment (James, 1981).

SERVING THOSE IN NEED

During the mid-20th century, under the leadership of Presidents Kennedy and Johnson, the government's commitment to mental health and the treatment of mental illness continued. Kennedy chose to focus on the problems of mental health and mental retardation, "because they are of such actual size and tragic impact and because their susceptibility to public action is so much greater than the attention they have received" (Kennedy, 1964). He called for a national plan to investigate causes, strengthen resources, and improve training and facilities. In a speech on proposed measures to combat mental illness and mental retardation, Kennedy stated:

> I have sent to the Congress today a series of proposals to help fight mental illness and mental retardation. These two afflictions have been long neglected. They occur more frequently, affect more people, require more prolonged treatment, cause more individual and family suffering than any other condition in American life. It has been tolerated too long. It has troubled our national conscience, but only as a problem unpleasant to mention, easy to postpone, and despairing of solution. (Kennedy, 1964, p. 51)

Funding for the recommendations of the commission was provided by the Community Mental Health Centers Act of 1963, which directed NIMH to set up requirements and regulations for the establishment of **community mental health centers.** Additionally, grants were to be made available for activities such as staffing, planning, initial operations, consultation, and education services. The idea behind this act was to provide diverse services to the population, including inpatient and out-patient care, emergency services, assistance to the courts, and services for the mental health of children and the elderly. By 1975, Congress had authorized over 609 multiservice centers (James, 1981).

Another response to the personnel shortage was the Scheuer Subprofessional Career Act of 1966, administered by the Department of Labor. The philosophical basis for the act was that poor people and minority group members, if trained appropriately, could provide effective mental health services. Programs were developed to train such people to be teacher aides, child care workers, corrections officers, and mental health workers. Most of the education was essentially in-service training, but some programs had links to vocational schools or community colleges.

During Kennedy's years as president, he set the tone for increased emphasis on the eradication of poverty in the United States. His vision brought much hope to populations that had despaired of changing their situations without assistance. Kennedy ignited the support of the nation to help the less fortunate. Following the assassination of Kennedy in 1963, Lyndon B. Johnson took the oath of office as president. Johnson assumed the legacy of Kennedy's commitment to the impoverished, but this was not a new role for him. Before his election to the vice presidency, he had spent 23 years as an advocate for those who had little hope for the future and no one to represent them.

Varying estimates are made of the number of poor people in America during the Johnson era. John K. Galbraith's (1976) well-known book, *The Affluent Society*, described a country in which people continuously improved their standard of living and the quality of their lives. Michael Harrington (1962) depicted the country very differently in *The Other America*. According to his research, 50 to 60 million Americans lived in poverty, a good many of them in isolated rural regions of the country, especially in the South and the Southeast, and others in large cities on the

West and East coasts. These poor people had few skills for employment, lived in substandard housing, and were malnourished and illiterate.

In 1964, Johnson ran for president on a platform addressing the social problems described by Harrington. He proposed a comprehensive network of social policies and program initiatives. The public response to positive government social intervention was overwhelming, and Johnson was reelected by a large majority. In his 1965 State of the Union address, he declared an "unconditional **war on poverty**" in order to create a "Great Society." Johnson believed the roots of poverty had to be attacked. Programs developed in the War on Poverty and Great Society initiatives included VISTA, the Neighborhood Youth Corps, the Job Corps, College Work Study, and Head Start. Their objective was to eradicate poverty by providing ways for the poor to improve their economic conditions. Many community action programs encouraged client participation in planning, delivering, and evaluating services.

Johnson also promoted the rights of the poor. For example, the Voting Rights Act of 1965 abolished the literacy tests that had been used to deny uneducated people the vote, and the Affirmative Action Order of 1968 and the Office of Economic Opportunity improved employment opportunities for minorities. Further evidence of the president's commitment were Medicare and Medicaid, amendments to the Social Security Act approved by President Johnson on July 30, 1965. **Medicare** (Title XVIII) provides health insurance for people over 65. **Medicaid** (Title XVIX) gives grants to the states to assist them in helping medically indigent citizens receive medical and hospital care.

THE HUMAN SERVICE MOVEMENT

Since the 1960s, the human service movement has experienced unprecedented growth, evidenced by the increase in the number of training programs, the increased size of the mental health delivery system, and the development of the human service administration at the federal level. In 1966, the first human service program was established at Purdue University, a two-year associate degree program that focused on the training of entry-level mental health workers.

Originally, a new type of human service worker was envisioned that was a cross between the professional with an advanced degree and the volunteer. A major assumption about the new workers was that their firsthand work experiences, coupled with education and training, would enable them to establish greater rapport and credibility with their clients. In addition, their firsthand knowledge of the problems would give them greater understanding of clients and their difficulties. The initial intent was for these workers to perform innovative roles such as client advocacy and client–community liaison, but in reality they came to perform more traditional roles such as direct care giving (Southern Regional Education Board, 1979).

NIMH continued its involvement with the movement during the 1970s. The New Careers branch of NIMH was established to provide leadership in the development of entry-level programs for disadvantaged persons. In 1975, this became the Paraprofessional Manpower Branch, which led the way in defining and developing the training for all levels of paraprofessional workers. There was much concern in the existing mental health system about who the new paraprofessionals would be, what jobs they

TABLE 2.5 | SUMMARY POINTS: HUMAN SERVICE MOVEMENT

- 1966—First human service program established at Purdue University
- 1975—Paraprofessional Manpower Branch defined training for human service workers
- 1970s—Mental health treatment shifted from institution to the community
- 1970s—Professional human service organizations established

would perform, and whether they would perform adequately. It was the responsibility of the Manpower Branch to address these questions.

In spite of the concern voiced by the other professionals in the mental health system, many of these newly trained human service workers were welcomed. During the 1970s, the number of clients served by the mental health system increased dramatically. New workers were needed, and the traditional ways of providing mental health services were not efficient or effective in meeting the changing needs. Highly skilled professionals with advanced degrees had been serving small numbers of clients. Human service workers could now provide the simpler direct-care services to greater numbers of clients while the highly skilled professionals worked with the more difficult problems and supervised the human service workers. **Deinstitutionalization,** a movement that began in the 1950s, called for transferring many institutionalized patients to the community for outpatient care. By the 1970s, a major segment of mental health treatment had shifted from the isolation of the institution to the complex environment of the community. As the concept of community mental health developed, different types of professional services were needed.

During this same time period, organizations that signaled a move toward professionalism emerged. Such organizations serve many purposes. They may regulate a profession or its workers, facilitate communication among its members, or foster excellence in research or service within the profession. Two organizations in particular were instrumental in the move toward a human service profession: the National Organization for Human Services (NOHS) and the Council for Standards in Human Service Education (CSHSE). Both are still active today. Their websites are at http://www.nationalhumanservices.org and http://www.cshse.org.

LATE-20TH CENTURY: REVISING THE SOCIAL WELFARE SYSTEM

The election of Richard Nixon as president in 1968 marked two important changes in the federal government's involvement in social reform: a decline in federal spending and a different way of managing human service programs. Both represented a return to more traditional values and a much more conservative approach to human services. Nixon's **New Federalism** called for individuals to assume responsibility for their own situations. Power, resources, and influence began to flow back to the states and local communities. The emphasis was on the development of self-help programs and the provision of services by the private sector.

With regard to human services, Nixon focused on a commitment to the family and a commitment to eradicating poverty. He believed that families were able to determine their own needs and should use aid as they determined best (Bowler, 1974). The Supplemental Security Income (SSI) program, which provided additional financial support for people needing assistance, translated this theory into practice.

President Gerald Ford's major impact on the human service delivery system was to continue the reduction of the federal government's involvement in human services. Ford supported an increased commitment by the private sector to support assistance to the needy. He had a major impact on human services through his 60 vetoes, which cut more than $9.5 billion that had been appropriated by Congress. Among the programs he vetoed were proposed improvements in federal aid to education, the school lunch program, and health care.

During his campaign for the presidency, Jimmy Carter discussed reorganizing the federal executive branch. Five departments (Health, Education, and Welfare; Agriculture; Justice; Labor; and Interior) were involved in the reorganization. Initially, the services had been divided into categories of federal funding rather than sets of human problems. One-third of these programs overlapped with each other or with programs in other departments. One major problem was in the Department of Health, Education, and Welfare; more than 300 of its programs crossed over into other departments. Another impetus for the reorganization was to fulfill a campaign promise by separating education programs from health and welfare services. The result was the creation of separate departments: the Department of Health and Human Services and the Department of Education. The use of the term *human services* denoted the wide variety of program services addressing human needs. The choice of the term clearly marks the point when human services became associated with a wide range of services, not restricted to those associated with mental health.

During the Carter administration, the President's Commission on Mental Health, chaired by Rosalyn Carter, found that between 10 and 15% of the population (20 to 32 million people) needed some form of mental health services at any one time. Unfortunately, the commission also discovered that many people did not have access to good, affordable mental health care. Further, there was a lack of support services for people with chronic mental illness, which included approximately 1.5 million people in mental hospitals, nursing homes, and other residential facilities. President Carter proposed and Congress passed the Mental Health Systems Act, which promised comprehensiveness, flexibility, and innovation by emphasizing services for people with chronic mental illness and by emphasizing prevention. It also attempted to address the shortage of mental health personnel in underserved areas, requiring people who received federal money for their training to work in an area with a personnel shortage for a period as long as the time they received financial support.

DISMANTLING THE WELFARE SYSTEM

From the 1930s to the 1980s, the government's social policy was to assume responsibility for citizens who could not provide a reasonable quality of life for themselves.

Voters elected presidents who advocated substantial reduction of the federal budget and decreased federal government involvement in human services—a stark contrast to the policies of the previous administrations.

One of the first signs of retrenchment came from California. On June 7, 1978, California voters passed Proposition 13, an amendment to the state constitution (Pilisuk, 1980). The goal of the legislation was to amend the property tax structure. One result was that less money became available to fund a variety of services, including social services. People were beginning to question the effectiveness and efficiency of the government; they did not want to pay for so much government intervention. When the proposition passed, its supporters predicted that there would be substantial reductions in the services offered by government, and an increase in resources available from private sources.

What actually happened was that fewer professionals were employed, but the number of people in need did not decrease. Human service workers, serving larger caseloads, felt overworked, ineffective, and devalued. Their jobs seemed to have lost what little status they had; voters had sent a clear message that the services they provided were not supported. Existing programs were cut back, and fewer new programs were funded, but the needs were as great as ever. Self-care, community support systems, and natural helping networks had to take up the slack. More people in need began to turn to neighborhood groups, churches, friends, and families for assistance.

The passage of Proposition 13 was an early sign of the changing attitude of the American public toward government spending for human services. In 1980, Ronald Reagan was elected president on a platform that called for establishing new priorities in human services, slashing government spending, and reducing the government's involvement in human services. One of Reagan's priorities was to return the administration of human services to the individual states, communities, and private sources. His reasoning was that it is not the government's function to provide such services and that government delivery of such services is not effective or efficient. He terminated a number of social programs and drastically cut spending on others. Those affected included "AFDC, childcare, school lunch and other nutrition programs, food stamps, subsidized housing, energy assistance, family planning, public and mental health services, alcohol and drug abuse counseling, legal aid, the Job Corps, and the like" (Trattner, 1999, p. 365).

Reagan's reelection in 1984 was another overwhelming victory. His second term continued to emphasize the economy, defense, and foreign policy (Ginsberg, 1987). The plight of the poor worsened during this period, and one result was a welfare reform bill designed to help single parents, particularly women, enter the job market. The Family Support Act was signed into law in 1988. Among the programs authorized was the JOBS program, which required single parents on welfare with children older than 3 years to work or be in training in order to receive assistance. The act also mandated new procedures for collecting child support payments and one year of support for child care and transportation so that single parents could work or participate in training. For the most part, though, both Reagan administrations largely ignored the plight of the poor and disenfranchised, focusing instead on defense spending and tax cuts.

TABLE 2.6	SUMMARY POINTS: LATE 20TH CENTURY—REVISING THE SOCIAL WELFARE SYSTEM

- The election of Richard Nixon in 1968 marked a decline in federal spending.
- Jimmy Carter established the Department of Health and Human Services in 1978.
- The state of California passed Proposition 13 in 1978, signaling less willingness to support social services with taxes.
- The Family Support Act passed in 1988, requiring education and training for welfare recipients.

As a result of Reagan's policy, there was a shift in service delivery. The number of nonprofit and private agencies in human services expanded, and human service institutions and agencies contracted out for services (Ginsberg, 1987). Reagan also advocated transferring federally owned housing and prisons to the private sector. Just as the labor market tends to respond to economic demands, the human service labor market reflects human service demands (Austin, 1983). During the 1960s and 1970s, the human service market was growing, and the number of opportunities for employment and for advancement increased. During the 1980s that growth slowed, although some opportunities did develop in the private sector with, for example, the privatization of correctional facilities and the development of employee assistance programs in private industry.

George Bush, Sr., Reagan's vice president, won the 1988 presidential election and claimed a mandate to continue many of the policies of the Reagan administrations. Generally, Bush's administration is noted for its emphasis on foreign policy and its lack of attention to domestic issues. In fact, because of the pressure of deficit spending, Bush and legislators agreed to slowly cut military spending. In 1990, military expenditures were cut, with the understanding that the money would not be shifted to support social programs. The most significant human service-related legislation of his four years was the Americans with Disabilities Act (ADA), which was passed in 1990. With little cost to the federal government, ADA was designed to get people into the workforce who otherwise would not be able to enter or who were kept out for other reasons, such as discrimination.

WELFARE REFORM

A declining economy, the growing gap between rich and poor, and the need for **welfare reform** all contributed to the election in 1992 of Democrat Bill Clinton, governor of Arkansas. One of his campaign pledges was to "end welfare as we know it." In 1996, The **Personal Responsibility and Work Opportunity Reconciliation Act** (PRWORA) replaced Aid to Families with Dependent Children, which was the primary welfare law sponsored by the federal government to provide aid to eligible mothers with children. This legislation ended the federal government's six-decade guarantee of aid to the poor. Under the former welfare program, eligibility for support was based on income and was regulated by the federal government.

| BOX 2.4 | HIGHLIGHTS OF THE NEW LAW |

The welfare reform bill signed into law by President Clinton makes the most dramatic changes in federal antipoverty programs in six decades. Following are highlights:

- Ends a 61-year guarantee of federal aid for poor children. Instead, Aid to Families with Dependent Children, the main federal cash welfare program, and smaller programs are folded into block grants that states will use to operate their own programs.
- Reduces spending by about $55 billion over six years, mainly by cutting food stamps and aid to legal immigrants.
- Imposes a five-year lifetime limit on welfare benefits. States can exempt up to 20% of their caseload for hardship reasons and set shorter time limits.
- Requires recipients to begin working two years after receiving welfare and mandates that 50% of single-parent families work 30 hours a week by 2002. States already running welfare work programs under federally approved waivers can continue the programs until the waivers expire.

- Reduces spending on food stamps, the federal coupons redeemed for food at supermarkets, by $28 billion over six years and allows able-bodied individuals without children to receive food stamps for only three months in any three-year period, unless they are working part time. Individuals can get another three months if they are laid off from work.
- Bars most federal aid, including Medicaid and cash welfare, to future legal immigrants for five years. Current immigrants cannot receive disability and food stamps during their first five years in the USA, and states have the option to deny other aid. Exceptions include refugees and immigrants who have generally worked for 10 years.
- Makes it more difficult for children with mental problems to receive federal disability payments—a program that has been widely abused, critics say.

Source: From "Highlights of the New Law," *USA Today*, August 23, 1996, p. 3A. Copyright © 1996, *USA Today*. Reprinted with permission.

POLICIES AND PROCEDURES

The key components in the reformed welfare system were state control, work requirements, time limits, and penalties. The states received federal funds in a block grant program called Temporary Assistance to Needy Families (**TANF**), and there was, and still is, flexibility concerning how the states spend their money. Each state receives a fixed amount of money each year, and they must also contribute to the welfare program. The state contribution is called the mandated maintenance of effort (MOE). Many states have used their TANF and MOE dollars to provide traditional welfare services, such as cash assistance, employment services, child care, and emergency assistance; however, some states have expanded their services. In additional, the goals of this legislation related to marriage and family formation and included promoting marriage, reducing the birth of children out of wedlock, and supporting two-parent families.

Human service professionals working within the framework of the new welfare-to-work law provide a mixed review of the experience. They applaud the new focus of moving clients off the welfare rolls and into meaningful work that will allow them to provide economic stability for their families. But they still see the difficulties that their

---

BOX 2.5	WEB SOURCES
	Welfare Reform

http://www.acf.dhhs.gov/news/welfare/

This site published by the Department of Health and Human Services describes current TANF guidelines, policies and procedures of welfare policy, and current state grant formulas and forms. It also links the reader to a history of welfare reform.

http://www.ncsl.org/statefed/welfare/welfare.htm

This site sponsored by The National Conference of State Legislatures describes research on welfare reform, current issues, and demographics from 50 state and gives evaluations of the new welfare policies.

http://www.acf.hhs.gov/acf_working_with.html#state

This site provides links to all state welfare websites. Following these links allows the researcher to explore the differences among the policies and the evaluation outcome efforts for state welfare policies.

---

clients have in gaining employment that will support their families. Using a case management approach to provide a multitude of services, they are able to help clients and their families meet basic needs; however, they are concerned about the rules and regulations of the program. The next section contains descriptions of the types of clients that human service professionals see as they work in the "welfare" arena.

THE FACES OF WELFARE TO WORK

With the implementation of the new law comes the responsibility of evaluating its outcomes. Conducting research about welfare has been challenging. The following three profiles of recipients, illustrate several of the job patterns of the welfare "leavers" (those who exit welfare) and welfare "stayers" (those who receive welfare). The job patterns include sustained employment, multiple employment, and no employment and on the welfare rolls (Pacchioli, 2003; Loprest & Zedlewski, 2006).

> "Silvia" is a welfare stayer who maintains consistent employment. This 18-year-old mother stays with her mother, who provides daycare for her children. She supports herself and her children with family support and some public assistance.
> "Mercedes" maintains several jobs. She is 41 and has three sons. She works 70 hours a week and still has difficulty paying her rent. Her father provides some support and gives her money for child care.
> "Nieves," a 21-year-old, has no job and depends on welfare. She takes care of her four children, her sister's three, and her mother. She has not been able to maintain consistent housing and has moved 11 times over the last three years. (Pacchioli, p. 7)

The stayers represent a set of individuals with characteristics that at least partially explain their difficulties in leaving the welfare rolls. They fall into two categories: (1) long-termers and (2) short-termers and cyclers (Moffit, Cherlin, Burton, King, & Roff, 2003). The long-termers, considered disadvantaged, have a low level of education and serious mental and physical health problems. They report high levels of domestic abuse or violence and low unemployment rates. Some are caring for family members who have physical illnesses or have disabilities. Many report that they could not find flexible employment. Janet represents one of these long-termers.

> "Janet" is a 40-year-old African American woman with three children. Other family members, such as her uncle and his family, live with her. She has received parenting services and is monitored by the department of human services. She was reported for child abuse and neglect, and she has a history of using and selling drugs (Moffit et al., 2003).

The short-termers and cyclers are women who use welfare services from time to time to meet specific needs, such as pregnancy or other emergencies. Some of them work and receive benefits. Many are in transition and intend to move off the welfare rolls. Gina represents one of the women in this category.

> Twenty-eight-year-old "Gina" exits the welfare program and then applies again. Her requests for services revolve around her pregnancies. She works full time when she is not pregnant. She lives with her three children but not with either of the two men who fathered them. Gina understands the welfare policies, and she does not remain on the rolls for any length of time. She can support herself and her children when she works as a medical assistant, when her mother cares for her children (Moffit et al., 2003).

These stories of women involved in the welfare system, either as leavers or stayers, help us understand the impact that welfare reform has had on their lives. Let's look at the successes and challenges of the recent welfare legislation.

EVALUATION OF WELFARE REFORM

Debate continues about the effectiveness of welfare reform. Is it really working? There are differing opinions concerning the success of Welfare to Work. Many say "yes, it is helping families become more self-sufficient," while others believe that still more women and children are living below the poverty line. So, what facts are known about what has happened to those staying on welfare, those who left welfare, and nonwelfare recipients who live at or below the poverty line?

- Marriage declined and cohabitation increased for both welfare leavers and nonwelfare populations.
- Immigrant welfare recipients remain on welfare longer than nonimmigrant recipients.
- Work training and efforts to remove barriers to work helped increase work and work-related activities for those on welfare and welfare leavers.
- Multiple barriers increased for Spanish speakers.
- There is an increase in income for current welfare recipients compared to welfare leavers and nonwelfare individuals.
- The number of nonwelfare individuals living below the poverty line has increased. (Loprest & Zedlewski, 2006a).

SIGNIFICANT CHALLENGES

As states implement the welfare legislation, they use different strategies to address family structure and demographics, family benefits (and caps), and the nature of the TANF program with regard to work. For example, TANF regulations allow states flexibility with regard to different types of family units and eligibility for benefits. The exception is the regulation that pregnant teens need to live in supervised settings. Under previous welfare legislation, it was difficult for two-parent families to receive welfare and teen mothers could receive aid. Today, following the TANF regulations, all states require that teen parents must live with families or in supervised settings. Half of the states count the income of stepparents and half of the states count the income of those cohabitating when determining eligibility for welfare. States will also allow two-parent families to be eligible for welfare, if they meet the eligibility standards (Loprest & Zedlewski, 2006b).

Under the previous welfare legislation, immigrants were eligible for welfare services. Under PROWRA, legal immigrants were banned from receiving welfare for five years if they entered the country after August 22, 1996. States were able to provide these immigrants services with state funds if they so chose, and currently, there are some states that are supporting legal immigrants with state funds.

Previously, AFDC provided additional support for families who had children while on welfare, but many states had "family caps" on the amount of welfare that a family could receive if the number of children in the family increased during the time the family was receiving welfare. The caps remain in many states (Loprest & Zedlewski, 2006b).

Most of the state welfare programs began a "work first" policy early in the implementation of the new legislation; hence many individuals with little training or education were placed in low-paying service sector jobs. But today some states are refocusing their efforts to find good jobs for their clients. A "good job" means higher pay, benefits, full-time work, and some opportunity for training or advancement. For example, the Annie E. Casey Foundation funded an initiative in six cities to provide training for welfare leavers to work in medical offices, administration, construction, and manufacturing. Workers in this program earned higher wages and remained in their employment longer than lower-waged workers (Annie E. Casey Foundation, 2006). This type of work supports research on the high job satisfaction of welfare leavers. Many are in service sector jobs with low pay and few benefits, yet they report positive work experiences (Scott, 2006). Most states, however, exempt mothers from work requirements if they have a child who is less than 1 year old.

One population disaffected by the legislation are nonresident fathers (Miller, 2006). There are new laws that allow the state to collect child support from noncustodial parents. The law, however, does not help these fathers gain employment skills, stable work, and benefits. PRWORA also does not provide support for these fathers to be with their children. Suggested services to these fathers might include mediation, parenting plans, and parental education as well as vocational services (Miller, 2006).

LEGISLATIVE CHANGES IN THE 21-CENTURY

There are several legislative changes that mark the federal involvement in human services. These include the passage of a prescription drug act and an expanded support of faith based human services.

The Medicare Prescription Drug, Improvement, and Modernization Act of 2003 (MMA) was passed to provide outpatient prescription drug benefits for individuals on

Medicare, Part D. Benefits are available to over 43 million people who enroll in private plans that offer coverage and are approved by Medicare (Henry J. Kaiser Family Foundation, 2006). This plan replaces Medicaid as a source of drug coverage. Implementing this new program has not been easy.

Although pharmacists and physicians believe that MMA has the potential to help their customers and patients, they also say the complicated regulations cause problems for customers and patients (Palosky & Levitt, 2006). Initial problems consumers and patients encountered included: (1) the prescribed drug was not on the chosen plan; (2) customers could not verify that they had enrolled in a plan, (3) customers who were receiving state Medicare could not access their federal plan; and (4) customers experienced serious medical problems because they could not fill prescriptions they needed. As the implementation of MMA matures, the hope is that most beneficiaries will receive adequate prescriptive drug coverage through Part D enrollment or other creditable sources such as drug coverage under employer or union plans.

To help Americans in need, President George W. Bush initiated an effort to bring faith-based agencies and organizations into partnership with the federal government by creating the White House Office of Faith-based and Community Initiatives. He also created **Centers for Faith-based and Community Initiatives (CFBCI)** in 11 federal agencies. The mission of the CFBCI in the Department of Health and Human Services is "to lead the Department efforts to better utilize faith-based and community-based organizations in providing effective human services" (U.S. Department of Health & Human Services[DHHS], 2006). President Bush stated:

> The paramount goal is compassionate results, and private and charitable groups, including religious ones, should have the fullest opportunity permitted by law to compete on a level playing field, so long as they achieve valid public purposes, like curbing crime, conquering addiction, strengthening families, and overcoming poverty (DHHS, 2006).

To reach this goal, CFBCI has developed technical assistance for faith-based organizations in terms of grant writing and service delivery to these organizations, trained departmental and agency staff on ways to develop collaborative efforts, modified governmental policies and regulations so that faith-based organizations can be competitive in securing funding, developed a grant opportunities notebook that outlines possible funding opportunities, and held regional conferences to support partnership efforts. The conferences are supported by 11 federal departments, including the Departments of Justice, Agriculture, Labor, Health and Human Services, and Housing and Urban Development, and agencies such as the Small Business Administration.

Several of the programs highlighted by the CFBCI are a Compassions Capital Fund, the Mentoring Children of Prisoners, and an Access to Recovery program, and a Prisoner Re-entry Initiative. To help faith-based organizations develop programs the DHHS CFBCI provides a "toolkit" that includes a description of best practices, information about establishing partnerships, supporting documents for grant acquisition and grant management, guidelines for outcomes measurement, information about potential revenue sources, and technical assistance. Bush views this effort as an eight-year process that began in 2002 with the Compassion Capital Fund and ends with an assessment of these efforts in 2009 (DHHS, 2006).

A FINAL THOUGHT

At this writing important issues remain unresolved. Among them are the war on terrorism, the partisan divide in the United States, the Social Security funding crisis, the balance of protection and civil liberties, abortion, health care, the war in Iraq, and the living wage. Although prescription drug coverage, the 2006 Voting Rights Act reauthorization, and attempts to improve education and to reform Social Security have received attention, a number of Americans have needs that continue to be unmet. In response, human service professionals have renewed their efforts to advocate for their clients and their profession.

KEY TERMS

AFDC

almshouses

asylums

Centers for Faith-based and Community Initiatives (CFBCI)

community mental health centers

deinstitutionalization

individualism

laissez faire

Medicaid

Medicare

The Medicare Prescription Drug, Improvement, and Modernization Act of 2003 (MMA)

National Institute for Mental Health

New Federalism

Personal Responsibility and Work Opportunity Reconciliation Act (PRWORA)

poor relief

probation

settlement house

Social Darwinism

Social Security

social workers

TANF

war on poverty

welfare reform

THINGS TO REMEMBER

1. Before the Middle Ages, people believed that mental illness was caused by evil spirits, and early forms of treatment focused on ridding the body of these spirits.

2. Until the 1500s, the Catholic Church was chiefly responsible for providing human services, and it was under the Church's guidance that many institutions were founded for the poor, orphans, the elderly, and the handicapped.

3. The decline of feudalism, the growth of commerce, and the beginning of industrialization made it necessary to find new ways of assisting those in need.

4. Pressures caused by the increasing number of poor in the cities created the need for a large-scale attack on poverty and prompted the passage of the Elizabethan Poor Law of

1601, critical legislation that guided social welfare practices in England and the United States for the next 350 years.

5. In the early years, the colonists used the English system as a model for their philosophy toward and services for the poor and needy. By the early 1800s, however, other philosophies prevailed, ones that discouraged and limited the provision of human services.

6. Major reforms during the late 1800s concentrated on improving the treatment of institutionalized mentally ill and children.

7. The Charity Organization Society, a forerunner of the Community Chest and the United Way, is an example of society's response to the needs of an expanding urban population.

8. A settlement house was a large house in a slum area that served as a community center,

sponsoring such activities as recreation; classes in English, cooking, and citizenship; vocational training; and child care.

9. President Franklin D. Roosevelt introduced the Social Security Act of 1935, which fundamentally changed the federal government's role in providing human services.

10. During the years John F. Kennedy served as president, he set the tone for increased emphasis on the eradication of poverty in the United States, bringing hope to populations that had despaired of changing their situations without assistance.

11. The emergence of human service training programs and the development of a human service philosophy mirror the historical events and presidential leadership from the 1960s to the present.

12. In his 1965 State of the Union address, President Lyndon Johnson declared an "unconditional war on poverty" and developed programs that attacked the roots of poverty in order to create a "Great Society."

13. The National Organization for Human Services and the Council for Standards in Human Service Education have been instrumental in the development of the human service profession.

14. The election of Richard Nixon as president marked a change in the federal government's involvement in social reform with a decline in federal spending.

15. During the presidency of Ronald Reagan, commitment to human services passed from the federal government to state and local governments, the private sector, and needy individuals themselves.

16. The first Bush administration supported the passage of the Americans with Disabilities Act, which provided guidelines to reduce the discrimination of individuals with disabilities.

17. Bill Clinton reformed the welfare system by proposing a new law that emphasized training, education, short-term support, and personal responsibility.

18. Welfare reform has decreased the number of families on the welfare rolls and increased the number of the families who are employed.

19. The Medicare Prescription Drug Bill and the faith-based and community partnership efforts are recent legislative changes to support those in need.

ADDITIONAL READINGS: FOCUS ON HISTORY

Beers, Clifford W. (1945). A *mind that found itself: An autobiography*. Garden City, NY: Doubleday, Doran.
    Clifford Beers writes of his experiences as a three-time patient in mental institutions around the turn of the 20th century.

Herrick, J. (Ed.) (2004). *Encyclopedia of social welfare history in North America*. San Francisco: Sage.
    This encyclopedia has 180 entries that provide information about the history of social welfare in the United States, Canada, and Mexico. Included are primary materials, a multinational perspective, suggestions for further reading, appendices, and an index with cross-references.

Jensen, L. (2003). *Patriots, settlers, and the origins of American social policy*. Cambridge, UK: Cambridge University Press.
    This book provides an account of the development of America's first entitlement policies during the first 100 years of the United States. It challenges the belief that the United States lagged behind other countries in developing national social programs.

Marshall, Helen E. (1937). *The forgotten Samaritan*. Chapel Hill, NC: University of North Carolina Press.

Marshall has produced a well-written biography of Dorothea Dix, humanitarian and reformer.

Seccombe, K. (2006). *"So you think I drive a Cadillac?": Welfare recipients' perspectives on the system and its reform.* (2nd ed.). Needham Heights, MA: Pearson, Allyn & Bacon.

Welfare recipients share their experiences with welfare and their views on its reform. Topics include their plans, hopes, and dreams for the future, as well as their perspectives on work

requirements, family caps, and other TANF features.

Trattner, Walter I. (1999). *From poor law to welfare state: A history of social welfare in America.* New York: Free Press.

Trattner gives an overview of social welfare in the United States from the colonial era to the present. He includes highlights of the mental health, child welfare, and public health movements, as well as beginnings of social welfare as a profession.

REFERENCES

Account Historians Journal. Retrieved September 21, 2006, from http://findarticles.com/p/articles/mi_qa3657/is_200206/ai_n9105176/pg_1.

Albee, G. W. (1961). *Mental health manpower trends.* New York: Basic Books.

Annie E. Casey Foundation. (2006). *Initiatives and projects.* Retrieved September 10, 2006, from http://www.aecf.org/initiatives/summaries.htm#1.

Austin, C. (1983). Case management: A systems perspective. *Families in Society: The Journal of Contemporary Human Services, 79,* 451–459.

Beers, C. W. (1945). *A mind that found itself: An autobiography.* Garden City, NY: Doubleday, Doran & Co.

Bowler, M. (1974). *The Nixon guaranteed income proposal: Substance and process in policy change.* Cambridge, MA: Ballinger.

Cranston, A. (1986). Psychology in the Veterans Administration. *American Psychologist, 41*(9), 990–995.

Friedrich, O. (1976). *Going crazy: An inquiry into madness in our time.* New York: Avon Books.

Galbraith, J. K. (1976). *The affluent society.* Boston: Houghton Mifflin.

Ginsberg, L. H. (1987). Economic, political and social context. In L. H. Ginsberg (Ed.), *Encyclopedia of social work* (18th ed.) (pp. xxxii–xxxvi). Silver Springs, MD: National Association of Social Workers.

Harrington, M. (1962). *The other America.* New York: Macmillan.

Henry J. Kaiser Family Foundation. (2006). *Medicare: Fact sheet.* Retrieved Spetember 10, 2006, from http://www.kff.org.

Irvine, H. (2002). The legitimizing power of financial statements of the Salvation Army in England, 1885–1892.

James, V. (1981, April). Mental health worker news: A forum for the mental health profession. *Bulletin: Council for Standards in Human Services Education, 4.*

Kennedy, J. F. (1964). Remarks on proposed measures to combat mental illness and mental retardation. *Public papers of the Presidents of the United States: John F. Kennedy* (January 1–November 22, 1963), 50–51. Washington, DC: U.S. Government Printing Office.

Loprest, P., & Zedlewski, S. (2006a). *Assessing the new federalism: Executive summary.* Washington, DC: The Urban Institute. Retrieved September 10, 2006, from http://www.urban.org/UploadedPDF/311357_occa73.pdf.

Loprest, P., & Zedlewski, S. (2006b). *Assessing the new federalism: The changing role of welfare in the lives of low-income families with children.* Washington, DC: The Urban Institute. Retrieved September 10, 2006, from http://www.urban.org/UploadedPDF/311357_occa73.pdf.

Macht, J. (1990). A historical perspective. In S. Fullerton & D. Osher (Eds.), *History of the human services movement, 7,* 90–9.

Marshall, H. (1937). *The forgotten Samaritan.* Chapel Hill: University of North Carolina Press.

Miller, M. K. (2006). Through the eyes of a father: How PRWORA affects non-resident Fathers and their children. *International Journal of Law, Policy and the Family, 20*(1), 55–73.

Moffit, R., Cherlin, A., Burton, L., King, M., & Roff, J. (2003). The characteristics of families remaining on welfare. *Welfare, Children, & Families. Policy Brief 02–2.* Baltimore: John Hopkins University.

National Institute of Mental Health (NIMH). (1971). *Mental illness and its treatment: Social issues resources issue series* (Vol. 1, Article 3; DHEW Publications No [HSM] 72–9030). Washington, DC: Author.

Neugebauer, R. (1979). Medieval and early modern theories of mental illness. *Archives of General Psychiatry, 36,* 477–483.

Pacchioli, D. (2003, January). Not by jobs alone. *Penn State Online Research, 24*(1). Retrieved September 5, 2003, from http://www.rps.psu.edu/0301/jobs.html.

Palosky, C., & Levitt, L. (2006). *News release: National survey of pharmacists and national survey of physicians.* Retrieved September 10, 2006, from www.kff.org/kaiserpolls/pomr090706nr.cfm.

Pilisuk, M. (1980, April). The future of human services without funding. *American Journal of Orthopsychiatry, 50*(2), 200–204.

Richmond, M. (1917). *Social diagnosis.* New York: Russell Sage Foundation.

Scott, J. (2006). Job satisfaction among TANF leavers. *Journal of Sociology & Social Welfare, 33*(3), 127–149.

Southern Regional Education Board (SREB). (1979). *Roles and functions for different levels of mental health workers.* Atlanta, GA: Author.

Trattner, Walter I. (1999). *From poor law to welfare state: A history of social welfare in America.* New York: Free Press.

U.S. Department of Health and Human Services (DHHS). (2006). *The center for faith-based and community initiatives.* Retrieved September 10, 2006, from http://www.hhs.gov/fbci/.

Zimbalist, S. E. (1977). *Historic themes and landmarks in social welfare research.* New York: Harper & Row.

CHAPTER **3** | # HUMAN SERVICES TODAY

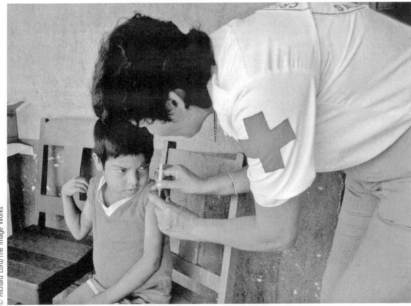

© Richard Lord/The Image Works

After reading this chapter, you will be able to:

- Document reasons for the expansion of human service settings.
- Identify areas of technology use in human services.
- Define "managed care."
- List the challenges presented by the international dimension of human services.
- Identify five significant trends in human services.

Self-assessment

- Explain why human service delivery has expanded beyond the traditional settings.
- How has technology changed the delivery of human services?
- Describe the impact that managed care is having on the human service delivery system.
- Why is it important to understand the international dimension of human services?
- How will the trends occurring in the next few decades affect human service delivery?
- Describe how religious diversity challenges and brings opportunities to a community.

One facet of the definition of human services is how and where services are delivered today. This chapter examines new settings, new skills, and recent trends in human service delivery. As you read this chapter, you will see that human services today has a much broader scope than ever before. It takes place in a variety of settings, addresses global human needs, interfaces with the managed care system, and reflects recent advances in communication and technology. Human services is also impacted by other changes such as terrorism, the growing number of individuals over 65, and the increasing diversity of the United States. This chapter examines each of these dimensions in more detail to help expand your definition of human services.

NEW SETTINGS FOR HUMAN SERVICE DELIVERY

One way to describe the broadening scope of human services today is to think about where services are delivered. In many instances, services continue to be delivered in agencies or institutional settings; but with a growing emphasis on making services accessible and comprehensive, service delivery in nontraditional settings has increased. Rural services, industrial and military settings, and schools are highlighted in this section.

INSTITUTIONAL AND COMMUNITY-BASED SERVICES

There has been a change in philosophy regarding the delivery of services in institutional settings and in the community. The difference in settings is an obvious factor. Earlier institutions were located in remote places because pastoral settings were believed to be peaceful and calming. These settings may also have been chosen because

BOX 3.1 | YOUTH IN NEED

Youth in Need (YIN) is a multiservice agency that serves children, youth, and families throughout Eastern Missouri. The precipitating event in 1974 for the founding of YIN was a teenage girl whose face was bruised from yet another beating. She was brought to the local jail, where at that time all runaway and homeless youth were housed with adult criminals. One of the founders of YIN, Reverend Earl Worley, described the beginning of YIN: "It was late at night and we knew we had talked about opening a youth shelter long enough. Looking at that young girl, we knew that we couldn't let down one more kid." Since that time, YIN has developed a number of programs to make children's healthy development and well-being the community's highest priority.

One of their programs, Street Outreach, is targeted to homeless and runaway youth who are living on the streets of St. Louis and surrounding areas. Staff travel streets and neighborhoods in a specially designed and stocked van to provide blankets, food, and clothing; most importantly, they are committed to help youth problem solve and locate needed resources. Their work is illustrated by the following case:

> We stopped to talk with a homeless teenager who was downtown near the library. He was upset. He had been in a number of shelters and transitional living programs but just hadn't been successful. He said, "I have a temper. I just want to go home. I've tried to call my dad's phone number." He had gone to the library earlier that day to call but didn't know how to make a collect call. So I gave him a cell phone, something we think is no big deal, and told him to call his dad. They hadn't seen each other in several years. He called: "Dad? It's me." And he started crying. It was a really great moment. It was just a cell phone but he had not known how to make a collect call or to get a phone card that some agencies have. His dad picked him up two or three hours later. It was a pretty rewarding experience—one I won't forget.

members of society did not like to be reminded of the existence of people with mental illness. Correctional facilities have been built in rural areas because the criminal population is considered dangerous to others. Again, people did not like to be reminded of this population. Now, however, in mental health, the trend continues toward downsizing institutions and increasing the number of **community-based services.** In the past, many people who were institutionalized could have functioned in the community with some professional support. The goal of community-based mental health care is to enable clients to interact with their environments in the least restrictive setting in which they can function.

Community-based mental health has changed the nature of service delivery. The focus of treatment has become health and wellness instead of illness. The process involves other social institutions such as schools, recreation facilities, and religious organizations. In addition, the psychological and medical treatment received by clients has been adapted for community-based care. Much human service work is in case management: The human service worker acts as planner, consultant, and liaison between the mental health agency, the client, and the other supportive institutions. Human service professionals also provide help for the families of people with mental illness.

A concerted effort has been made in community-based services to extend the office to the community. Many agencies now include outreach programs that send staff throughout neighborhoods and communities to work with clients where they live, shop, work, or "hang out." Youth in Need is a St. Louis area multiservice agency that reaches homeless and runaway youth on the streets. Box 3.1 profiles this effective program.

Community-based care in corrections is designed to take individuals from prisons and local jails and place them in the community within supervised, planned programs. These programs link educational services, counseling, substance abuse treatment, and employment assistance. In these programs, much of the responsibility falls to the client to take the initiative in using available services.

Schools are now a site for human service delivery in many communities. Teachers encounter the problems of children and youth each time they enter the classroom. They ask: "Can learning occur in an environment characterized by gangs, dropouts, teenage pregnancy, substance abuse, AIDS, and violence?" Predictions for the future do not offer much hope.

A partnership between human services and education is important to meet the complex needs of children and families. School-based services or **full-service schools** are popular terms that describe the creation of an array of integrated support services in schools where children, youth, and families need to be successful (Kronick, 2005). This movement melds quality education and support services. What services are provided in full-service schools? The answer depends on several factors such as the needs of students and their families, the viability of school reform, and the cooperative efforts of local agencies. Dryfoos and Barkin (2006) suggest that the integration of educational, health, and social welfare services may provide support for vulnerable children growing up today.

Examples of other nontraditional settings for human service professionals are malls, funeral homes, and hospitals. Increasingly, graduates are finding that their generalist knowledge and skills transfer to virtually any setting where people may experience problems or need support or assistance. There is every indication that nontraditional settings will increase.

HUMAN SERVICES IN RURAL AREAS

Interest in providing services in rural areas is increasing. Two factors account for this interest. First, historically those living in rural areas, which are losing population, have been disadvantaged, experiencing a steady erosion in their quality of life. They are more likely to be elderly, be members of disadvantaged minorities, lack the kinds of opportunities available to metropolitan counterparts, and need the help of human service agencies and professionals. Evidence also suggests, however, a growing pattern of relocation to rural areas and small towns, which is a reversal of 20th-century migration trends from rural to urban areas.

Small towns and rural areas are attracting those who see advantages in living where there are lower crime rates, opportunities for professional advancement, and larger labor pools with lower wage expectations. Thus, an increasing number of people who are not disadvantaged live in rural areas; indeed, they may have significant wealth. They include property owners, professionals, and business people. Those who are living in rural poverty and those who are not disadvantaged may experience similar problems, such as mental illness, family conflicts, and physical limitations, that require the help of social service agencies and helping professionals.

A second reason for the interest in human services in rural areas is the difficulties or barriers in providing accessible and adequate services. Recruiting and retaining trained health care and helping professionals, the large geographic distances between clients and providers, the cost of services, the maintenance of confidentiality, the isolation, and the coordination of care are all problematic in rural areas. Another significant barrier is the community stigma attached to having problems and receiving services. This negative perception may prevent individuals and families from getting the professional help they need. In some cases, individuals seek informal help from the extended family, the church, and social clubs, particularly when formal support systems are lacking.

The provision of mental health services is particularly problematic in rural areas. In addition to the problems mentioned, mental health problems often remain undiagnosed. Rural primary care providers such as physicians and nurse practitioners are likely to care for those with mental health problems and encounter difficulties in referring them for specialized care. Here again, distance, stigma, and costs are among the barriers that prevent successful referrals.

Recently, new models have emerged for delivering services to rural clients. They represent attempts to meet the unique needs of this population by providing child welfare services, meeting transportation needs, using members of the community for social support, providing home-based care, targeting the identified needs of clients, and asking about clients' needs and preferences. In addition, educators now recognize that service provision in rural areas requires academic preparation that focuses on creative solutions to improve options, improvisation to meet needs, collaboration with a range of other professionals and informal supports, and the building of an infrastructure to provide needed supports to rural residents and communities.

HUMAN SERVICES IN INDUSTRY AND THE MILITARY

Traditionally, human services has been associated with people in financial need, particularly those who are unemployed or who are labeled as poor. Today's employers recognize that workers who are physically and psychologically well are more productive employees. Industry has learned to identify signals that indicate when an employee needs assistance: tardiness, absenteeism, ineffective job performance, and inability to cooperate or communicate with others. Many companies now encourage their workers to seek help.

Industry's initial interest in human services began when drug and alcohol abuse among employees showed alarming increases. The federal government was instrumental in establishing guidelines for treating this problem. The Federal Comprehensive Alcohol Abuse and Alcohol Prevention, Treatment and Rehabilitation Act (the Hughes Act) was passed in 1970 and created the National Institute on Alcohol Abuse and Alcoholism. The act was significant for the field of human services because it established an approach that was different from the treatment for people with mental illness. The act required federal agencies to have alcohol abuse and prevention programs available to employees—programs now well-known as **employee assistance programs** (EAPs).

EAP services are offered to employees of most major corporations. Some address broad needs of workers, such as counseling for abuse, personal issues, and marital problems; encouraging wellness with diet counseling, exercise, stress management, and personal awareness education; and developing work-related skills through such programs as employee orientation, management development, human relations training, team building, organizational development, and preparation for retirement.

Most professionals who provide this support have baccalaureate and master's-level training. The scope of human services has once again expanded beyond the fundamental provision of basic assistance.

Passage of the **Americans with Disabilities Act** (ADA) has also had a significant impact on business, industry, and other employers. Signed into law by President George H. W. Bush on July 26, 1990, ADA was patterned after the 1964 Civil Rights Act. The intent and spirit of ADA was, and continues to be, to enable people with disabilities to have access to goods and services—including employment—that is equal to the access available to citizens without disabilities. ADA is nondiscriminatory legislation, not affirmative action legislation. The act affects almost 50 million Americans with disabilities and focuses on employment, public services, access to goods and services, and telecommunications.

A priority of the administration of George W. Bush is the New Freedom Initiative that has as its purpose the elimination of the barriers that prevent people with disabilities from participating fully in community life. Under the auspices of the Office on Disability, this initiative provides a comprehensive, government-wide framework to achieve that goal. For a person with disability, quality health care may mean the difference between living independently in the community or living in an institutional setting.

The overwhelming majority of the nation's employers openly embrace ADA's equal access and reasonable accommodation tenets. If a candidate is qualified for a particular job and can perform the essential job functions, that person has the same opportunities as anyone else. The employer must make alterations to the work setting to account for the disability. Through mediation, alternative dispute resolution, arbitration, and litigation, case law is further defining and clarifying ADA's parameters. The integration and acceptance of people with disabilities has increased greatly in the short period since passage of the act, but more remains to be done.

Another nontraditional setting for human service delivery is the military. Meeting basic human needs in the military is different from accomplishing the same in a civilian setting, partly because of the atmosphere of discipline and commitment to the organization. In 1881, the American Red Cross began providing social services to the military out of a concern for the health and welfare of the men and women in uniform. A medical orientation characterized military social service until 1976, when the Service to Armed Forces (SAF) was developed to help the military better serve the families of military personnel. Field offices were established in military hospitals and military installations to assist communication between service personnel and families. The field offices provide a team of professionals, including a human service worker, to counsel military personnel (Masi, 1982). In January 1999, the Navy also announced a new program, LIFElines, that links personnel and families by e-mail. This program was part of a $3.4 million Quality of Life program that promotes a national model leading the way in human resources support services.

Operation Iraqi Freedom (OIF), launched in March 2003, reminded us that war can be traumatizing for some military personnel and their families. OIF has become the largest sustained ground operation since Viet Nam. Soldiers exposed to combat may develop mental disorders, such as posttraumatic stress disorder, depression, and generalized anxiety. In fact, about one-third of U.S. military personnel who have returned home are receiving mental health services (Gardner, 2006).

TABLE 3.1 | SUMMARY POINTS: SERVICE DELIVERY SETTINGS

- Human service delivery continues in traditional settings such as social service agencies and institutions.

- Mental health, corrections, and family services are examples of community-based service delivery.

- Rural human service delivery faces many barriers including distance, cost, confidentiality, and shortages of professionals.

- The Federal Comprehensive Alcohol Abuse and Alcohol Prevention, Treatment and Rehabilitation Act prompted the establishment of employee assistance programs in the workplace.

- The Americans with Disabilities Act ensures equal access to goods, services, and employment for people with disabilities.

- Full-service schools integrate education, health, and social welfare services.

The U.S. military has several programs to screen war veterans as they return stateside. One program gives veterans a half-day schedule so they can reconnect with their families; the other part of the day is spent with their soldier buddies. A second program is the Post-Deployment Health Assessment to screen for both physical and mental health problems.

THE IMPACT OF TECHNOLOGY

Technology continues to change the delivery of human services. Human service providers are expanding the ways that they use technology to help their clients both directly and indirectly. Technology is used in the areas of communication, information management, service delivery, and professional development. Development in technology is dynamic, and continued change is the norm. Administrators of services, direct service providers, and clients are all "customers" of the computer systems that continue to emerge and we expect growth in the creative use of technology to continue occurring at a rapid pace.

The primary goal for using technology in the human service delivery system is to provide services more effectively and efficiently. For many human service professionals, use of technology has already helped them provide better quality services in a more cost-effective manner. As these technologies become more interwoven in our lives, they will be used simply because they represent the standard way of doing business. One pervading ethical concern about the increased use of technology is the protection of confidentiality. As paper and face-to-face communication has shifted to technology-driven methods, protection of the client and the helping activity must continue to be ensured. In Chapter 9, confidentiality as it relates to technology is explored in more detail.

COMMUNICATION

Computer technologies and the advances in satellite communications support the ways many interactions occur in human service settings. **E-mail** continues to be one way human service professionals communicate and share information and files with colleagues, whether they are in the same building or across the state, nation, or sometimes, globe. Human service professionals also use distribution lists and Listservs to share ideas and concerns regarding ethics, treatment, managed care, and funding. Instant Messaging (IM) and SMS (Text Messaging) are two new ways that individuals are communicating with each other. IM typically represents communication from computer-to-computer, while Text Messaging is typically between cell phones. Both of these methods of communications allow individuals to communicate synchronously. The advantage of using IM and Text Messaging is the ability to send and receive messages instantaneously.

Another way human service professionals in distant locations can communicate with each other is by **teleconferencing.** Many large organizations find this technology a cost-effective way to conduct meetings and to talk with each other about service delivery, new programming for clients, and ways to learn new information and skills. For example, Nunavut is a Canadian territory created in 1999, that is approximately two million square kilometers and extends from the Hudson Bay to the North Pole. The Inuit comprise 85% of the approximately 29,000 people living in the area. There are 28 settlements and none are accessible by road (Government of Nunavut, 2006). The Department of Health and Social Services is committed to providing a broad range of services to its constituencies by using clinics, clients' homes, outpost camps, and teleconferencing (Department of Health and Social Services, 2006). This is but one example of how teleconferencing is used to stay in touch with other professionals and also to provide services.

Cellular phones and pagers are standard issue for many human service professionals providing direct services to clients. These devices also allow professionals to be available at all times. A case manager working with child abuse cases says, "I carry my cell phone 24/7 because I deal with children and their families. I need to be available— they need me." (Jennifer Robertson, personal communication). These devices also provide security to many workers when they are in dangerous or isolated situations.

Communications also occur through the **World Wide Web** using individualized web pages. In this way, many individuals and organizations can provide information to those online. For example, many organizations are using the Web for organizational visibility, direct services, community education, advocacy, and securing resources. Web pages provide Internet users with phone numbers and e-mail addresses of help lines and relevant offices, as well as information about programs, special conferences and events, and organizational information such as mission and agency structure. Agencies provide online services through chat rooms, e-mail counseling, and online support group meetings. Advocacy efforts involve promoting awareness and support on policy and legislative issues and helping the community find other resources it needs.

Organizations are also using the Web to reach their members and to recruit potential new members, donors, and volunteers. As an example, the web page for the National Organization for Human Services (http://www.nationalhumanservices.org) offers information about the organization, with links to its role and mission, the board of directors, the regional organization, and membership.

The World Wide Web is a powerful multicultural tool used to connect people to other people. As you will read later in this chapter, increasing one's understanding of cultures, human diversity, and related ethics is necessary given the rapidly changing demographics of the United States and the world (Chapter 9). The Web allows the sharing of stories, histories, choices, reflections, and interactions that reach beyond what has been traditionally available in books, periodicals, or classrooms. **Web logs** (blogs) are sites where individuals can post their diaries, journals, thoughts, and opinions about their experiences of or ideas about a particular subject. Numerous blogs focus on human services. An example is the *Washington Post* site on local human services entitled "Focus on Fairfax." One can read entries about current events such as legislative cuts to services, the latest research, and services to populations in need (Focus on Fairfax, 2006). Blogs provide an opportunity for public information sharing and debate.

Just as technology supports better communication, it also offers an improved way of managing information. There are many ways in which computers and their software help manage information within the human service delivery system.

INFORMATION MANAGEMENT

Using computer technology, managers coordinate information from a variety of sources and then organize the data to facilitate planning, decision making, and reporting. Information can also be managed to support evaluation and help tie service delivery to outcomes and cost. The information entered into a human service database can include a client's name and other relevant demographic data (age, gender, race, and marital status), prior use of the human service delivery system, intake information and assessment results, problem identification, treatment plans, treatment records of services provided, and evaluation of those services according to outcomes reached and client satisfaction.

In addition, in this environment of managed care, the information system may also include service costs, payment, the cost of each service delivered, and a record of the interaction with the managed care organization. The interaction record may show the kinds of services authorized by frequency, duration, and definition of the service provider. One advantage of a management information system is its ability to transfer information electronically across organizations and among workers. This feature benefits both human service professionals and clients in several ways. First, the client and the professional save the time and energy required to generate the data for a second or a third time. If the data represent intake or initial assessment information, the professional can review it with the client and request additional information to ensure accuracy. Second, work can begin with the client much earlier because, in some cases, much of the information gathering is complete. Access to broad information gives the human service professional a more comprehensive review of a client's experience within the service delivery system.

Just as technology supports human service work using management information systems, it also helps to provide services to clients.

PROVIDING SERVICES TO CLIENTS

The services available through new models of service delivery range from computer programs that assess client knowledge or skill and recommend a plan of action to actual counseling online in real time. A telecommunications system was set up by the state of Maine to assess patients and clients in rural areas for both medical and

BOX 3.2	WEB SOURCES

Find Out More about Human Services on the Internet

The following websites illustrate the wide range of Internet sources for human service professionals.

http://www.psychservices.psychiatryonline.org/cgi/content/full/55/4/460

This is a book review of a text, *Human Services Technology*, written by Hy Resnick and published in 2004. It outlines the latest ways in which technology supports service delivery and professional practice.

http://www.apa.org/topics/rights/

This American Psychological Association website details the expectations that mental health patients may have for services within the managed care environment. Guidelines for quality care and patient rights are outlined.

http://www.counseling.org/Resources/CodeOfEthics/TP/Home/CT2.aspx

This website is for the American Counseling Association's 2005 Code of Ethics. Within the code, ACA outlines the ethical guidelines for using technology in counseling.

---

behavioral health needs (Lea et al., 2005). There are both institutions and homes that are using these teleconferencing services. Specific services include mental health, diabetes management, and pediatrics. There is a mobile telemedicine boat that also serves islands off the coast of Maine. Future uses project videoconferencing in areas such as domestic violence and case management for juvenile offenders on probation.

Many software programs and tools are available to teach clients specific knowledge or skills to enhance their daily living or increase their vocational potential. Many of the programs are designed for clients who are experiencing difficulties. One such program, "Talking It Out," helps adolescents deal with their conflicts. Using the computer software, teens communicate with each other about their conflicts. The program serves to mediate the issues and teach conflict management skills (Resnick, n.d.). Another program uses distance art therapy to help clients cope with traumatic illness (Collie, 2004). This program invites clients to use drawing (by computer) to explore their illness and the issues surrounding it.

Technology has also influenced the delivery of counseling services. In many programs, the client uses an interactive computer program followed by a discussion with a human service professional of the client's responses. One such interactive multimedia system, developed by the Beck Institute for Cognitive Therapy and Research, computerizes cognitive therapy and is used at the Norton Psychiatric Clinic in Louisville, Kentucky (Gunthert, Cohen, Butler, & Beck, 2005). One component of the treatment is a computer program that asks clients to take a test about symptoms of depression. It helps clients see the thinking that leads to depression. Using the program allows clients to reflect about alternative ways of thinking and implementing alternative solutions and behaviors.

Counseling and other support services are also provided online. This allows human service professionals to be available via e-mail or the Web to work with individuals who are experiencing specific difficulties, thereby increasing access to services. Proponents of online counseling believe that without this venue, many people would not be able to benefit from the knowledge and care of helpers. Others, however, express concerns about confidentiality, informed consent, and competence. Nevertheless, the number of participants receiving services online continues to grow. Certain sites also provide medical consultation and child-care advice. Thus, the phrase "the doctor is always in" reflects the constancy of the Internet and its easy accessibility.

Because of the prevalence of **E-therapy**—online or Internet therapy—and the accompanying concerns of members of the professional community, there are guidelines for those clients who wish to use such therapy. These guidelines address the following types of questions: Are you a good candidate for online therapy? How do you find a credentialed professional? How do you make an appropriate choice among professionals? How do you locate online counseling websites and compare? How do you ensure confidentiality? (ABC's of Internet Therapy, 2006). The American Counseling Association includes guidelines about computer technology in its Code of Ethics (American Counseling Association, 2005). These include understanding the limitations of the client, determining if technology is an appropriate counseling methodology, and explaining to the client the limitations of the computer counseling services.

Online chat forums also help to provide support to those in need. They address a range of topics and are accessible on many networks. One example is a chat group for police officers in Chicago. The purpose is for members of the force to get to know one another in an informal environment (http://ponetwork.com/chat.html). A second example is the discussion network developed by the Nebraska Network for Children and Families to focus on elder care (http://www.answers4families.org/). It provides an opportunity for those providing care for Alzheimer's clients, those providing assisted-living services, and those caring for older people. There are both Listserv and discussion formats available for those who need social support.

PROFESSIONAL DEVELOPMENT

Professional development is an important aspect of lifelong learning, and technology makes it easier for human service professionals to take advantage of the latest information about populations being served as well as the knowledge and skills of emerging best practice. One way this information is available is by CD-ROM. Most compact discs of interest to the human service professional can be found in a local university or city library. One advantage of using these CDs for research is the easy access to current information.

Another advancement in professional development is the availability of software that facilitates skill development. Programs are available to teach interviewing, problem solving, rehabilitation counseling, decision making, counseling, crisis counseling, organizational assessment, case management, and many other skills. Much of the software is interactive and uses simulation as the primary instructional tool. In teaching problem solving in case management, many programs use simulated cases of individuals with severe problems and difficulties. Students and practitioners are asked to identify and prioritize needs, and to choose alternatives and outcomes. Most programs provide the client's current status and other, more detailed information about client history.

Pod casting is a relatively new way to deliver audio and video training materials to human service professionals. Pod casting allows users to access information by subscription; in other words, the audio and video transmissions are delivered to the user without the user seeking the transmission. This method of delivery provides

TABLE 3.2 | Summary Points: Uses of Technology

- Communication in human services is enhanced by e-mail, Listservs, teleconferencing, and the World Wide Web.

- Telemedicine, management systems, and care networks are examples of information management systems.

- Direct services to clients by means of technology include assessment, counseling, information, and education.

- Technology allows human service professionals to utilize the latest information about practice, client groups, and skill development.

---

up-to-date information to the user quickly and efficiently. For example, the National Institute of Health (2006) provides live audio reports on human service-related issues such as diabetes, addiction, obesity, and heart disease.

In summary, human service professionals are currently using many technologies to improve the ways they communicate with each other, expand the ways information is managed, provide services to clients, and engage in professional development. We predict that technology will continue to have an impact on the profession during the 21st century.

MANAGED CARE

Managed care has had a profound effect on the delivery of human services. Its influence is felt by both client and human service professional as they work together to plan and provide services. Today, managed care organizations administer a large percentage of the group health insurance as well as mental health care, childcare, corrections, and other social services. We now look at managed care and how it has affected the delivery of health, mental health, and other services.

Managed care is a term used to describe a set of tools or methods designed to manage resources and deliver human services, especially in the areas of health care and mental health. It developed from public demand for accountability of service delivery and from rising costs in health and mental health care. Although the American public was seriously concerned about the cost of health care in the 1980s, today there is continuing attention on managed care and its responsibility for deterioration of care (Dorfman, 2006). Prior to the use of managed care to allocate resources and services, most care was provided on a **fee-for-service** basis. In other words, a health or human service professional would provide a specific service and charge a standard rate. The payment for these services would come from the client, an insurance provider, or the agency or organization supporting the client care.

The Influence of Managed Care

Managed care is defined as a

plan to control employer's health care cost through the introduction of practice guidelines or protocols for health care providers, and to improve the methods used by employers and employees to select health care providers. The goal of the plan is to create a financial accounting system in order to manage the impact of medical treatment on the patient's clinical response and quality of life (Barron's, 2006).

In the case of human services, managed care influences the delivery of services to clients within the social service network with **external reviews, standards of good practice,** and a **continuum of care.**

The external review is used in several ways to monitor and communicate to service providers what they can provide and still receive financial coverage for providing. For example, one type of review authorizes the expense of needed services for a client. For the human service professional, this means that before a service can be provided and before the professional can be reimbursed or paid, the managed care organization reviews the requested service and asks questions such as these:

- How do you define the problem?
- What treatment do you recommend?
- Why do you recommend this treatment?
- Do you have any evidence that supports using this treatment?

A guiding principle for managed care review is to approve the lowest level of care that will meet the client's needs. In other words, if hospitalization has been recommended, the managed care reviewer asks, "Could the client also be treated in the home?" If 10 weeks of therapy is recommended, the question is, "Will four weeks be adequate?" If the client needs a vocational assessment, psychological assessment, physical assessment, and a social history, managed care reviewers may recommend conducting the physical and the psychological assessment first before determining whether the others are needed.

Another component of the external review is related to the provision of good quality services. The previous set of questions is asked prior to service provision; questions are also asked *after* service delivery. These questions focus on effectiveness of care, cost effectiveness, accessibility, safety of care, and satisfaction of client. Other considerations surround quality of care, and many of those focus on fair treatment of the client, such as the ease with which the client can access the services, the meeting of client expectations, the attention to and fair disposition of client appeals and grievances, and client satisfaction. Satisfaction within the service delivery system extends beyond the client to families of clients and to the human service professional. One issue that has surfaced within the professional, client/patient, and political context is "patient rights" within the managed care context.

The Substance Abuse and Mental Health Services Administration's Center for Mental Health Services (2006) developed standards of care for managed care systems. These focus on how managed care organizations interface with consumers. The principles of quality of care include:

- Treat all people with respect and dignity
- Be based on "best practices"
- Develop delivery and data collection systems to address unique developmental needs of children and families
- Ensure services are tailored to individual needs and preferences
- Provide services in the least restrictive and most natural setting

- Provide mechanisms for disputes of resolutions
- Provide services within a continuum of care
- Include multiple services for children

The American Psychological Association (2006) has published the *Mental Health Patient's Bill of Rights* that lists the rights that patients should expect when receiving mental health services. The rights are explained in detail with an emphasis both on the rights and on the appropriate questions the client can ask the managed care professional when discussing benefits and services. The **Mental Health Patient Bill of Rights** covers issues such as the right to know, confidentiality, choice, determination of treatment, nondiscrimination, and treatment review.

Continuous review is another way managed care interfaces with service delivery. In continuous review, there is periodic dialogue between human service providers and the managed care personnel about the status of the client and the effectiveness of the services. The purpose of this review is to identify any problems with the assessment, the treatment plan, or its implementation. Another purpose of the review is to remind those providing services to plan adequate and effective treatment. Many professionals believe that both quality of care and reasonable cost should guide decisions about service. The following case illustrates what one client experienced:

> Jimmy Jones, a 14-year-old, single, white male, has recently been truant from school and was caught fighting with other students. His difficult behavior began about the time his father, with whom he has a close relationship, was diagnosed with cancer. Jimmy's doctor recommended that he see a counselor who specializes in working with adolescents to help him cope with his father's illness. After an initial visit with the counselor, 10 visits are authorized by the Jones's insurance company. Part of the authorization requires the counselor to file periodic progress reports. After the tenth visit, a review of the case will determine whether additional visits will be authorized.

Managed care also affects the way we think about and deliver services to specific client populations. Because managed care emphasizes appropriate services for clients and matching services to specific outcomes, both managed care personnel and human service professionals are working to develop standards of best practice for meeting specific client needs. In the past, because of the complexity of problems that client's experience, some human service professionals have had difficulty stating clearly the appropriate services for addressing the needs of their clients—needs that stem from poverty, unemployment, illiteracy, juvenile delinquency, child abuse, and other difficulties. Further complicating the task of developing standards is the complexity and large number of problems that many clients face. When practitioners and managed care personnel work together to define best practices, clients are more likely to receive quality treatment. One example of effective partnerships is occurring in the field of gerontology and managed care. The University of Tennessee Medical School is working with managed care organizations to provide support to the caregivers of Alzheimer's patients, including preventative mental health support in an attempt to avoid future mental health problems. The treatment helps meet the needs of the Alzheimer's patient, supports the caregiver, and conserves financial resources.

Another important concept for delivering human services within the managed care environment is *continuum of care*. Continuum of care describes an integrated system of settings, services, professionals, and levels of care and services. The client moves from site to site as the needs dictate, and receives appropriate care as needed. There are many examples of continuum of care. For the elderly, this continuum may include physician services, emergency services, acute care, skilled nursing facilities, outpatient centers, home care programs, day treatment programs, mental health services, and family/community support (American Dietetic Association, 2006). Continuum of care applied to the homeless population moves these individuals from living on the streets to self-sufficiency. Goals for clients include getting housing, receiving job training, developing independent living skills, and receiving mental health services. Some also receive substance abuse treatment, and individual and family counseling. When working with the homeless, there is always a balance between length of care and moving clients to self-sufficiency.

What would a continuum of care look like for children and adolescents? The most intensive treatment is inpatient/acute psychiatric care. This level of treatment is appropriate when children and youth need constant supervision, medical intervention, and therapy. Many times clients receive these services when there is a probable threat of violence to self or others. A less-intensive level of treatment would be outpatient services. Children and youth in this category would receive multiple services, such as psychiatric services, counseling, group therapy, and social skills training. At the other end of the continuum is home-based therapy, which is appropriate when children and youth are in troubled situations that can be addressed with brief, short-term interventions.

As you can see, managed care is influencing the way all human services are delivered by introducing or emphasizing such concepts as external review, standards of best practice, and continuum of care. These in turn affect the way human service professionals do their work.

MANAGED CARE AND THE HUMAN SERVICE PROFESSIONAL

Managed care has affected the daily work of the human service professional, especially in providing direct service. This interaction has required a shift in the roles and responsibilities of the professional in three ways: an emphasis on case management responsibilities, increasing demands for documentation, and the growing use of gatekeepers.

Today, more human service professionals than ever are using case management in providing services to their clients. With an emphasis on cost-effective service delivery, coordination of care through a case manager has emerged as a method to better ensure efficiency and high-quality service. The purpose of case management, as discussed in Chapter 1, is to oversee the comprehensive care of a client. It can include (1) assessment, (2) planning, coordinating, and monitoring of treatment, and (3) evaluation. Human service literature describes two types of case managers. One is a case manager in a human service organization who assumes many of the responsibilities just listed; the other works for a managed care organization. The following examples illustrate their different responsibilities.

Chris Bachman, a rehabilitation counselor, has a caseload of 70 clients. Chris works with each client to develop a plan of services, some delivered by Chris himself but most provided by professionals at other agencies. Chris monitors the delivery of services, authorizes payment on behalf of his agency, and evaluates with the client the services received.

Tasha Jones is a case manager who works for Healthcare, Inc., a managed care organization that has clients in five counties. Her major responsibilities include external utilization review and resource allocation. Her contact with human service professionals like Chris Bachman is through applications, forms, or phone calls. She has never met a client or a human service professional in person.

As more services are regulated and directed by managed care organizations, the need for the services of both types of case managers will grow. Another influence of managed care is the increased documentation associated with service delivery. The workload for many human service professionals has doubled as they use the managed care external review process. A request for services can include an initial assessment, a detailed description of the client's problem, a service plan, a periodic assessment of the implementation of the plan and status of outcomes, requests for reimbursement, and termination of clients. Often the documentation required for the managed care process is different from that required by the agency. Thus, unless the managed care organization has established the same information system as the organization, the professional may have two systems of documentation to maintain.

Another change that has emerged is an elaborate gatekeeping function for initial screening of clients. **Gatekeeping** in the managed care system, especially in the area of mental health, is a method used to control access to services. Often, to receive mental health services, clients must have a referral from a physician. The purpose of this physician referral is to decrease the utilization of mental health services, but the result has been to increase the client load of the physician who must sign the referrals. Gatekeeping also occurs when a special service, not considered part of the standard of good practice, is needed or recommended. The client is not free to take the initiative to seek that service but must have the permission of and referral from the primary caretaker—in most cases, the physician. At times, the introduction of the gatekeeper to mental health services places hardships on both the client and the human service professional. Clients see this visit to the physician as a barrier to getting services, and they often encounter physicians who are not sympathetic to their nonmedical problems. Sometimes they must wait to see the physician, and this wait delays their receiving the mental health services they need. For human service professionals, the gatekeeper is another layer of bureaucracy between them and their clients. On a positive note, however, many of these professionals are working with the gate-keeper physicians to help them understand the mental health needs of their clients.

THE INTERNATIONAL DIMENSION

Any discussion about human services today without considering its international dimension would be difficult. Everyone on the planet is drawing closer as a result of technological advances in transportation and communication.

Today, people travel the world in a matter of hours rather than days or weeks. Advances in communication keep us instantly informed about developments throughout the world by satellite, e-mail, and faxes. The information superhighway has no

TABLE 3.3 | SUMMARY POINTS: MANAGED CARE TERMS

- **External reviews**—evaluation of a request for services prior to service delivery
- **Standards of good practice**—specification of outcomes, relationship of outcomes to services, and efficient and effective service delivery
- **Continuum of care**—integrated system of settings, services, professionals, and levels of care

borders, with users in most countries around the globe. The world is becoming a smaller place when we consider factors other than physical distance. Thus, we need to know what is happening internationally in terms of human services—the recent changes that have occurred, the challenges that remain, and the lessons from other countries about service delivery.

Thoughts about future trends trigger a global alarm. Calculations by the world's biggest supercomputer at the Hadley Center in England project the following:

- Thirty million people will be hungry in 50 years because it will be too dry to grow crops in large parts of Africa.
- An additional 170 million people will live in countries with extreme water shortages.
- Malaria, one of the world's most feared diseases, will threaten larger areas of the world—including Europe—by 2050 (Patz et al., 2005).

A closer look at the challenges of international human services and their implications for the United States and for you as a human service professional help us understand their very serious nature now and provides insights about future problems.

CHALLENGES IN INTERNATIONAL HUMAN SERVICES

Global population began to increase rapidly in the 20th century, a situation aptly described by the term *population explosion*. This was not a worldwide phenomenon but occurred almost entirely in the developing countries of Africa, Asia, and Latin America. The dramatic contrast in growth between the more developed and less developed countries continues to increase. Today, 99% of the world's population growth is in developing countries. For instance, developing countries add about 80 million people per year to the world's population compared to the 1 million added in developed countries. Middle Africa, followed by western Africa, is expected to be the fastest growing region in the first half of the 21st century, with its population growing 193% by 2050. Limited health care, particularly in rural areas; education, poverty, social unrest, and literacy are challenges in these countries.

Another challenge for the 21st century is international migration. In 2005, there were approximately 191 million migrants worldwide, up from 176 million in 2000. Women account for 49.6% of the 2005 estimate. In fact, this number of migrants would constitute the fifth most populous country in 2005 (International

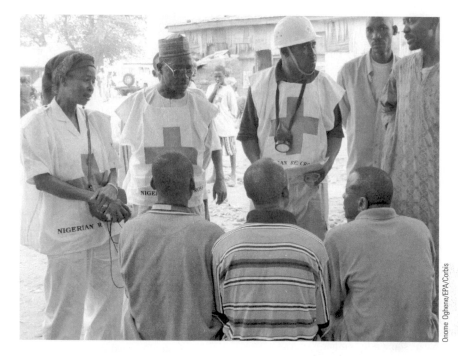

Onome Oghene/EPA/Corbis

Organization for Migration, 2006). Approximately 75% of this number are in 12% of the countries in the world, with most moving from one less-developed country to another. For both countries of origin and countries of destination, this movement raises major socioeconomic issues. These numbers are only a small percentage of the estimated global migration that also includes refugees, guest workers, and illegal foreigners.

Another challenge is **urbanization,** a long-term global trend that is most pronounced in poor countries that are least able to cope with its pressures. Today, a third of the world's population—about 600 million people—do not have the means to meet their basic needs, such as clean water and sewage disposal. Mumbai (Bombay), the largest city in India, has a population of 15.1 million. By 2015, it will be the second-largest metropolis in the world, with 27.4 million people. In Mumbai, between 200 and 250 families arrive each day, hoping for a better life in the city. Many begin their lives there as pavement dwellers because there is no other place to live. Land is scarce, and rooms and apartments are full. The newcomers may remain on the sidewalks for the rest of their lives, or they may move to a slum dwelling. In either case, clean water, electricity, paved paths/roads, and working community toilets are often nonexistent. Although slum living represents upward mobility in many developing countries, slum dwellers complain about the gangs, high rent, drugs, violence, sewage, and floods.

The challenges in international human services continue to be great. The plights of refugees and migrants, those with AIDS, the homeless, drug users, and the displaced in the aftermath of natural disasters—in addition to the problems discussed here—are some of those challenges.

BOX 3.3	INTERNATIONAL FOCUS
	A Liberian Refugee

Monique Kolubo-Simpson is an American-Liberian who fled Liberia in 1990 after her life was threatened by rebel forces. She retuned there because of her love for her country and to be near family and friends. In 2004, her life was threatened again when the rebel soldiers attacked her village. She was frightened for her life and once again fled.

She began the day that she left home like any other. She had heard stories of fighting in the area, but she did not realize how dangerous the situation had become until she looked out the window of her home and saw long lines of people leaving the village with only what they could carry. The fighting reached their village as her family decided to leave; already homes were being destroyed and people were being shot in the cross fire. Her father took charge and ordered the entire family to leave. Monique looked back at her home just before she left and grabbed her watch. She thought it might be valuable at some point in her journey.

Instead of fleeing on foot, her family was able to leave by car. As they headed for the American Embassy, they were stopped at a checkpoint. Since it was a peacekeeping checkpoint, they were allowed to go through with little hassle. Further down the road the car was stopped at a rebel checkpoint. They complied with the rebels by answering their questions and letting them search the car and their belongings. Finally they were released, only to be stopped again at a rebel checkpoint headed by a 16-year-old rebel soldier. This stop was terrifying, but finally they were allowed to proceed.

They reached the embassy where they stayed with little food and bare sleeping quarters. For days no one knew if they would be rescued before the rebel soldiers took the embassy. Finally, a helicopter came to evacuate them. As Monique left the country, she had two primary thoughts. She continued to worry about her friends who had left the country by foot, and she was glad that she would not have to live through the war.

Source: Adapted from U.S. Committee for Refugees and Immigrants. (n.d.). A refugee from Liberia—Monique Kolubo-Simpson. Retrieved February 24, 2004, from http://refugeesusa.org/meet_amer/refugee_liberia.cfm

Influences on the United States

How does the international dimension of human services affect the United States? Although most information in this book concerns human services in this country, we must also be aware of its international dimension. Immigrants to the United States increase our awareness of those nationalities that have become or are becoming part of our population. In the early history of the country, immigration was limited primarily to Europeans; 100 years ago, 90% of the immigrants to the United States came from European countries. During the last 30 years, however, the wave of immigration has been primarily non-European, including Chinese, Japanese, Filipinos, Koreans, Vietnamese, and Indians. Since 9/11 the United States has experienced an increase in immigrants from predominantly Muslim countries in the Middle East, North Africa, and Asia. In 2005, for example, more people (96,000) from Muslim countries became legal permanent U.S. residents than in any year in the previous two decades (Elliott, 2006).

Another interesting ethnic development is the recognition of **multiracial** individuals. Tiger Woods, the golf professional, has mixed ancestry that includes Caucasian, Black, Indian, and Asian. Another well-known individual who has affirmed his mixed ancestry is the actor Keanu Reeves, who is Hawaiian, Chinese, and Caucasian. The 2000 Census was the first attempt in this country to identify multiracial individuals. Today, approximately one-third of U.S. residents now claim minority status, and approximately 2.4% of the population identify themselves as members of more than one race, a figure that is expected to increase.

Another important consideration of population in the United States in 2005 is the 36 million foreign-born people (Population and Diversity, 2006). The fastest growth in this group has been in southeastern states. Of the five million new arrivals to the United States between 2000 and 2005, 58% settled in the six states that traditionally attract the largest number of immigrants: California, Texas, Florida, New York, New Jersey, and Illinois.

Today and in the foreseeable future, the United States must grapple with numerous issues related to diversity. Who is a minority? Should changes in immigration laws reduce illegal immigration rates? What efforts should be employed to control immigration? Do immigrants take jobs from unemployed citizens? Are immigrants entitled to public education and other benefits? Should English be the official language of the United States? What impact will these ethnic shifts have on Medicare and Social Security? And what about terrorism and civil liberties? While these questions are debated throughout the United States, we continue to be part of the global community and play a role in the international human services discussed earlier.

Some human service professionals work as service providers or volunteers in other countries, particularly developing countries. Others are employed by UN agencies, the World Bank, or the Peace Corps or volunteer for shorter periods with religious groups, such as the Missionaries of Charity, or nonprofit organizations, such as Cross-Cultural Solutions or the Red Cross.

Many other human service professionals elect to remain in the United States. Given the population projections, it is increasingly likely that these helpers will work with people of very different backgrounds from them. The Latino population presents an example of the complexity of the situation. In the United States, this group is growing almost five times faster than that of non-Latinos and by 2010 is expected to be the nation's largest minority. Although ethnic groups from Spanish-speaking countries such as Mexico, Nicaragua, and Argentina are referred to as Latino or Hispanic, those cultures and customs are as diverse as the English-speaking populations. It would be a mistake to assume that they are a uniform, cohesive group that is culturally homogenous. Hispanic or Latino communities are found in Miami, Spanish Harlem, and migrant labor camps, and each is culturally, ethnically, and geographically diverse, making an awareness and appreciation of each group's uniqueness necessary for effective human service delivery.

TRENDS IN HUMAN SERVICES

Human services will be different in this century. We know that change occurs rapidly. In this chapter, you have read about changes already taking place that impact service delivery today. The utilization of technology, managed care, and the diverse and nontraditional settings for helping activities will continue to impact human services, but other trends will influence what and how services are delivered and to whom. It is appropriate that as part of our discussion of human services today, we devote some thought to the future. It will come quickly. To trigger your thinking about the future, we discuss five major trends to conclude the chapter.

BOX 3.4   INTERNATIONAL FOCUS
Kevin Burns—A Peace Corps Experience

Namaste. This common Nepali greeting is derived from the literal meaning, "I salute the god within you." I am working in Nepal as a Peace Corps volunteer. I have been here about 18 months. It has been quite an experience for me. My first experience in Nepal was a week in Kathmandu, the capital of Nepal. We left for Tansen, a beautiful town in the mid-hills of Nepal, to begin our training. In Tansen during training, I lived with a host family that did not speak much English. They were very nice. Days were spent studying about the culture, learning the language, and learning the technical aspects of my upcoming job. Here I learned how to eat the typical way of the country: lentils and rice with vegetables *(dal-blaat)* for lunch and a big plate of rice for supper.

After our training we returned to Kathmandu for a week, and then I traveled to my post of two years—Mechinagar Municipality. It is located in the Teria on the Eastern border with India. I work in the new community development branch of the municipality. My job description says I will be working with programs in health, sanitation, education, income generation, and local organization coordination. While I have been doing my work, I have not always felt productive, but I have learned an enormous amount about living in another culture.

The community development section is brand new. I work with the community development coordinator. I have learned that in the work it is important to "drink tea." I also began to understand the importance of understanding how things work here, the culture, and even the importance of drinking tea—milk tea with sugar. Whatever you do, wherever you go, whether you visit a friend or an office, tea is served.

Our office is implementing a UNICEF urban out-of-school program with nonformal education and skill training for local youth who are not in school. We also have been working on improving local health care services. Other activities include women's literacy classes, an expanded local saving and credit program, and programs involving the local marginalized ethnic groups.

I live in three rooms of a family's house. I now have a Nepali mother, Ama, and father, Buwa. I am their new youngest son. They are a nice family. Ama doesn't speak any English and her Nepali is too fast. It has been

only recently that I have begun to understand her (sometimes). The house is located on the main road between the two bazaars. My rooms are downstairs in a two-story cement building. The family has a garden out front and chickens in the back. The housing here is usually either brick and cement, wooden with bamboo walls and tin roofs, or all bamboo huts with thatch roofs. In my neighborhood there is a mixture of all three. Away from the area is farmland, although 40 years ago this was a dense, malaria-infested jungle.

The cow is the most sacred animal in Nepal. It is a crime to kill one here. In early India the sacredness of cows helped during a famine because, if people ate the cattle, then the farm productivity would drop and only make the famine recovery worse. I think most Americans think of Buddhism in Nepal, but that is because most people know little about the mountain culture, which is more than just Buddhist. Nepal is the birthplace of Buddha. Over 85% of Nepalis are Hindu, with about 10% Buddhists and 2% Moslem. Hindus here also incorporate Buddhism in their worship, so it is an interesting mix. Hindus do not believe in one all-powerful God, but there are over 330,000 different gods and goddesses.

I am slowly learning to speak and read Nepali, which has a different alphabet from our Western one. Actually there are over 20 separate languages spoken in Nepal (maybe up to 100 dialects). The national language—Nepali—is spoken by most everyone. One of the first things I learned when I arrived was that I know very little about how to help here. Nepal is poor; it ranks in the bottom ten of the lowest per capita income in the world. According to UNICEF, about 50% of the children in my area are malnourished. The literacy rate here is about 40%, which is up from 2% in 1945. In my district, which is the country's largest agricultural producer, 80% of the land is owned by 20 families.

Looking at Nepal through the eyes of the United States can be depressing. Don't forget we spent many years dealing with the same issues that Nepal is beginning to tackle such as child labor, equal rights, and others.

Source: Kevin Burns, Peace Corps Volunteer, 2000. Reprinted with permission.

AGING IN AMERICA

Growth and change of the elderly population in America rank among the most important demographic developments of the 20th century and will continue their importance in the 21st century. This development has serious implications for the next 50 years. The population in the United States aged 65 and over is expected to double in size within the next 25 years. The number of those 85 and older is also increasing. The Hispanic population of older adults is expected to grow from 2.2 million in 2004 to over 15 million by 2050. By 2028, this population is expected to be the largest racial/ethical minority among older people (U.S. Census Bureau, 2005). It is not just the numbers that cause concern, however; some current trends among the elderly will be accentuated—and will impact human service delivery.

This group will have increasing education levels, include more minority elderly, and include more women than men. Many will be reasonably healthy and live independent and active lives, although there will still be a great disparity in terms of income and health status in certain segments of the population. The health of older Americans is improving. Poor health is related primarily to chronic conditions such as arthritis and heart disease (U. S. Census Bureau, 2005). Real median income for older citizens fell 2.8% for men and 3.6% for women, and incomes are expected to continue to decline. But education is positively correlated with better heath, higher income, and a more prosperous retirement. The most vulnerable are older single women with low incomes, baby boomers with less education, and minority groups with low economic status. Those aged 85 and older are also at risk. Life expectancy, medical advances, and improved health and lifestyles make the 85 and older population the fastest-growing age group in the United States. The changes in the American family, particularly divorce, may result in less support for members of the aging population, because the numbers of elderly living alone is increasing (U.S. Census Bureau, 2005).

These changes in the population will present challenges for human services during the next 50 years. There will be a significant number who are troubled by poor health, dependency, and the inability to perform simple tasks. Additionally, those who are in good health will not escape the transition from active and independent living to some form of assisted living. Addressing these needs will present challenges for human services and society at large, particularly in the areas of income assistance, health care, housing alternatives, employment issues, leisure opportunities, and environmental modification. Three such issues—housing, depression, and confronting death and dying—are introduced here.

HOUSING   Living arrangements for those 85 and older are determined by several factors: financial assets, ability to care for self, social support, cultural values, access to social services, and types of housing available. The types of living arrangements vary; four alternatives are presented here (Kinsella & Velkoff, 2001).

First, many individuals own or rent their own homes, and their first choice is to "age in place." Services such as mobile meal delivery or home health care make this possible. Often in the United States, older Americans do not choose the second alternative, living with their children; they want to remain independent and fear they will be a burden. When parents do live with their adult children, as an alternative to independent living, mutual consent contributes to a successful co-existence. A third choice, **assisted living,** is a relatively new choice for those 85 and older. The number of individuals choosing this option is increasing, because level of care can be matched to individual need. Assisted living environments offer a combination of personal space and social services to meet the needs of their clients. An increasing number of older adults live in institutions (U.S. Census Bureau, 2005). More women than men use nonfamilial institutions, and the likelihood of an institutional stay increases with age (Kinsella & Velkoff, 2001). Although a stigma about nursing home care exists, trained professional staff, broad programming, hygienic and safe conditions, and support from governmental services contribute to quality care.

DEPRESSION   Just as important as the living arrangements for the aging population are the mental health issues that many of them face. One important issue is depression. According to the National Institute of Health (2006), over 6.5 million individuals over the age of 65 experience depression. Many individuals have experienced episodes or times of depression throughout their lives, but for others, this first occurs in the 80s or even 90s. There are several difficulties in diagnosing depression in those over 65, mostly related to stereotypes about aging, culture, values, and lack of knowledge about the disease. Many individuals believe that depression is just a natural part of the aging process and goes hand in hand with decline in later years. An assumption is made that the difficulties associated with getting older are just part of the aging experience and that it is natural to feel stressed and "down." Others, aware of the stigma related to mental health, hide their depression or refuse to seek treatment. Many older people or their families simply know little about the disease and do not recognize when it is present. Fear of the treatment itself or the cost of treatment also keeps many people from seeking help.

There can be serious consequences for not seeking help from depression, such as suicide or a higher mortality rate. While depression is linked with "bereavement, sleep disturbance, disability, prior depression, and female gender" (Furness, 2003, p. 1147), the highest rate of suicide is for older white males. In addition, many individuals experience depression after a stroke or heart attack or related surgery.

CONFRONTING DEATH AND DYING   Although many members of the aging population do not experience depression, sadness and grief over loss are inevitable. These emotions are natural and predictable reactions to leaving home, deterioration of health, developing a disability, and losing independence and the ability to care for one's self. Death of a spouse and the process of dying present special challenges. According to Erikson (1963), in the final stage of life—ego integrity versus despair— one comes to terms with both the meaning of life and the place of death within the experience of living. For most individuals over 65, several issues around dying and death, such as care for a loved one, require social support and social services.

Bereavement is the "loss of someone to whom a person feels close and the process of adjusting to it" (Papalia, Olds, & Feldman, 2004). One of the most difficult losses for those over 65 is the death of a spouse. The survivor is likely to experience a wide range of emotions, such as denial, disbelief, confusion, shock, sadness, and despair. In addition to emotional turmoil, adjustments to daily living require new skills in order to perform roles previously assumed by the former spouse (paying bills, washing clothes, cooking, home and auto repairs) and require revising social connections as a widow or a widower. During this time the survivor works through stages of grief that include shock and disbelief, preoccupation with the memory of the dead person, and resolution (Hiller & Barrow, 2007). Older widows are more likely to seek out social support during this time, while widowers tend to isolate themselves. However, both older female and male survivors have more coping skills than younger survivors and often deal with death and loss more effectively.

In recent years, attempts have been made to make the dying process more humane both for the dying spouse and for the survivor. Attention to the psychosocial needs as well as the medical needs has expanded services beyond physicians and hospitals to social support networks and home and family. Hospice care provides patient-centered care to patients and their families, with the focus on providing palliative care by keeping the patient comfortable, pain free, and within a familiar setting. Although hospice services are typically provided in the patient's home or the home of a family member, hospitals or hospice centers also offer these services. In each of these settings, medical professionals, social service professionals, and the family form a team to serve the patient's needs. Support is also available for the family members.

Human service professionals play a major role in assisting those 65 and over as they grapple with the issues of the aging process. Because of this, the need for a variety of social services and human service professionals will expand in the coming decades.

AN EMPHASIS ON DIVERSITY

Typically, when we think about **diversity,** it is the ethnic makeup of our country that comes to mind. In fact, earlier in this chapter you read about the changing demographics of both the United States and the world, and how those changes will impact human services. It is accepted today that as you enter the human service profession you will encounter clients who are different from you. You will also be working with other helping professionals who are different from you. For example, at an agency in Miami, a team of human service professionals represents a variety of countries: Spain, Cuba, El Salvador, Romania, and the Dominican Republic. Not only do the members of the team differ in the countries where they were raised, but they also speak different languages, come from different economic backgrounds, are different ages and genders, and entered the United States under various circumstances.

You can prepare for working relationships such as these by learning about multicultural counseling, reading the plethora of books that address ethnic diversity, and increasing your awareness of other cultures through travel, interaction with other students, and television, books, and movies. Diversity, however, has a much broader connotation than ethnic diversity, and it is an understanding of this more-sweeping concept that will help us address the challenges of 21st-century problems.

Diversity is inherent to the American way of life. The term *diversity,* broadly conceived, is used to refer to many demographic variables, including age, color, disabilities, gender, national origin, race, religion, and sexual orientation (Office for Equal Opportunity and Diversity Management, 2003). America draws strength from its diversity; for example, contributions from racial and ethnic minorities have enriched all our lives. During the 21st century, emphasis will be placed on the broader definition of diversity. Since 9/11, there is a growing awareness of differing

BOX 3.5	WEB SOURCES

Find Out More about Older Adults

The following sites will help professionals who are working with older adults or children of older adults:

http://www.aarp.org

This website has articles on current issues for the 50+ population: computer tips and technology updates, volunteering, and recent survey information on attitudes about death and dying. It also covers travel and education opportunities, legislative issues related to seniors, and other relevant articles and links.

http://www.agingwithdignity.org

This is the site of Aging with Dignity, a privately funded, nonprofit organization that advocates for the needs of elders and their caregivers, with a particular emphasis on improving care

for those facing the end of life. Founded in 1996 by Jim Towey, this organization has developed a document called *Five Wishes*, which allows people to communicate their preferences in terms of care and treatment should they become seriously ill.

http://www.elderweb.com

This website provides information about long-term care for older adults, with excellent links on legal, financial, medical, and housing issues.

http://www.estateplanninglinks.com

This website contains links to other sites on estate planning, elder law, and tax-related issues for both the layperson and the professional.

spiritual beliefs, and issues surrounding homosexuality have sparked debate in Congress and in state legislatures.

The Ethical Standards for Human Service Professionals (National Organization for Human Services, 2000) recognize "an appreciation of human beings in all of their diversity" as a basic tenet of human service delivery. Specific standards further address "the respect, acceptance and dignity" due each client (#2), the need to be advocates "for the rights of all members of society, particularly those who are members of minorities and groups at which discriminatory practices have historically been directed" (#16), and the provision of services "without discrimination or preference based on age, ethnicity, culture, race, disability, gender, religion, sexual orientation or socioeconomic status" (#17). Human service professionals are also "knowledgeable about the cultures and communities within which they practice" (#18), and they are "aware of their own cultural backgrounds, beliefs, and values" (#19). Although there is concern about service delivery within the limit and scope of one's professional knowledge and skills (#26), human service professionals engage in continuing education, professional development, and supervision in order to work effectively with culturally diverse groups (#21). This, then, is the challenge of the 21st century: to develop the knowledge, skills, and self-awareness to be effective in delivering human services.

Both the changing demographics and the ethical standards that address diversity give additional importance to understanding the concept of "worldview." Each person has a worldview that affects thoughts, decision making, lifestyle, and behavior; it also encompasses our attitudes, values, and opinions. Most importantly, it affects how we see each other and the world. It is a critical concept for human service professionals. Individuals who are different from you racially, ethnically, or in other ways will probably have a different worldview than you do. This may result in the helper attributing negative traits to the client (Sue & Sue, 2003). Another consequence is the influence worldview has on the helping relationship, for example, the client's view of the helping process and the helper, and the helper's approach to problem assessment and the choice of interventions. The challenge for human service professionals is to become aware of and understand their own worldview, to expand their worldview to become effective cross-culturally, and to be sensitive to the worldview of their clients. We will explore three areas of diversity. As you read this material, think about your worldview and its impact on service delivery with these potential clients.

RACIAL AND ETHNIC DIVERSITY   Racial and ethnic diversity often come to mind first when the word *diversity* is mentioned. According to Federal classifications, African Americans (blacks), American Indians and Alaska Natives, Asian American and Pacific Islanders, and white Americans (whites) are races. Hispanic American (Latino) is an ethnicity and may apply to a person of any race (Surgeon General's Report, n.d.). This example reflects the reference of the term **ethnicity** to a common culture, heritage, and shared meaning. It may include religious groups (e.g., Jews), country of origin (e.g., China), or any other facet passed from generation to generation (Brammer, 2004). These terms are important in the United States where the ethnic and racial structure is changing. In 1998, non-white groups accounted for 28% of the population. The 2000 census puts the number of non-whites at 30%, and by mid-century, the percentage is expected to be almost 50%. It is both statistics and our ethical standards that require us to learn as much as possible about minority worldviews. There will not be enough minority helpers for each racial or ethnic group to have its own.

We must also be sensitive to the fact that equal opportunity underlies the American belief system, yet racial and ethnic minorities bear a greater burden from unmet mental health needs. As a result, they suffer a greater loss to their overall health and productivity (Surgeon General's Report, n.d.). There are many reasons for this: the cost of care or services, societal stigma, fragmented services, and the client's fear and mistrust of treatment. Other barriers may come from the helper's lack of awareness of cultural issues, bias, or inability to speak the language. Whatever the barriers, the fact remains that equal access to services has not been achieved.

RELIGION   Diversity in the United States also embraces religious differences. In fact, the United States has been called the most religiously diverse nation in the world, primarily because it is a nation of immigrants. America was already home to Native American traditional spiritualities when the colonies were settled by those who established different Protestant churches. During the 19th and 20th centuries, the immigration of Roman Catholics, Jews, and people who practiced Chinese religion, Islam, and Sikhism further diversified religion in the United States (Robinson, 2003). Most recently, a 1965 change in immigration law was the most significant development in bringing about cultural change, particularly in increasing religious diversity (Buck, n.d.). The Hart-Celler Bill ended a closed-door policy in place since the 1920s, replacing national and ethnic quotas with quotas based on occupation and family reunification. As a result, the settlement of significant communities of Muslims, Hindus, Buddhists, Sikhs, and Jains occurred. Today, of those 18+ years of age in the United States, 76.5% are Christian (Catholic, Baptist, Methodist, Lutheran, etc.). Other religions (Jewish, Muslim/Islamic, Buddhist, etc.) total 3.7%. Those specifying no religion comprise 14.1% (U.S. Demographics for Religion, 2003).

Religious diversity brings both challenges and opportunities to a community. As a challenge, religious difference is a main factor in social conflict on local, national, and global levels as shown by the political impact of religious fundamentalism and ethno-religious groups. Some object to the presence of other religious groups in their communities, citing the vandalism and violence against certain groups, the negative stereotypes, discrimination, and ignorance.

Religion is an area of strongly held beliefs and emotions. Those who see diversity as an opportunity or strength are also intense about their beliefs. They cite the richness of significant religious holidays and observances and the increasing number of ecumenical and interfaith organizations as positive forces in religious diversity. They also believe that religious diversity facilitates a dialogue that enables the exploration of new and old questions. How has America dealt with religious difference historically? What are today's challenges for communities, schools, and public institutions?

SEXUAL ORIENTATION   Another emotional diversity issue is sexual orientation. This is now a regular topic on radio and television talk shows, and increasingly in casual conversations. Because these interchanges frequently involve public policy, legal issues, and religious beliefs, they become intense and often polarizing. Misconceptions and fear contribute to heightened emotions.

Perhaps the most prevalent misconception is that homosexuality is a disease. Neither the American Psychological Association nor the American Psychiatric Association consider homosexuality to be an emotional or mental disorder. There are serious issues that confront people in a sexual minority such as gay, lesbian, bixsexual, and transgendered (LGBT), particularly the social stigma they experience. This segment of the population often does not have the same basic rights as other citizens. In many states and cities, a person within the LGTB community can legally be denied housing, employment, and public accommodation on the basis of sexual orientation. These inequalities, coupled with the desire for equal rights and equal protection of those rights and the inability to offer financial and legal security to their families, have led many to be involved in civil rights issues.

How do we work with those who are different from us? All people are shaped by the culture in which they were raised, including those who consider themselves the dominant culture in the United States (Okun, Fried, & Okun, 1999). What do you know about your own culture and how it is perceived by others? Are you open to learning about others whose worlds are different?

The ability to work effectively with diverse groups means establishing relationships based on the trust and respect for others, increasing our awareness and knowledge of other ways, listening without judgment, and appreciating the worldview of others. The challenge to human service professionals in the 21st century is to take the lead to work effectively with others, whether that is a client, a neighborhood, a regional population, or other professionals.

TERRORISM

September 11, 2001, has become a defining moment in the 21st century. Americans everywhere will always remember where they were and how they heard about the bombing of the World Trade Centers, the crash into the Pentagon, and the aborted flight in a field in Pennsylvania. For many Americans, the terrorist attacks on this date changed their perceptions of the world and their place in it. Suddenly, we joined much of the world as a victim and a site of terrorist activity.

Terrorism is defined in the Code of Federal Regulations as "the unlawful use of force or violence against persons or property to intimidate or coerce a government, the civilian population, or any segment thereof, in furtherance of political or social objectives" (Federal Emergency Management Agency, 2003). The goals of terrorists are to create fear among the public, convince citizens that their government is powerless against terrorism, and receive publicity for their causes. Generally, terrorism is categorized as domestic or international.

The distinction between these two is not where the act occurs but the origin of the responsible individuals or groups: The bombing of the Murrah Federal Building in Oklahoma City was an act of domestic terrorism, whereas the acts of 9/11 were international in origin. The events of 9/11 changed our lives in many ways. Everyday reminders of how life has changed are longer lines at airports; concrete barriers; a greater police presence in cities; a color-coded, five-level threat system; and increased emphasis on biological weapons research. Our language has changed as well. Anthrax, weapons of mass destruction, "dirty bombs," smallpox, "watch lists" of suspected terrorists, homeland security, and biological warfare have become part of the national discourse.

Terrorism has affected the work of human service professionals. Because terrorist acts are random, unprovoked, and intentional, people immediately feel helpless. Acute stress, trauma, and unsuccessful efforts to understand something that is beyond normal comprehension may result in fear, helplessness, vulnerability, and grief. Human services professionals will encounter both short- and long-term consequences as individuals and as helpers.

SHORT-TERM CONSEQUENCES   Many people are impacted by a terrorist attack. The American Psychological Association (2001) divides these people into three categories: (1) survivors of past traumatic events, (2) people who personally witnessed or were victims of the terrorist act, and (3) those who experience traumatization from learning of friends, family, and others who were subject to the violence or from exposure to repeated media accounts. Symptoms include recurring thoughts of the incident, isolating one's self, survivor guilt, and feeling the loss of control over one's life. In the event of an attack, there may be significant injuries, confusion, panic, strained health and mental health resources, and extensive media coverage.

Human service professionals can provide assistance to those who are coping with trauma from terrorism as well as other crises. Crisis intervention skills, discussed in more detail in Chapter 7, are helpful in the moment—remaining calm, checking for injuries, and activating support networks. Human service professionals can help victims understand delayed reactions of fear and helplessness, the importance of maintaining one's routine, the sharing of feelings and concerns, and learning what has happened and what is being done to combat terrorism.

LONG-TERM CONSEQUENCES   For others, the effects of terrorism may be longer term. Fear or hatred of foreigners, called *xenophobia,* is heightened following an act of

> **BOX 3.6** | WEB SOURCES
>
> *Resources for Coping with Traumatic Events*
>
> http://apahelpcenter.org/articles/article.php?id=22
>
> This is a brochure from the APA website, entitled "Managing Traumatic Stress: Tips for Recovering from Disasters and other Traumatic Events."
>
> http://mentalhealth.samhsa.gov/cmhs/Traumatic Events/default.asp
>
> This site provides information for those who work in diaster relief, encouraging them to deal with their own responses before and while they are helping others.
>
> http://www.bt.cdc.gov/masscasualties/copingpub.asp
>
> This site defines a traumatic event, outlines the symptoms and signs of PTSD, presents ways you can help others cope, especially children.
>
> http://www.nimh.nih.gov/publicat/violence.cfm
>
> This National Institute of Health website offers a comprehensive section entitled "Helping Children and Adolescents Cope with Violence and Disasters."
>
> http://familyinfoserv.com/crisis.html
>
> This Family Information Services website contains resources for families, children, and parents.
>
> http://www.ojp.usdoj.gov/ovc/publications/infores/cat_hndbk/welcome.html
>
> This site, in response to 9/11 helps individuals understand the nature of terrorism and how to cope with the phenomena.

international terrorism and can become a social and psychological danger. Diversity in a community or population may increase the fear generated by terrorism, particularly if distrust exists. For others, concern about the possibility of future terrorists acts increases stress and anxiety in daily lives.

Human service professionals can address the fear in both cases. For example, diversity is often an opportunity for strength and knowledge. Those who have past experiences with terrorism can be a support to those who are having their first experience. Second, the fear of future incidents can be alleviated by preparation. The random, sudden nature of terrorism causes fear and helplessness. Feeling a sense of control over some aspects of one's life can help. The American Red Cross (n.d.) suggests steps to restore a sense of control and calm, such as creating an emergency communications plan, selecting a meeting place, and assembling a disaster supplies kit. Other resources on coping with traumatic events are listed in Box 3.6.

NEW ROLES AND SKILLS FOR CLIENTS AND HELPERS

As the 21st century begins, one well-accepted change is the role of the client in the helping process. For many years, the client was a passive recipient of services—accepting the decisions, following the direction of a helper, and generally assuming little responsibility for what occurred in the process. With the recognition of clients' rights, the emphasis on consumer satisfaction, and the advent of welfare reform, the participation of the client in human service delivery has increased greatly; in many instances, the client becomes actively involved in the helping process.

This change has necessitated efforts on the part of human service professionals to engage the client as a partner in the helping process. Establishing a collaborative relationship calls for skills that promote a climate of trust and a sense of partnership. Taking time to get to know the client, considering the client's point of view, and exploring client expectations are part of this process. Once a relationship exists, the client becomes an active participant in assessing the problem and the situation, collecting information, determining a course of action, and evaluating the process. As a result of these actions, the client shares responsibility for the success or failure of the endeavor.

For human service professionals, this shift in the client's role has some benefits. First, the client shares the responsibility with the helper for the effectiveness of the helping process. Being actively engaged in the process increases the likelihood that the client will follow through on whatever tasks are necessary and will be more satisfied with the results. Second, the establishment of a relationship with the client also impacts the client's satisfaction. Having a good relationship with the helper means that clients believe that the helper listened, spent time with them, and provided follow-up services. Finally, clients have much to teach the human service professional about themselves, their problems, and the services they need. Ignoring these aspects of service delivery leads to ineffective and inefficient services. These are important lessons for helpers that will carry over to their work with other clients.

Just as the client assumes a new role in the helping process, 21st-century human service professionals need different helping skills. Advocacy, a skill recognized, accepted, and taught as a human service skill, will continue to be emphasized in the future. Another skill, selling, may be more nontraditional. Both advocacy and selling will be critical for successful service delivery in the future.

As human services changes, there may be both positive and negative reactions. It is possible that services will become more streamlined yet less available, and cost containment will save money but become an overriding factor in limiting treatment and other services. It is even possible that legislation unfair to some groups or individuals will become law. These possibilities make vigilance on the part of human service providers particularly important as they look out for the interests of their clients.

Advocacy means speaking out on behalf of clients or those who cannot speak for themselves. It frequently involves clients, their families, the community, and other professionals. Direct advocacy efforts may take many forms: empowering clients to act; improving environments; acting on behalf of a client by writing letters, filing forms, and so forth; informing clients about programs, services, and policies; and guiding a client through choices and changes. There are also situations that require advocacy on a larger scale. Are needed services provided? Are they available and accessible? Is the public policy fair and equitable? In these instances, a human service professional may act as a spokesperson to inform the public and legislators about what exists or what is needed. It may also be necessary to act as part of a collaborative effort for common agreement or support about an issue. The advocacy role of the human service professional is discussed more completely in Chapter 6. As you think about the future and the skills you will need to be an effective service provider, you also will want to think about how to prepare for this role.

A more nontraditional skill that is receiving attention is **selling.** Initial responses to this skill may be objections to sales as pushy, competitive, aggressive, manipulative, and fast-talking, whereas in reality many salespeople are professional, respectable people who do a good job selling because they believe it is a helping profession. According to recent sales literature, a new model of selling has emerged, one that is compatible with human service values and easily integrated with such practice (Futrell, 2005).

TABLE 3.4 | SUMMARY POINTS: TRENDS

- The effect of urbanization in poor countries will continue to create difficulties in meeting the basic needs of people.
- Demographic shifts in the United States raise questions about immigration policies, language, employment, and entitlement programs.
- One important shift is the growth and change of the elderly population, which indicates an increase in the number of elderly as well as changes in their characteristics.
- Clients will remain active participants in human service delivery.
- Advocacy and selling are examples of helping skills that are becoming increasingly important.

The new model of sales emphasizes a relationship approach to selling that focuses on the "we" in the relationship and the development of a partnership that is characterized by flexibility, two-way communication, and the resolution of concerns. The following quote illustrates how selling occurs in human services:

> We interview them, talk about our program a bit, and talk about why they were referred to us. So you think our program has something to offer you? Do you think there would be any benefit to us helping you? Could we work together? And 90% say yes. We are pretty good at selling our program. It is a sales job that is a part of health care that isn't discussed too often. It is selling that needs to go on, particularly with getting people into a program. (Jan Cabrera, personal communication)

This quote is from the director/case manager of an intensive case management program in Los Angeles, which assists patients with severe mental illness who are living in this community and which provides "cradle-to-grave" comprehensive services. The human service professional must have the client "buy in" so the client will volunteer to participate and then use the services available.

CONSERVATISM

Modern political **conservatism** emerged in the 19th century in response to the political and social changes of the times, discussed in Chapter 2. Conservatism at that time meant preserving the power of the king and aristocracy, maintaining the influence of landholders against the rising industrial bourgeoisie, and continuing the ties between church and state ("Conservatism," 2003). By the 20th century, conservatism meant advocating economic laissez-faire and opposing extending the welfare state, and was supported primarily by manufacturing and professional groups who wanted to maintain the then status quo.

For the last 50 years, conservatives have offered policies that emphasize freedom, market solutions, and the dangers of big government. George W. Bush, the 43rd U. S. president, has embraced the principles of "compassionate conservatism," insisting that society can improve the lives of all Americans without government support or entitlements. To that end, recasting social welfare policies has been an administration priority. Examples of proposed changes that reflect this conservative philosophy are the federal funding of charitable work by religious groups, greater reliance on private health plans to treat the elderly, tightening welfare restrictions, and managed care prescription drug coverage for Medicare recipients.

What exactly does this trend mean for human service professionals and the clients they serve? Human service agencies and organizations may be affected in different ways, depending on their relationship to federal and state governments, their funding sources, and their missions. Human service educators recognize that their field continues to change rapidly and that innovative approaches to traditional helping may be needed to meet the demands of service delivery in the 21st century. It is also important to retain those traditional skills that are effective. As human service professionals, our challenge is to stay abreast of both societal trends and new developments in order to provide quality services to those who need assistance.

KEY TERMS

advocacy

Americans with Disabilities Act

assisted living

community-based services

conservatism

continuum of care

diversity

e-mail

employee assistance programs

E-therapy

ethnicity

external reviews

fee-for-service

full-service schools

gatekeeping

managed care

Mental Health Patient Bill of Rights

multiracial

selling

standards of good practice

teleconferencing

terrorism

urbanization

web logs

World Wide Web

THINGS TO REMEMBER

1. Human services are delivered to populations in a variety of settings, including rural areas, industry, the military, schools, and other community-based settings, all of which increase the number of clients who can be reached.

2. Schools have become a site for service delivery, as teachers and human service professionals share the same clients.

3. The trend toward providing more services in community-based settings and less in institutional ones is helping to serve clients in the least restrictive environment.

4. Community-based services were first used with clients with mental illness who were deinstitutionalized; now, populations receiving community-based services include those in the criminal justice system, the developmentally disabled, and the elderly.

5. The barriers to service delivery in rural areas include shortages of workers, the large geographic distances between clients and providers, the cost of services, confidentiality issues, and coordination of care.

6. Technology has begun to change the way human service professionals meet their responsibilities, particularly in the areas of communication, information management, service provision, and professional development.

7. Communication avenues used by human service professionals include e-mail, Listservs, the World Wide Web, cellular phones, and teleconferencing.

8. Computer technology is available to help human service professionals manage information and use data to make decisions about planning programs, establishing costs, and reporting.

9. Technology is being effectively used to provide services to clients, including diagnosing and assessing, teaching new skills, and assisting those with disabilities or impairments.

10. The increased use of managed care organizations is dramatically changing the delivery of human services through the use of external reviews, the demand to develop standards of best practice, the need for better information management, and an emphasis on a continuum of care.

11. Managed care standards, developed for accountability in health and human services, provide needed services efficiently and effectively.

12. As technological advances draw the world closer, we become more aware of the human service challenges in an international context, such as increases in the global population, international migration, and urbanization.

13. In the international context, many individuals live in large cities in poor countries, where they struggle to meet basic needs and have little access to housing, sanitation, and nutritious food.

14. Among the trends in the United States that will influence future human service delivery are the growth and change of its elderly population, the increasing diversity of clients and professionals, the increasingly active participation of clients, and the development of new and, in some cases, nontraditional skills.

ADDITIONAL READINGS: NEW TRENDS

Deparle, J. (2004). *American dream: Three women, ten kids, and a nation's drive to end welfare.* NY: Viking Adult.
The author, a *New York Times* reporter, presents an informed examination of the challenges, successes, and failures involved in welfare reform by following one extended poor family from the end of slavery through the close of the millennium.

Kongstvedt, P. R. (2003). *Managed care: What it is and how it works.* Sudbury, MA: Jones & Bartlett. This handbook describes the origins, varieties, and future prospects of managed care. Issues discussed include reimbursement, network management, Medicare and Medicaid, regulation, and accreditation.

Kronick, R. F. (2005). *Full service community schools: Prevention of delinquency in students with mental illness and/or poverty.* Springfield, IL: Thomas.
This book is based on the application of full-service school principles to three inner-city elementary schools. Culture and self-efficacy, a systemic perspective, the Appalachian experience, and juvenile justice and the rights of children are topics integral to meeting the needs of the children in these schools.

Moorehead, C. (2006). *Human cargo: A journey among refugees.* NY: Holt.
As an experienced writer about human rights for 25 years, the author presents an overview of the fate of refugees who are either searching for a better life or seeking asylum after persecution, rape, torture, and genocidal massacres.

Snowdon, D. (2002). *Aging with grace: What the nun study teaches us about living longer, healthier, and more meaningful lives.* New York: Bantam.

The results of tracking the lives of 678 elderly nuns to assess the effects of aging offer insights into how to live healthier lives now. The author and researcher is one of the world's leading experts on Alzheimer's disease.

Williams, M. A. (2001). *The 10 lenses: Your guide to living and working in a multicultural world.* Sterling, VA: Capital Books.

This book is a tool to help readers understand the 10 human mindset "lenses" through which we view race, culture, and ethnicity in our world.

REFERENCES

ABC's of Internet Therapy. (2006). *Talk to a therapist on line.* Retrieved September 23, 2006, from http://www.metanoia.org/imhs/.

Administration on Aging. (2006). *Mental health.* Retrieved October 10, 2006, from http://www.aoa.gov/eldfam/healthy_lifestyles/mental_health/mental_health.asp.

American Counseling Association. (2005). *2005 Code of ethics.* Retrieved October 10, 2006, from http://www.counseling.org/Resources/CodeOfEthics/TP/Home/CT2.aspx.

American Dietetic Association. (2006, September). *Journal of American Dietetic Association.* Retrieved September 30, 2006, from http://www.eatright.org/cps/rde/xchg/ada/hs.xsl/media_9483_ENU_HTML.htm.

American Red Cross. (n.d.). *Home.* Retrieved October 11, 2006, at http://www.redcross.org/.

American Psychological Association. (2001). *Coping with terrorism.* Retrieved September 11, 2003, from http://www.apa.org.

American Psychological Association. (2006). *Mental health patient's bill of rights.* Retrieved September 30, 2006, from http://www.apa.org/topics/rights/.

Baldor, L. C. (2003, September 14). Government missing goals on illegal aliens. *News Sentinel,* p. A6.

Barron's. (2006). *Managed care.* Retrieved September 30, 2006, from http://www.answers.com/topic/managed-care.

Brammer, R. (2004). *Diversity in counseling.* Belmont, CA: Brooks/Cole/Thomson.

Buck, F. (n.d.). *Religious diversity works to define 21st century America. FACSNET.* Retrieved October 1, 2003, from http://www.facsnet.org/issues/faith/williams.php.

Bumiller, E. (2003, September 7). 9/11/01, 9/11/02, 9/11/03: Who won? *New York Times,* 14.

Collie, K. (2004). Interpersonal communication in behavioral telehealth: What can we learn from other fields? In J. Bloom & G. Waltz (Eds.), *Cybercounseling and cyberlearning: An encore* (pp. 345–365). American Counseling Association and ERIC Counseling and Student Services Clearinghouse.

Conservatism. (2003). In *Columbia encyclopedia* (6th ed.). Retrieved October 14, 2003, from http://www.encyclopedia.com/html/cl/conservatsm.asp.

Department of Health and Social Services. (2006). *Government of Nunavut.* Retrieved October 11, 2006, from http://www.gov.nu.ca/hsssite/hssmain.shtml.

Dorfrman, S. (2006). *Preventive interventions under managed care: Mental health and substance abuse services.* U.S. Department of Health and Human Services. Retrieved September 30, 2006, from http://mentalhealth.samhsa.gov/publications/allpubs/SMA00-3437/default.asp.

Dryfoos, J., & Barkin, C. (2006). *Adolescence: Growing up in America today.* New York: Oxford University Press.

Elliott, A. (2006, September 10). More Muslims arrive in the U.S., after 9/11 dip. *New York Times,* p.1.

Erikson, E. (1963). *Childhood and society.* New York: Norton.

Federal Emergency Management Agency (FEMA). (2003, February 11). *Hazards.* Retrieved September 11, 2003, from http://www.fema.gov/hazards/terrorism.

Focus on Fairfax. (2006). *Washington Post.com.* Retrieved September 23, 2006, from http://blog.washingtonpost.com/fairfaxfocus/human_services/.

Furness, G. (2003). Depression in the elderly could improve public health: risk factors for depression among elderly community subjects: A systematic review and meta-analysis. *American Journal of Psychiatry, 160*(6), 1147–1156.

Futrell, C. M. (2005). *ABC's of relationship selling.-* Boston: McGraw Hill.

Gardner, A. (2006). Study found most did so within two years of return. *Healthfinder*. National Health Information Center. Retrieved September 6, 2006, from http://www.healthfinder.gov/news/newsstory.asp?docID=531267.

Government of Nunavut. (2006). *Our land*. Retrieved September 23, 2006, from http://www.gov.nu.ca/Nunavut/English/about/ourland.pdf.

Gunthert, K., C., Cohen, L. H., Butler, A. C., & Beck, J. S. (2005). Predictive role of daily coping and affective reactivity in cognitive therapy outcome. *Behavioral Therapy, 36*(1), 77–88.

Hiller, S. M., & Barrow, G. M. (2007). *Aging, the individual, and society*. Belmont, CA: Wadsworth/Thomson Learning.

International Organization for Migration (IOM). (2006, September 14). *Global estimates and trends*. Retrieved September 14, 2006, from http://www.iom.int/jahia/Jahia/cache/offonce/pid/254.

Jansson, B. S. (2001). *The reluctant welfare state*. Belmont, CA: Wadsworth/Thomson Learning.

Kinsella, K., & Velkoff, V. A. (2001). *An aging world: 2001*. U.S. Census Bureau, Series P95/01=1. Washington, DC: U.S. Government Printing Office.

Kronick, R. F. (2005). *Full-service community schools: Prevention of delinquency of students with mental illness and/or poverty*. Springfield, IL: Thomas.

Lea, D. H., Johnson, J. L., Ellingwood, S., Allan, W., Patel, A., & Smith, R. Telegenetics in Maine: Successful clinical and education service delivery model developed from a three year pilot project. *Genetics in Medicine, 7*(1), 21. Retrieved September 23, 2006, from http://www.liebertonline.com/doi/abs/10.1089/153056203763317620?journalCode=tmj.

Masi, D. (1982). *Human services in industry*. Lexington, MA: Lexington Books.

National Institute of Health. (2006). *NIH radio*. Retrieved September 23, 2006, from http://www.nih.gov/news/radio/index.htm.

National Organization for Human Services. (2000). *Code of ethics*. Retrieved October 11, 2006, from http://www.nationalhumanservices.org/.

Office of Equal Opportunity and Diversity Management. (2003, August 15). *Home*. Retrieved October 1, 2003, from http://www.doi.gov/diversity/workforce_diversity.html.

Okun, B. F., Fried, J., & Okun, M. L. (1999). *Understanding diversity*. Pacific Grove, CA: Brooks/Cole/Thomson.

Papalia, D. E., Olds, S. W., & Feldman, R. D. (2004). *Human development* (9th ed.). Boston: McGraw Hill.

Patz, J. A., Campbell-Lendrum, D., Holloway, T., & Foley, J. A. (2005, November 17). Impact of regional climate change on human health. *Nature, 438*, 310–317. Retrieved October 11, 2006, from http://www.nature.com/nature/journal/v438/n7066/full/nature04188.html.

Population and Diversity. (2006). *International information programs*. U.S. Department of State. Retrieved September 14, 2006, from http://usinfo.state.gov/scv/history_geography_and_population.

Resnick, H. (n.d.). *Talking it out: A computer based mediation software for adolescents*. Retrieved September 23, 2006, from http://www.krisbosworth.org/documents/talking_it_out.pdf#search=%22%22talking%20it%20out%22%20software%22.

Robinson, B. A. (2003, September 30). Reacting to religious diversity: Religious exclusivism, pluralism, & inclusivism. *Ontario Consultants on Religious Tolerance*. Retrieved October 1, 2003, from http://www.religioustolerance.org/rel_plur.htm.

Substance Abuse and Mental Health Services Administration. (2006). *Principles for systems of managed care*. Retrieved September 30, 2006, from http://mentalhealth.samhsa.gov/publications/allpubs/MC96-61/default.asp.

Sue, D. W., & Sue, D. (2003). *Counseling the culturally diverse*. New York: Wiley.

Surgeon General. (n.d.). *Office of the Surgeon General*. Retrieved October 11, 2006, from http://www.surgeongeneral.gov/.

U.S. Census Bureau. (2005). *Dramatic changes in U. S. aging highlighted in new census, NIH report*. Retrieved October 10, 2006, from http://www.nia.nih.gov/NewsAndEvents/PressReleases/PR2006030965PlusReport.htm.

U.S. demographics for religion. (2003, August 15). Sacramento, CA: Instructional Systems. Retrieved October 1, 2003, from http://www.teachingaboutreligion.org/Demographics/map_demographics.htm.

MODELS OF SERVICE DELIVERY

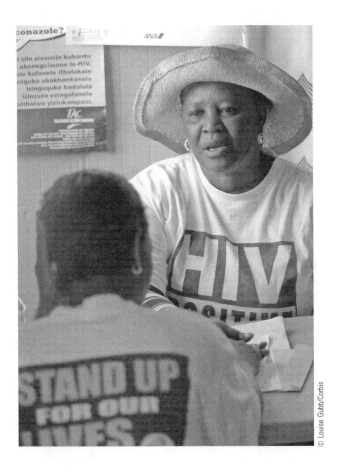

CHAPTER 4

© Louise Gubb/Corbis

After reading this chapter, you will be able to:

• Define three models of service delivery.
• Trace their development.
• Illustrate the use of these models in human service delivery today.
• Apply the three models to a human service problem.

Self-assessment

• Outline the differences among the medical model, the public health model, and the human service model.
• What principles of the medical model and/or the public health model are present in the human service model?
• Compare the treatment of mental illness in the three service delivery models.
• List the key factors that contributed to the development of the human service model.
• Describe how the three models might coordinate services to address a human service problem such as teen pregnancy.

In developing a definition of human services, we have discussed its various character-izations, briefly traced the history of service provision, and explored recent develop-ments, emphasizing human services today. Another approach to defining human services is to examine the way it benefits service recipients. This chapter describes three models that represent different orientations in service delivery: the medical model, the public health model, and the human service model. The chapter concludes with a case that illustrates the interaction of these models.

In this chapter, you will meet clients who have received services delivered in the context of these three models. The cases of Robert Smith and Ralph Jones illustrate services provided by the medical model. Sean O'Reilly was a recipient of services provided by the public health model. Susan, her husband, Ted, and children, Matthew and Justin, illustrate the complexities of client needs, needs that may require multi-faceted, long-term intervention.

All three models are used to deliver services today, and depending on the problem, an integration of all three models may be most effective. In practice, some agencies may prefer one over the others, and one model may be more effective than the other two in some situations. Workers may be skilled in following one particular model, but they are likely to be working closely with practitioners who follow the other models. Therefore, you should know the characteristics of each model, its historical development, and how it is used. To help translate this information into human service practice, we examine a relevant social problem from the perspective of each model.

Each of the three models of service delivery has certain philosophical assumptions that guide its practice. These assumptions reflect beliefs about the causes of problems, their treatment, and the role of the professional in the model. To illustrate, we consider the nature of mental disorders from the perspectives of each of the three models.

The medical model is based on an orientation developed by the medical profession; it assumes that mental disorders are diseases or illnesses that impair an individual's ability to function. The disease or illness, in this case the mental disorder, has an organic basis and responds to medical interventions such as medication, laboratory studies, and physical therapies. Often the individual, or **patient,** receives treatment from a physician in a hospital or medical clinic.

The public health model resembles the medical model in its diagnosis and treatment process, but the models differ in recipients of services and methodologies of treatment. Whereas the medical model emphasizes individuals, the public health model focuses on *groups* in the population who may be identified by geography (community, country, region, or state), types of problems (abuse, poverty, specific illnesses), or specific characteristics such as age (children, the elderly). This model views mental disorders as the result of malfunctions or pressures created by the environment or by society. The mental disorder is evaluated for its impact not only on the individual but also on society at large. In addition to treating the individual, this model emphasizes preventing the problem through supporting activities such as use of films, speakers, school programs, and pamphlets, all aimed at educating the population about the problem.

The **human service model** is concerned with the interaction between the individual and the environment, stressing the need for balance between the two. Although recognizing both the medical and the public health perspectives, this model focuses on the interpersonal and environmental conflicts that may result from the problem (in this case, a mental disorder). Perhaps the individual (or **client** or **consumer**) has problems resulting from genetic predispositions, biochemical imbalances, faulty learning, lack of insight into behavior that may be inappropriate, a physical or mental disability, and/or influences from the social environment. Whatever the situation, the client is experiencing interpersonal and emotional difficulties that affect behavior. Treatment in this model encompasses services to both the individual and the environment through work with the client as well as the people and the institutions with which the client is involved. An important consideration in the model is the focus on client strengths rather than inadequacies. Each model provides a different perspective on the same problem. We now look at the development of each one.

THE MEDICAL MODEL

DEFINITION

The **medical model** sees the person coming for help as an individual whose problem is a disease or a sickness. The individual is "sick" or "ill," not healthy. Often called *patients,* these individuals depend on the physician or service provider to prescribe a treatment or cure for the "disease." Historically, this model can be summarized as a system that involves the following elements: symptom–diagnosis–treatment–cure (Reinhard, 1986).

The medical model, with a history that includes shamans, medicine men and women, and witch doctors, is perhaps the oldest of all treatment models. In fact, other models used it as they were developing. For example, in Chapter 2 we discussed the beginning of the new profession of social work at the turn of the 20th century. Mary Richmond, author of *Social Diagnosis* (1917), used the medical model to describe social casework. Believing that the presenting problem was rooted in the individual, she suggested that pauperism was a disease. The friendly visitor,

BOX 4.1	INTERNATIONAL FOCUS

Models of Service Design

Thinking about models of service design in developing countries, Howard N. Higginbotham (1979) suggested three basic models of service design today: traditional psychiatry, the public health approach, and the village system. He believed that the "the first model, traditional **psychiatry**, is similar to North American or European psychiatry, which has not been modified for use in non-Western settings." The focus of this model includes using residential facilities that means that recipients must travel to find help. Residential services range from long-term confinement or therapy like farming or doing daily chores. New admits and long-term clients may receive psychotropic medication and electroconvulsive shock therapy (ECT); few patients receive traditional **psychotherapy**.

The second model is a public health approach to services where prevention and training volunteers or paraprofessionals is emphasized. Patients are helped outside a residential settings using consultation with family and education of the patient and the family and other community resources.

Because the Western models have not worked well in developing countries, the village system has emerged as a viable option to treatment for those with mental illness. It uses native healers, therapeutic relationships, psychotropic drugs, and the natural therapeutic elements of the village, which include confession, dancing, and rituals.

Source: Adapted from "Culture and Mental Services," by Howard N. Higginbotham. In Anthony J. Marsella, Roland G. Tharp, and Thomas Ciborowski (Eds.), *Perspectives on Cross-Cultural Psychology*, pp. 205–236. Copyright © 1979 by Academic Press.

therefore, became a social physician whose duty was to heal the complex conditions of poverty (Zimbalist, 1977).

The corrections field also adopted the medical model during the 1930s, when its emphasis shifted from punishment to treatment. The change was based on the assumption that criminal behavior was the result of physical or environmental aspects of an individual's life, requiring treatment (Clear, Cole, & Resig, 2005). Theoretically, prisons were to become therapeutic communities, where inmates would be rehabilitated to reenter society. Unfortunately, budget constraints limited this change to one of name only: Departments of prisons became "departments of corrections," but punishment continued to be the reality. Structurally, the system already included parole, probation, and the indeterminate sentence. All that remained to complete the incorporation of the medical model was the addition of a classification system to aid in diagnosis and treatment (Clear et al., 2005).

HISTORY

As mentioned in Chapter 2, institutions developed as a way to meet the needs of some segments of society. Asylums were established primarily to care for people with mental illness, shifting care from the local community to rural institutions and replacing local financing with state funding. Responsibility for the care of people with mental illness rested with the medical profession.

Psychiatry emerged as a discipline at the end of the 18th century when Philippe Pinel became head of the Hospice de Bicêtre and later of Salpetriere (mental institutions in France). Some mental disorders had been recognized as such early on, but Pinel's removal of chains from patients and other humane acts emphasized the belief that pathological behavioral disorders had organic origins and that their treatment belonged to medicine. Accordingly, those diagnosed as mentally ill were to be treated as patients by physicians in hospital settings, just like other patients with medical problems. Pinel, hoping to create a science of mental disease, is credited with introducing the medical model into psychiatry by stressing the clinical diagnosis and appropriate medical treatment. (See Box 4.2.)

Until the end of the 19th century, insanity was socially defined: "An insane was a person whose behavior for pathological reasons was so disturbed that he had to be segregated in special institutions" (Pichot, 1985, p. 10). With the emergence of psychiatry as a medical specialty, a body of knowledge was established to explain the nature and causes of insanity. The discovery and application of the most effective treatments became a priority. Insanity became medically defined, meaning that the institution of treatment had to be a hospital instead of a prison, and the care of the patient would be handled by a physician, not a warden.

After the middle of the 19th century, use of the medical model to treat mental illness dominated. By the end of the century, however, the medical model was changing. A new school of thought rejected medical treatment and advocated psychotherapy for treatment of people with mental illness. The new philosophy was based on the assumption that diseases of the soul were completely separate from diseases of the body. Psychiatry concerned itself with the medicine of the soul; psychosis was the disease of the soul, and **neurosis** was the disease of the nerves (Pichot, 1985). Sigmund Freud's work reflected this orientation.

Early in his career, Freud was a researcher and clinician in biology and neurology; he made outstanding contributions to both fields. He used the scientific method, insisting that medical problems of mental illness be studied in the rigorous laboratory setting. Later, Freud rejected his earlier training and revolutionized the study and treatment of mental illness. He developed a method of therapy commonly known today as the **psychoanalytic method.** In this method, the clients/patients share all thoughts with the therapist. The therapist interprets this material to explain to patients the nature of their repressions and the influence of these repressions on their present problems. Freud also developed a theory of neurosis and one of the normal mind, based on the assumption that mental disorders were psychologically rooted.

Although Freud's impact was profound, psychoanalytic theory did not completely change the medical model or become the preferred method of treatment, for several reasons. First, its success was difficult to evaluate and to document. Second, it required too much time and expense to be a viable treatment for large numbers of people.

The treatment of people with mental illness continued to develop in the 1940s; however, more psychiatrists and improved treatment were needed. A common treatment during this decade was electroconvulsive or **electroshock therapy.** This treatment involved administering an electric shock of 70 to 130 volts to the brain, leaving the patient unconsciousness and/or in convulsions. On regaining consciousness, the patient sometimes experienced confusion and memory loss, but problem behaviors diminished after several weeks of treatments. Electroshock therapy was effective with depressed individuals, but it was used less successfully to treat other mental disorders. Its abuse during the 1960s resulted in negative perceptions of this treatment method, and these perceptions contributed to the growing popularity of psychotropic medications.

BOX 4.2 | PHILIPPE PINEL

Philippe Pinel (1745–1826) is famous in the history of medicine and mental health. In revolutionary France, Pinel courageously campaigned to secure a new status for persons with mental illness as people suffering from disease rather than being possessed by demons or manifesting the consequences of sin. Pinel argued, practiced, and taught that such persons require medical care rather than persecution or punishment, and that they are entitled to be treated with respect as persons and citizens. This was a revolutionary idea.

Pinel was born into a modest family of surgeons in southwestern France. Initially trained as a cleric and destined for service in the church, he decided to study science in Toulouse. By 1773, he had acquired a doctorate of medicine, but he continued his studies for four more years in Montpellier under Barthez. Sickness and health became his lifelong concern, and he systematically applied himself to learning all he could about medicine from ancient as well as contemporary sources. He acquired the education of a classicist and a humanist in addition to his extensive knowledge of the practice of medicine in his day. He moved to Paris in 1778 and supported himself by translating scientific and medical works and teaching mathematics.

Though extremely shy, he became a member of an important group of reformers and medical thinkers called the Ideologues. Benjamin Franklin tried to convince Pinel to go to America. However, Pinel was a patriot and wished to help modernize medicine in his own country. His interest in insanity derived from the suicide of a seriously depressed friend and patient in 1783. In 1792, apparently because of his connections with the Ideologues, Pinel was appointed Physician of the Infirmaries to the Hospice de Bicetre, a huge Parisian custodial institution for indigent ailing men.

During this time, Pinel published three significant works: *Philosophical Nosography* (1798), *Treatise on Insanity* (1801), and *Clinical Medicine* (1802). The first book would serve for years as a text for the classification of diseases; the second would lay the foundation for modern psychiatry; and the third, published in three successively enlarged editions, would spread his methodology and fame among the next generation.

In 1794, Pinel transferred to the Hospice de la Salpetriere, an institution that housed nearly 7,000 destitute women. He administered, practiced, and taught in this hospital for 30 years, applying the principles that gave him the reputation as a founder of modern psychiatry.

In medical practice, Pinel practically invented the role of the full-time resident physician who teaches and trains students, interns, and fellow researchers in a hospital ward. Along with other reformers, he argued for national curricula, standards, and diplomas for medical education. Pinel insisted that such education should be conducted in French and based on clinical practice and observations. He viewed the natural sciences as "accessories" to the practice of medicine.

With regard to mental health, Pinel is often given credit for what he learned from the uneducated but experienced and successful Keeper of the Insane at Bicetre, J. P. Pussin (1746–1811): namely, that the mental patients could be managed without cages, chains, or cruelty. Pinel brought Pussin to Salpetriere in 1802 to aid him in caring for the many unruly patients. Pinel combined Pussin's practical management principles with his own medical knowledge to develop his famous "moral method" for treating mental illness. This method assumes that mental illness is due to some imbalance in the patient, which the physician can treat and rectify. The crux of this method is extensive observation and knowledge about the patient. This knowledge makes possible detailed therapy, which the physician must carefully supervise. Pinel's approach is a far cry from bleeding, beating, purging, and imprisonment, which had been the usual methods of treating the insane.

Pinel's methods and publications made him well known, and students flocked to him. Among them were the future leaders of French medicine. Pinel's concern for humane treatment of persons with mental illness was realized in France and made that country a world leader in the enlightened treatment of mental illness. When Dorothea Dix traveled in Europe in the late 1850s, extending her great American crusade to reform in the treatment of the insane, she had only small changes to recommend to the French, and to the Turks in Constantinople who had been trained by the French.

Source: Used by permission of H. Phillips Hamlin (1985).

Psychotropic drugs, which act on the brain, are now among the most widely used treatments for mental disorders. Many human service professionals work with clients taking psychotropic medications and need to be knowledgeable about the drugs their clients are taking. The science of the preparation, uses, and effects of drugs is pharmacology. The branch of pharmacology of most interest to human service professionals is **psychopharmacology,** which focuses on "the psychological effects of drugs and the use of drugs to treat symptoms of mental and emotional disorders" (Ingersoll & Rak, 2006, p. 3).

One example of the necessity for knowledge about psychotropic drugs is on-label and off-label prescriptions. On-label means that the drug has been approved by the Food and Drug Administration (FDA) to treat a specific disorder; however, many psychotropic drugs are prescribed off-label. This means that they are not specifically approved by the FDA for a certain disorder. Rather, the medical professional believes, based on case studies and other evidence, that the drug will help the condition or disorder the client has. Neither label guarantees a drug is totally safe or effective for everyone.

Psychotropic medications can be divided into four major classes: antipsychotic drugs, antidepressant drugs, antianxiety drugs, and lithium salts. **Antipsychotic drugs** are effective in managing psychotic disorders such as bipolar disorder (colloquially known as manic depression) and schizophrenia. Although these drugs do not cure psychosis, they help to control certain psychotic behaviors such as suspiciousness, hallucinations, and impulsiveness. Haldol (haloperidol), Stelaxine (trifluoperazine), Thorazine (chlorpromazine), Clozaril (clozapine), and Mellaril (thioridazine) are well-known examples of antipsychotic medication.

Antidepressant drugs, the second class, relieve depression. There are two kinds of antidepressant drugs: the tricyclic antidepressants and the monoamine oxidase inhibitors. Human service workers will most likely come in contact with widely used tricyclic antidepressants such as Elavil (amitriptyline) or Tofranil (imipramine); however, Prozac (fluoxetine), Paxil (paroxetine), Luvor (fluvoxamine), and Zoloft (sertraline)—antidepressants unrelated to tricyclic or monoamine oxidase inhibitors—have become increasingly popular in recent years because of fewer side effects. These drugs are selective seratonin reuptake inhibitors (SSRIs).

The most widely used psychotropic medications by far are the **antianxiety drugs,** *sedatives,* and *hypnotics.* Prescribed to relieve anxiety, fear, or tension, these medications may be classed as barbiturates, benzodiazepines, or antihistamines. Benzodiazepines such as Valium (diazepam), Klonopin (clonazepam), Xanax (alprazolam), Tranxene (clorazepate), and Librium (chlordiazepoxide) are especially popular because they reduce anxiety without reducing overall performance.

The final class of psychotropic medication is **mood stabilizers.** They include lithium carbonate, calcium channel blockers (Calan, Isoptin), and anticonvulsants (Tegretol, Epitol). Used primarily in the treatment of bipolar disorder, these drugs are particularly effective in preventing the mania state, which is characterized by symptoms of extreme irritability, talkativeness, grandiose ideas, exaggerated self-esteem, and increased involvement in risky activities such as spending sprees or reckless driving.

Psychotropic medications have revolutionized mental health by facilitating deinstitutionalization, but the effects have not always been positive. For example, critics

TABLE 4.1	POSSIBLE SIDE EFFECTS OF PSYCHOTROPIC MEDICATIONS

Antipsychotic Drugs	Convulsions
Feelings of heaviness	**Antianxiety drugs**
Sluggishness	Drug tolerance
Weakness	Stumbling gait
Faintness	Slurred speech
Drowsiness	Drowsiness
Dizziness	Conjunctivitis
Tremors	Dry mouth
Seizures	Constipation
Tardive dyskinesia	Urinary problems
Loss of muscle tone	**Mood stabilizers**
Antidepressants	Toxic warning signs (nausea, tremors, muscle spasms)
Dry mouth	
Blurred vision	Thyroid disorders
Constipation	Renal toxicity
Urinary retention	Nausea
Lowered or raised blood pressure	Vomiting
Agitation	Diarrhea
Raised temperature	Sedation
Hallucinations	Confusion

say that antianxiety drugs mask symptoms so that individuals avoid dealing with the real problem. Clients who take major tranquilizers over a long period of time may suffer dangerous side effects, such as tardive dyskinesia, a neurological disorder characterized by abnormal, involuntary mouth or tongue movements. Table 4.1 lists other common side effects of the four major categories.

Today, those who deliver services in the medical model face several challenges. One is that the symptom–diagnosis–treatment–cure process more realistically leads to cure *or* control. Particularly with psychiatric illnesses, controlling the symptoms and making the patient functional are the guides for treatment. Complicating this issue are the numerous new drugs that appear with frequency. There are now many drugs that do not fit neatly into the four categories of psychotropic drugs just described. For example, the serotonin drugs (Prozac, Paxil, and Zoloft), which do not fit in one category, are broadly prescribed today to treat bulimia, obsessive-compulsive disorders, and anxiety disorders.

BOX 4.3 | WEB SOURCES

Find Out More about Psychotropic Medications

www.npi.ucla.edu/mhdd/INFO/modules/psychotropicmedsoverview.html

This site outlines psychotropic medications, their uses, and frequently asked questions about them.

www.cqc.state.ny.us/

New York State has prepared a website that offers the latest information on best practices, client/customer services, what's new, and other topics about quality care for the mentally disabled. "Could This Happen in Your Program?" provides a number of cases to challenge and spark reflection and discussion among direct-care staff about policies and practices.

www.applesforhealth.com/psymedchild1.html

This site describes the current information on the safety and efficacy of medications for children and adolescents with mental disorders. Data by NIMH provide advanced knowledge of the effects of psychotropic drugs on children.

www.mental-health-today.com

This site provides current articles about mental health treatment and psychotropic medications.

www.mentalhealth.com

This site provides an extensive list of psychotropic medications, their descriptions, indications, contraindications, warnings, adverse effects, dosage, and research findings.

A second challenge is determining who controls medical services. Is it the physician, the patient, insurers or managed care organizations, employers, and/or the government? To varying degrees, all seem to have a role. For example, the intrusions of government become greater each year. Although it is sometimes difficult medically to separate the organic and psychiatric states, it has happened at some state government levels; that is, diagnosis and reimbursement guidelines have differentiated physical and mental conditions. A second example is the impact of managed care discussed in Chapter 3. Typically, in a managed system, physicians receive a fixed amount per patient to take care of medical problems. A small part of the capitation fee is for behavioral health care. Once again, physicians are faced with an arbitrary separation between physical and psychiatric conditions. They also grapple daily with wanting to do the right thing but at the same time contain costs. Achieving this balance is difficult when physicians attend to the "whole" patient, which includes a consideration of the patient's environment and social circumstances. In some instances, physicians have lost their right to choose which drugs to prescribe because managed care staff overrule their recommendations in favor of less expensive medicines.

The past 30 years have demystified psychiatric illness and made its acceptance widespread. The future may include new perspectives. One may be an awareness that we treat mild disease too aggressively. A second perspective is that in some cases it is society that is malfunctional, not the individual—that is, society places people in situations that are not normal but expects them not to behave abnormally. For example, think about the malfunctional mother who has a full-time job as well as responsibility for the home and the children. The problem may not be that she is malfunctional but that society's expectations are unrealistic.

TABLE 4.2	SUMMARY POINTS: HISTORY OF THE MEDICAL MODEL

- Individual is "sick."
- Recipient is called *patient*.
- 18th-century Philippe Pinel removes chains of mentally ill.
- Pinel stresses clinical diagnosis and treatment.
- Psychiatry emerges as a medical specialty.
- Mid-19th-century psychotherapy emerges as treatment.
- Freud develops psychoanalytic method.
- Electric shock is introduced in the 1940s.
- Psychotropic drugs become the most widely used treatments.

CASE STUDIES

One obvious example of the medical model's application to human service problems is its use in treating mental illness. Two illustrative case studies follow. The case of Robert Smith describes the mental illness and treatment of a man in the late 1870s. This narrative not only illustrates the orientation of the medical model but also expresses the attitudes of that time toward mental illness. The case of Ralph Jones represents the use of the medical model over 100 years later. The use of the medical model in the second case is especially reflected in the prescription of medication and other physical treatments for Ralph's illness. In both cases, note that the clients are considered ill and that their treatment reflects this diagnosis.

ROBERT SMITH

Robert Smith was the fourth of six children and the third son. His family, third-generation immigrants from England, lived in Philadelphia. Robert was quiet and withdrawn as a child, and while he did the work the family found for him, he was never very energetic in seeking it out.

The Smith family was relatively poor. Their fortunes improved somewhat during the Civil War, when they were able to find employment in the war-related metal industry, but after the war they descended again into poverty.

In his late 20s, Robert began to have episodes of "mania," as a doctor later called it. While still usually quiet and withdrawn, Robert would become violent and aggressive if crossed by members of his family or neighbors or if frustrated by events. These episodes of mania cost him his job, and soon the family was having to watch him all the time. During an episode, he would sometimes attack anyone who tried to communicate with him; when the episode passed, he would again become withdrawn and listless.

When Robert's aggressiveness began to be expressed toward the neighbors as well as toward family members, the family began to seek help for him. They took him to physicians, who examined him but did not know what to do for him. By the time he was 32, Robert Smith's behavior had become so distressing that his family was desperate. He had been arrested more than once for destroying property in the neighborhood and threatening neighbors. His family had only barely kept him out of prison. His father took him to the county commission, which, after hearing the testimony of the family and the local sheriff, agreed to send him to the Blockley Almshouse in the fall of 1875. Blockley Almshouse was a huge collection of buildings maintained by the city of Philadelphia for its insane poor. When it was time for Robert to go there, the combined efforts of several family members and neighbors were necessary to overcome his resistance and subdue him.

At first, Robert was kept in the general hospital to recover from the injuries he had received in resisting the move to Blockley. Then he was transferred to a crowded asylum building, where he was nominally under the care of Dr. Isaac Ray, whom he actually never saw except from a distance. Robert had to sleep on a night bed put on the floor in a corridor. When his violent episodes occurred, he was put in a straight waistcoat, which reduced his ability to attack other patients or attendants. The ward was generally noisy and turbulent. There was little chance for a good night's sleep, nor was there anything much for the patients to do during the day except to excite each other, creating almost continual disturbances.

After a year in Blockley, and weeks in a straitjacket, Robert became less violent and more depressed. Cold-water treatments seemed to reduce his violent episodes while he was in Blockley. His family noticed that he had lost weight and they became worried about his physical health. They found the hospital dreary and depressing, but they were reluctant to have Robert discharged because they were afraid of what he would do outside. They were torn by their desire to get help for him and their concern that conditions at Blockley were unhealthy.

In the fall of 1876, the Smiths decided to move to Albany, New York. Because Robert seemed more manageable, if not better, they decided to take him with them. He made the journey all right, but the new environment seemed to bring on upsetting manic episodes such as he had had in Philadelphia. Within months, the family was again trying to decide what to do with him.

The business they had joined, begun by Mr. Smith's oldest brother, was modestly successful, so the family's financial resources were improved. When Robert's condition worsened, his family took him to a well-known local physician. After futile attempts to treat Robert, the doctor suggested that they take him to the Lunatic Asylum for the State of New York at Utica. The physician assured them that this asylum was a reputable one, much better than Blockley, and he signed a Certificate of Insanity, which helped them get Robert's admission to the asylum approved by a justice of the court.

In the early summer of 1877, Robert was taken to Utica by his father, uncle, and two older brothers. They traveled by boat, a short distance up the Hudson River, and then west on the Mohawk, a journey of some 150 miles.

The Smiths were impressed and encouraged by the asylum at Utica. They were shown the ward where Robert would stay; it was large, cheerful, and well furnished with large windows. None of the other patients were in straitjackets, and the Smiths were told that Dr. Gray, the superintendent, did not believe in mechanical restraints. Rather, he believed in an organized regimen of treatment that involved engaging the patients' minds and bodies in healthy activities, such as walking, bowling, gardening, and the mechanical arts.

Robert improved somewhat at Utica. The frequency and intensity of his manic episodes decreased, and within a year he was able to go home on a parole of about six months. However, he was never able to remain outside the asylum longer than that because his mania would return and intensify. He spent most of his remaining life in the asylum at Utica and died in 1890 from pneumonia, which he caught after a bout with influenza (Hamlin, 1985).

RALPH JONES

Ralph Jones has had a hard life. The third youngest of seven children, he apparently witnessed the suicide of his natural mother when he was 6. His natural father was either unable or unwilling to keep the family together, and all the children were sent to foster homes and orphanages.

Ralph was adopted at age 10 by a minister and a psychiatric social worker. He had a hard time getting along with them. He began dealing and using drugs when he was about 13 years old, abusing pot, phencyclidine (PCP), acid, and alcohol. He may have become an alcoholic by the age of 16. Ralph says that his adoptive parents were kind to him, but he just could not seem to do what they wanted, and after a while relations between them became very strained. At 16, Ralph was brought to the local youth program at the mental hospital because of his drug problems and violent acting out.

He did not complete high school but managed to get a GED while studying mechanics at a local vocational school and living in a group home. Ralph served 18 months in the Army. He was discharged with partial disability, caused by an injury to his left leg which he incurred playing football.

Ralph tends to be violent and lacks self-control when he has been drinking. Because of this behavior, he has lost many different jobs. Once, while drunk, he robbed and assaulted an elderly man in Florida—a crime for which he spent one year in jail. Also, he has been in several accidents, suffering injuries to his head and his back. He complains frequently of back pains.

Within the last five months, Ralph has been in jail twice and also in the state mental hospital. He was jailed on charges of driving while intoxicated. While there, he committed acts that were taken to be suicidal gestures. The first time, he cut his wrists superficially, and the second time, he slashed his throat with a razor blade. Both times, Ralph was brought straight from the jail to the mental hospital. The second incident occurred only three days before his jail term was to be completed.

A case review was undertaken after three weeks at the mental hospital. Admission notes were reviewed: Ralph was unclean, nonverbal, depressed, and lacking in judgment. He claimed to be suffering from alcohol withdrawal at the time of admission. The doctor who admitted him said that Ralph looked "psychotic" at the time.

A number of features of Ralph's situation came out during the case review. During his previous stay at the mental hospital, he had received shock treatments and was heavily sedated most of the time. He was given Thorazine, a tranquilizer used to control psychotic behaviors and calm patients down, and another drug to counter the side effects of Thorazine. The two psychiatrists he saw noted that he was uncooperative and lacked understanding of his suicidal, violent, alcoholic, abusive behavior.

Today his situation remains complex. First, Ralph admits to several suicide attempts or gestures, dating back to when he was 18, but he is not willing to talk about them other than to say that he is depressed all the time.

Second, he has a fiancée, whom he plans to marry within a year. She visits him regularly, dominates communication between him and the staff when she is around, and believes that he would be better off discharged. Also, she reports that he is well behaved, even gregarious, around her family. Ralph has virtually no other social contacts. She has been encouraging him to go to AA meetings and accompanies him when he does attend. In a conversation with a social worker, Ralph said he was afraid that she would press charges for a beating he gave her eight months ago.

Third, Ralph's contacts with his siblings and adoptive family have been minimal. He says he would like to live with his adoptive family, but they absolutely refuse to have anything to do with him. He has had no contact with any of his siblings in over two years.

Fourth, Ralph apparently does well at skilled manual work and is only about one term short of completing training as a mechanic at a vocational school. When asked about his plans for the future, he says that he wishes to complete his schooling, get a job, and then get married.

Fifth, he was married in his late teens and fathered two children (ages 7 and 8 now) before getting divorced at age 22. However, it is unknown where this family is and what connection, if any, he has with them.

Finally, it seems clear that Ralph is a depressed, angry person who can be dangerous to himself and others. His antisocial tendencies seem to have been established early in his life, and they are exacerbated by his alcohol problem. It is not at all clear that he has even begun to work through what was perhaps the central trauma of his childhood, his mother's suicide.

Two weeks ago Ralph was discharged and placed in a community halfway house. Ten days later he was readmitted to the mental hospital (three days ago) after he beat his roommate and then slashed his wrists. The treatment team, composed of a case manager, a nurse, a physician, a social worker, a psychologist, and a teacher, is not sure whether Ralph should be discharged again so that he can pursue the goals he articulates. The team is not convinced that he can handle life outside the hospital. The alcohol problem remains and seems to precipitate actions dangerous to Ralph and others; yet he still has goals, and apparently his fiancée remains supportive. If he were to establish a relationship with someone at a mental health center to secure help for him at his lowest points and if he were to attend AA meetings and stop abusing alcohol, some members of the treatment team believe that he might be able to get his life together and be placed in the community again (Hamlin, 1985).

These case studies describe two treatments of mental illness. As you answer the following questions, you will come to understand better the characteristics of the medical model.

- What problems did Robert Smith face? Ralph Jones?
- What treatments did Robert receive? Ralph?
- Why are these treatments classified as part of the medical model?

THE PUBLIC HEALTH MODEL

DEFINITION

Public health is a concept that is sometimes difficult to define. One challenge in defining it is its multidisciplinary nature, which leads to difficulty in understanding it as a whole and defining its operations. We can approach the definition of public health in three ways. One is to define it by examining its historical development, achievements, and health successes. The next section will provide a brief review of this perspective. A second approach is to examine its goal, which is to provide the opportunities and conditions for health as a basic human right. This goal is reflected in its mission: to fulfill society's interest in assuring conditions in which people can be healthy (Committee Study of the Future of Public Health, 1988). Because the concept of health has changed during the 1800s and 1900s, a third approach to defining public health reflects its dynamism and adaptability. For example, until the past few decades, health has meant the absence of disease and disability. Today, health has a more positive meaning—the capacity to live fully, which entails maintaining the physical, mental, and social reserves for coping with life's circumstances in a way that brings satisfaction (Seligman, 2004).

The terrorist attacks on September 11, 2001, presented new challenges for public health. Many people feared a bioterrorist attack was next, and the government's basic lab facilities, computers, personnel, and training were found to be lacking. This state of affairs prompted the rebuilding of the nation's public health system. "Dirty bombs," plague, anthrax, and smallpox have become part of our consciousness as serious threats to the population (Spake, 2003).

The **public health model** bridges the medical and human service models but is more obviously linked with the medical model. Diagnosis and treatment of individuals through the use of medicine and surgery are the core of clinical medicine. Physicians have delineated parts of the body (anatomy), how they function (physiology), their disorders (pathology), and the agents of disease (etiology). Their goal is to combat disease by repairing the breakdown of the "machinery" (Seligman, 2004). Those physicians who are cognizant of social, environmental, and biological factors and see disease as it affects populations have moved toward the public health model.

Public health is sometimes not separable from human welfare. Improving public health means improving education, nutrition, safe food and water supplies, immunization, and maternal and child health. It is particularly difficult to dissociate ill health from poverty.

In conclusion, a number of characteristics of the public health model distinguish it from the other two service delivery models. The public health model, like the medical model, is concerned with individuals who have problems, but it extends the concept of heath care beyond the traditional medical model. In the belief that individuals' problems may be linked to other social problems, the public health model serves larger populations rather than just individuals. Societal control is a prime concern of the public health model, as it attempts to solve many of society's social problems. In summary this model approaches social conditions by collecting data from the public and from examining individuals with problems.

The public health model applies a multicausal approach to studying the causes or origins of problems and emphasizes **prevention**. The preventive component also distinguishes this model from the medical model. The general aims of the American public health service system include not only a more equal distribution of health care services to all segments of the population (including the elderly, people with disabilities, and the impoverished) but also identification of social, nondisease problems and methods of attacking their causes and contributing factors. This is also the case in southern Africa, where HIV continues to spread. Public health efforts focused on prevention combine education about abstinence, condoms, and fidelity. The objective of the public health model is to improve the present and future quality of life and to alleviate health problems that have consequences for society in general.

HISTORY

Communicable diseases, poor sanitation, and lack of medical knowledge have been community health problems since ancient times. During the colonial period in North America, smallpox, yellow fever, and cholera were major health problems. Laws such as the Massachusetts Poor Law of 1692 gave local authorities the power to remove and isolate the afflicted. By the end of the 18th century, establishment of the first dispensaries and the first local boards of health had laid the foundations for voluntary organizations and public health agencies.

In the early 1800s, people migrated from the country to urban areas around burgeoning industrial plants. Severe disease outbreaks resulted from the poor nutrition, overcrowding, filth, and excessive work requirements of the inhabitants living in these slums. Lemuel Shattuck, a Boston city councilman, prepared a report financed by the Massachusetts legislature that presented the first plan for an integrated health program in the United States. The 1850 Shattuck Report in the United States precipitated both a sanitary awakening and social reform that constituted public health at that time (Afifi & Breslow, 1994).

The report declared the need for improved sanitation and disease control in Massachusetts and recommended establishment of state and local boards of health, collection of vital statistics, institution of sanitation programs, and prevention of disease (Shirreffs, 1982). Although widely ignored at the time, Shattuck's report has come to be considered the most farsighted and influential document in the history of the public health system (Committee Study of the Future of Public Health, 1988). By 1868, Massachusetts had established the first state public health department in the country.

The social philosophies of the early 19th century also impacted public health as they reflected two beliefs about disease. The first was that disease was providential. Like poverty and natural disasters such as floods, disease occurred as a result of God's wrath toward an individual. Therefore, the obvious solution to the problem was improved behavior. The second belief linked disease to the disorderly and filthy cities with their unpaved streets, poor drainage, untethered animals, and outside privies. Intuitively, people realized the impact of environmental factors on disease. Many believed that the solution was to eliminate dirt and filth to create a healthier environment.

A second important event was the organization in 1861 of the U.S. Sanitary Commission, the first major public health group in America. It is significant to the public health movement because its efforts were primarily preventive; it alerted the public to the benefits of preventive sanitary measures. Appalled by the poor conditions in army camps and hospitals, a group led by Dr. Henry Bellows, Louisa Schuyler, and Dr. Elisha Harris organized this voluntary citizen effort. A central focus of the commission was to unite all voluntary groups to aid governmental agencies in meeting the physical and spiritual needs of men in uniform. Initially, their efforts were directed toward teaching proper personal hygiene and inspecting and supervising living arrangements in camps and field hospitals. Their later efforts included recruiting nurses, distributing supplies, and assisting in communication between soldiers and their families.

Prevention emerged as a major component of the public health movement when Dr. Louis Pasteur and Robert Koch demonstrated that germs—not God or dirt—cause disease. The "golden age of public health" (1890–1910) included the discovery of causes for typhoid, tuberculosis, and cholera. Personal cleanliness, inoculations, serums, and hygienic laws became the basis of reform, and preventive medicine developed beyond research and lab diagnosis. Preventive medicine included a social focus, with well-organized public health education programs (Trattner, 1999). Today, the Public Health Service is part of the Department of Health and Human Services. It focuses on interventions aimed at disease prevention and health promotion that shape a community's overall profile.

Industrialization and its spread around the world during the 19th and 20th centuries stimulated the problems of communicable disease; these were followed by the difficulties that accompanied epidemics of chronic disease—coronary heart disease, cancer, diabetes, and chronic obstructive lung disease. Public health responded to the

BOX 4.4	PUBLIC HEALTH SERVICES

The Public Health Service has a distinguished history that dates back to the late 1700s, when many merchant seamen arrived ill and unattached in American port cities that had little capacity to care for them. In 1798, adopting the British tradition of caring for sick mariners at public expense, Congress enacted a measure, which President John Adams signed into law, that provided for "the temporary relief and maintenance of sick or disabled seamen." The first hospital dedicated to the care of merchant sailors was a building purchased near Norfolk, Virginia, in 1801. The first public hospital actually built with tax revenues, however, was in Boston.

Since that time, almost 200 years ago, the Public Health Service has grown to prominence as a federal enterprise dedicated to promoting and protecting the public's health, with a mandate that often embroils its agencies in controversy. The eight agencies of the Public Health Service are the Agency for Health Care Policy and Research, the Agency for Toxic Substances and Disease Registry, the Centers for Disease Control and Prevention (CDC), the Food and Drug Administration (FDA), the Health Resources and Services Administration, the Indian Health Service, the National Institute of Health (NIH), and the Substance Abuse and Mental Health Services Administration.

Source: From "Health Policy Report: Politics and Public Health," by John K. Iglehart, 1996, *Health Policy Report*, *334*, p. 203.

first set of problems and has made strides toward controlling the second. A third group of problems that has emerged in the past two decades consists of HIV/AIDS; domestic, school, and street violence; and substance abuse.

Many changes have occurred in public health over the years. In 1789, the Reverend Edward Wigglesworth assessed the health of Americans and produced the first American mortality tables. By 1900, influenza, pneumonia, tuberculosis, and gastrointestinal infections were the main causes of death in the United States. Average life expectancy at birth was 47 years. This last statistic has seen a phenomenal rise, with life expectancy at birth extending to 68 years by 1950, a change attributable to improvements in diet and sanitation and the development of antibiotics and vaccines. By 2004, life expectancy had grown to 77.9 years. Today, leading causes of death are heart disease, cancer, and stroke. The leading health problems are chronic diseases (National Center for Health Life Statistics, 2006).

The Healthy People Initiative, begun in 1979 and reformulated each decade, is the prevention agenda for the United States. It is a national effort to provide a vision for improving the health of all Americans and to guide decisions and actions. Led by the Public Health Service, the initial objectives for 1990 were established in 1980 and expanded for 2000 to include topics such as HIV infection and cancer. Objectives for *Healthy People 2010* were developed through a broad consultation process that involves many different people, states and communities, professional organizations, and other health-oriented groups. Focus areas include chronic kidney disease, disability and secondary conditions, health communication, medical product safety, respiratory diseases, and vision and hearing. You can check the progress of *Healthy People 2010* on its website (http://www.health.gov/healthypeople).

The major challenge has been to shift the national emphasis to prevention, with some of the following successes: Since the 1970s, stroke death rates have declined by 58% and coronary heart disease death rates have declined by 49%; a 32% decline in the death rate from car crashes is attributed to the increased use of safety restraints. Unfortunately, cases of AIDS, tuberculosis, asthma, and birth defects have increased.

TABLE 4.3 | SUMMARY POINTS: HISTORY OF THE PUBLIC HEALTH MODEL

- The model fulfills society's interest in assuring healthy conditions.
- Massachusetts Poor Law of 1692 empowered governments to act to promote healthy conditions.
- Local boards of health were established by the end of the 18th century.
- English Public Health Act of 1848 was passed.
- Shattuck (1842) and Chadwick (1850) reports apprised citizens of public health problems.
- The U.S. Sanitary Commission was established in 1861.
- Massachusetts established the first state public health department in 1868.
- By the 1900s, public health adopted a social focus.
- In 1979, the Healthy People Initiative was established.
- *Healthy People 2010* is being implemented.

The Internet has also greatly influenced health care. Health information has proliferated so rapidly that no one knows for certain how many World Wide Web health sites exist. This type of information can be a powerful tool in coping with diseases or maintaining one's health, but oftentimes fast and easy access does not equal accuracy of information. Knowing who puts out the information, checking for frequent updates, and looking for conformity to the Health on the New Foundation's Code of Conduct (HON Code) are clues to the accuracy of information.

CASE STUDIES

The following case study illustrates historical problems that are the primary focus of the public health model. It tells of Sean O'Reilly, who lived in the 1850s in New York City. The study illustrates the living conditions that called attention to public health concerns in America. Especially in larger cities, the problems of immigrants living in poverty greatly challenged public health professionals. The second case study illustrates a major public health effort today.

SEAN O'REILLY

Sean O'Reilly, age 25, was the first member of his family to emigrate from Ireland to America. He joined the great numbers of Irish who came to America in the wake of the potato blight that devastated Ireland in the middle of the 1840s. His journey, in a wooden sailing vessel from Liverpool, took 40 days. The voyage was very difficult. Like most poor immigrants, he traveled in steerage, a lower deck below the water line, reserved for third-class passengers. The space was four to six feet high and lined with two berths of wooden bunks. The floor was crowded with baggage, water, and cord wood. The only fresh air for the steerage area came from the hole in the deck for the hatchway.

After the six-week crossing, Sean emerged from steerage looking pale, weak, and 20 pounds lighter than when he started. He had not succumbed to cholera or dysentery,

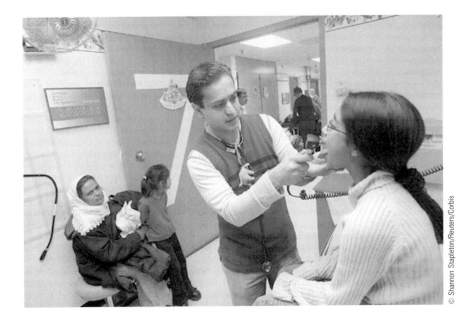

© Shannon Stapleton/Reuters/Corbis

as had several other passengers. The starvation, filth, and crowded conditions he had encountered during the passage to America were just a continuation of the hardships he had experienced in Ireland, which had driven him to emigrate.

The ship docked in New York. Even though Sean did not feel well, he was not eligible for medical treatment from the Marine hospital on Staten Island, as he did not have a communicable disease. Nor did he have enough money to enter Bellevue, the city hospital. He ignored the "runners" who accosted him on board, trying to get him to travel to other cities for a "small" fee. He left the ship and joined hundreds of other new arrivals, mostly Irish like himself, in search of a place to live and a job.

Although Sean had been a farmer in Ireland, he felt that the land had somehow rejected him. He wanted to stay with other Irishmen, near the sea, so he decided to remain in New York City. Sean found work before he found lodging. The first night, he slept in an alley, and the next day he joined a construction gang, moving earth to build roads in the city. The men he met at work suggested that he live with them in a tenement building that housed other newly arrived Irish immigrants. His first Saturday night in America, he was invited to and attended a "kitchen racquet" (get-acquainted party) organized by the family who lived downstairs.

Housing was the most difficult problem Sean faced; laborers' jobs, the sort of work he could do, were plentiful but irregular. Slum lords who took advantage of immigrants in dire need of housing crowded families into small, filthy, dimly lit, poorly ventilated tenements situated on narrow, unpaved streets with inadequate drainage. Partly because there was no integrated health program or municipal board of health, the city was disorderly, dirty, and disease ridden.

From the time he landed, Sean became part of the considerable Irish community in New York. He shared two rooms with a family of six. His living conditions never significantly improved. He held several jobs constructing roads, buildings, and sewage ditches. The jobs involved long hours, hazardous working conditions, low wages, and frequent short periods of unemployment.

Any money he made beyond bare living expenses went to the church and to his small account in the Emigrant Industrial Savings Bank of New York. This account enabled him to bring his family to America through the system known as "one bringing another," in which each immigrant worked and saved for a prepaid ticket for the next member of his family to come to America. By the late 1850s, most of Sean's family had joined him in New York.

REMOTE AREA MEDICAL VOLUNTEER CORPS

Remote Area Medical (RAM) Volunteer Corps is a charitable organization with no paid employees, which uses an airborne force of volunteers dedicated to serving mankind and providing free health care, veterinary services, and technical and educational assistance in remote and rural areas in the United States and around the world. Its history is deeply rooted in the adventuresome nature of its dreamer, designer, and founder, Stan Brock. He lived for many years in the Amazon region of Guyana, South America, where he managed the world's largest tropical ranch. The only medical care was many days' walk away in Georgetown, the nearest city. After ranch owners acquired a small aircraft, he would transport sick or injured people and fly in basic medical necessities. He became a sort of "jungle quack," doing his best to get aid to the rain forest dwellers. When he left there to co-host the Wild Kingdom television series, he traveled extensively, still discovering people who were medically helpless all over the world. He vowed that some day he would find a way to take medical care to people who had none.

The vow became reality when RAM was incorporated in March 1985 and subsequently received tax-exempt charity status by the Internal Revenue Service. Since then, there have been as many as 34 yearly expeditions, serving thousands of people and animals on a conservative budget amounting to over $7.5 million. There is a medical record on every person and animal treated.

RAM has used the services of over 3,500 volunteers from throughout the United States, Canada, Europe, and South America. RAM volunteer health care delivery teams consist of physicians and surgeons of all specialties, nurses, dentists, dental assistants, optometrists, opticians, technicians, veterinarians, and administrative and logistical support personnel who travel to destinations as far away as India or who work here in the United States. Team members pay their own expenses and are asked to procure medicines and other supplies. A team might have as few as 10 members or as many as 40.

RAM teams go only where they are invited. Word of mouth, an expedition nearby, a news article, and often unknown sources familiarize a group or community with its services and frequently generate invitations. The team carefully assesses the area's needs, visits the site, and when appropriate, arranges an expedition. In addition to activity in this country, RAM has programs underway in Guatemala, Haiti/Dominican Republic, India, and South America. Foreign expeditions can be ten days to three weeks in length, during which team members might treat as many as 4,000 patients.

RAM medical services run the gamut from a basic blood pressure check to full scale surgery. Operating teams repair cleft lips and palates, remove cataracts, correct eye muscle problems, and perform trauma surgical procedures. Internal medicine, family practice, or emergency specialists provide treatment for skin disorders, intestinal parasites, tropical diseases, and routine ailments and injuries. Dental teams offer emergency extractions and restorative work. Eye care professionals check visual acuity, examine for ocular disease, and dispense free eyeglasses. Thousands of pairs of eyeglasses a year are secured from the Lions Club Eyeglass Recycling program and carried overseas. In this country, RAM's portable optical lab enables skilled technicians to make new glasses to prescription on site. All providers strive to educate patients, their family members, and the community about the basics of oral and physical health, first aid, hygiene, food handling, clean water, animal management, and self-care.

Remote Area Medical is unique in the scope of services it offers, the frequency with which teams are dispatched, its local and international focus, the variety of destinations selected yearly, and the success of its multifaceted mission. It is truly a relief organization by people of the world for people of the world.

The following questions will help you clarify the role of public health today.

- How do the public health problems in the last case study compare with those Sean O'Reilly encountered?
- How do these two case studies illustrate what you have read about the history of the public health model?
- How do the solutions in public health in the 1850s differ from those today?

THE HUMAN SERVICE MODEL

DEFINITION

A primary focus of the human service model is to provide services that help individuals solve their problems. As Table 4.4 shows, this model differs considerably from the medical model and the public health model. According to the human service model, problems are an expected and even necessary part of everyday life. They occur because human existence is a complex process, involving interaction with other individuals, groups, institutions, and the environment. The human service model considers the problem of the individual within the context of the environment. If an individual must be temporarily removed from the environment to provide effective treatment, then treatment within the context of the environment will continue once the individual reenters that environment.

Individuals are one of the *clients* or *consumers* of the human service system. Clients can include smaller groups such as families, larger geographic populations such as neighborhoods or communities, and populations having problems in common such as the homeless and substance abusers.

The primary method of treatment or service is **problem solving,** a process focused on the here and now that maximizes the identification and use of client strengths. The first phase, problem identification, is critical to the entire process. Correctly identifying the problem, be it uncontrollable anger, unemployment, chronic tardiness, housing, or substance abuse, for example, focuses the process on resolution. Incorrectly identifying the problem may result in client frustration, the perception of the helper as ineffective, and a continuing problem. For these reasons, human service professionals take time to build a relationship with their clients, fully explore the problem or situation that the client is experiencing, and identify any strengths or resources that the client may have.

Once the problem is accurately identified and client strengths determined, some type of intervention may occur. The goal of the intervention varies depending on

TABLE 4.4 | AN OVERVIEW OF THREE MODELS OF SERVICE DELIVERY

	View of the problem	Who is the client?	Who is the worker?	Where does the treatment occur?	Method of treatment	Goal of treatment
Medical	Individual has a physiologically based illness or disease	Individual who receives services is called *patient*	Trained professional in health sciences (physician, nurse, dentist, psychiatrist)	Office Institution	Diagnosis Treatment Behavioral prescription Medication Psychoanalysis	Return individual to prior state
Public Health	Individual, groups, and society have disease or illness. Environmental and social pressures also contribute to problem.	Individuals and special populations or geographic areas (community, neighborhood, state, nation) can be clients	Public health training combines medical knowledge with community action skills	Office Community	Medical diagnosis Prescription Education Mobilization of resources Advocacy for special populations	Prevention Social action
Human Services	"Problems in living" may be internal, environmental, and/or intrapersonal	Individuals, families, special populations, and environment can be clients	Volunteer Paraprofessional Entry-level human worker who works with abuse, rehabilitation, education, etc. Professionals (rehabilitation or mental health counselor, social worker, psychologist)	Offices/agencies/institutions serving individuals, families, children Community	Problem-solving process	Enhance client's well-being, quality of life Teach client problem-solving skills Prevention

the problem. Generally, problems occur in one or more of three areas: emotions, thoughts or beliefs, and behaviors. Problems that deal with feelings or emotions such as feeling inferior or lacking self-awareness may respond best to strategies that encourage the verbal and nonverbal expressions of feelings or sensory imaging (Okun, 2002). If problems relate to how one thinks, for example, solving problems or interpreting situations, then learning coping skills, reframing, or restructuring may be helpful. Violence, a habit like smoking, and self-defeating actions are examples of behavioral problems that may respond to strategies such as reinforcement, contracts, and homework assignments. More complex problems like eating disorders, phobias, and depression may be a combination of all three areas and consequently, require an intervention that addresses all areas.

Identifying strengths follows the same process of enumerating emotions, thoughts, or beliefs and behaviors that have helped the clients succeed in the past. The client is encouraged to match personal strengths to identified problems as a way of planning interventions.

The problem-solving approach is used in this model for several reasons. First, the process provides a systematic way of thinking about complex situations. Problem identification suggests ways to describe situations in clear, understandable terms, encouraging the client and the worker to prioritize the problems that need to be addressed and discouraging impulsive, reactive behaviors. As a part of this approach, client strengths focus on the positive rather than deficits, an encouraging approach for clients. Second, the effectiveness of the process can be assessed at each stage. If the worker or the client discovers new information or if the problem or the environment changes, then the process can be revised. Third, clients can learn this problem-solving process and use it themselves when they no longer require services. Clients have the opportunity to improve their own problem-solving skills by working with a human service worker to solve problems and by rehearsing the behaviors under the worker's direction. Fourth, the outcomes of the process support the philosophy of human services by fostering client self-esteem and sense of personal responsibility as clients work successfully through the process. In addition, the results of the process improve the quality of life for the client. Fifth, the approach is a tool for identifying other problems that may occur and determining strategies to prevent future problems.

PHILOSOPHY

In its broadest sense, the philosophy of human services was solidified during the 1940s. It included the following beliefs:

- People had the right to expect their society, through its technology and other resources, to prevent their deprivation and provide for their basic human needs.
- The society, through its government, had the irrevocable responsibility for providing people with adequate human services.

The community health movement, directly related to deinstitutionalization contributed to the development of a human service model. Community mental health centers often were modeled after other public health efforts. Bringing services to those

TABLE 4.5 | SUMMARY POINTS: THE PROBLEM-SOLVING PROCESS

- Process focuses on here and now
- Phases or steps range from three to six
- Process begins with problem identification and identifying client strengths
- Process then moves to decision-making stage
- Process terminates in implementation
- Evaluation is important throughout the process
- Meeting people's needs comprehensively and effectively requires an understanding of the "whole person" and his [or her] relationship to [the] environment
- Meeting the "whole person's" needs means that the resources of many disciplines should be cooperatively mobilized for him [or her]

Source: Adapted from *Human Services Today*, by K. Eriksen, p. 53. Copyright © 1981 by Reston Publishing.

in need within the framework of community health helped broaden the definitions of care, services, recipients, and goals of intervention. At about the same time the medical field began to recognize of the goals of the human service field. The medical profession began stressing patient responsibility for diet, exercise, recreation, and rest. A third factor contributing to the growth of the human service model was the support of President Jimmy Carter, who publicized the fact that Americans did not have access to adequate mental health care. This was attributed to residence, gender, race, and age. Carter's understanding of the mental health dilemma reflects the human service philosophy of the 1940s, with its emphasis on both the responsibilities of society and the importance of working with the whole person.

Most authors agree that a model of human service delivery should include the following characteristics or themes (Burger & Youkeles, 2004; Eriksen, 1981; Harris, Maloney, & Rother, 2004; Mehr & Kanwischer, 2004):

1. The **generic focus** is critical in both human service training and delivery.
2. Services should be accessible, comprehensive, and coordinated.
3. The *problem-solving approach* emphasizes the here and now. Included in this approach are the acts of helping the client solve the problem and teaching the client problem-solving skills while building on client strengths.
4. Taking into consideration the impact of social institutions, social systems, and social problems, the model works with the person and the environment.

TABLE 4.6 | SUMMARY POINTS: HISTORY OF THE HUMAN SERVICE MODEL

- 1940s—Development of human service philosophy occurs.
- 1950–1990—Community mental health movement expands definition of "good care."
- 1960s—Medical profession recognizes importance of human service goals.
- 1990s—Human service educators recognize common human service themes.

5. Treating the *whole* person is best accomplished when the worker recognizes client needs in relation to others and to the environment.
6. Human services is *accountable to the consumer*. Clients are active participants in the human service model, making decisions, taking action, and accepting responsibility for themselves.

CASE STUDY

The following case study illustrates several concepts you have read about in this chapter. It presents four possible clients who are experiencing problems and who have different perspectives on their problems. This situation also illustrates both the individual and the family as clients. Let us focus first on the human service model of service delivery.

Consider yourself the human service professional who has received the following case. As you read it, think about these questions:

*   How have Susan, Ted, Justin, and Matthew solved problems in the past?
*   How do you think each person in the case study will define the problems?
*   As you consider problem solving as a systematic way of thinking, how would you as a human service professional approach the problem Susan faces?
*   Identify any strengths of any of the four individuals that might be helpful in addressing problems.
*   How will the themes and characteristics of human services guide your work with this case?

SUSAN AND TED

Susan and Ted met in college, where she was studying to be a teacher and he was studying to be an engineer. Ted was from an upper-middle-class family; Susan, from a religious, working-class family. Even while they were dating, Ted was a heavy "social drinker," but Susan ignored his drinking. She wanted to marry a man with a college education and have a large family. She came from a small, close-knit family and had only one sister. She remembered her family as having few luxuries while she was growing up, but much love and nurturance. Ted's family was also small, but not close. Ted had no contact with his family, even though they lived in the same town as the university.

During Ted and Susan's sophomore year, Susan's grades began to fall. She was on a partial scholarship and was in danger of losing it. She dropped out of school and moved out of the dorm into an apartment with Ted. Then Susan became pregnant. Ted dropped out of school and got a job as a draftsperson for a small local firm. They married.

Leaving behind a happy, carefree life without responsibility, they now faced an uncertain future. Susan tried to be the "perfect wife" her mother had been. She was determined to work before the baby was born and assume the role of homemaker. Ted began drinking heavily. He lost several jobs during Susan's pregnancy and often took his anger out on her by hitting her and keeping her constantly tense and fearful. He turned to drugs, and the relationship deteriorated further.

After losing several more jobs, Ted had to take a menial, low-paying job just to make ends meet, and his resentment increased. He spent more time away from home, leaving Susan with only the money she was earning for food or transportation.

She was alone and depressed but did not confide in her family, because she did not want to upset them.

Often Ted was away for days. As Susan's pregnancy progressed, he became more violent. Once, he beat her so badly that he cracked two of her ribs and broke her nose. He also attempted to strangle her. She told no one and lied to her doctor, coworker, and friends about the injuries. Ted "came to his senses" and tried to make amends, but he began drinking heavily once again and in a fit of rage kicked her in the stomach, bringing on labor. Susan delivered a son in the sixth month of her pregnancy. Justin weighed 3 pounds, 2 ounces, and had difficulty breathing. He was placed in an intensive-care nursery for six weeks before his parents could take him home. During this time, Susan worked and Justin continued to be sickly, suffering from chronic ear infections and colic. Ted had trouble adjusting to his new son, so Susan quit her job and took care of him alone.

Justin had many health problems and was constantly under the care of physicians. He was often hospitalized with pneumonia and severe dehydration. When Justin was 14 months old, Ted deserted them. Susan had no money, no job, and no car. She turned to her parents for a small loan and got a job in a department store making minimum wage. She had to work, but it angered her to leave Justin with a babysitter. Being a single parent was difficult. By the time she paid the rent, the bills, and the babysitter, there was no money left. She was desperately unhappy but determined to make the best of things.

Several months later, Ted returned. He had a new job making good money and was ready to "work things out." He continued to drink and he still beat her, but she now wanted him at any cost. He soon learned this fact. One year later, Susan had another son, Matthew. At this point, Ted and Susan bought a house in a small town near the university and proceeded to raise their family. For Ted, this consisted of nightly bouts with the bottle in front of a television set and of forcing himself sexually on Susan. The years passed, and Susan continued to put up with his drinking and rapes. Eventually, Ted's drinking became uncontrollable, and he started abusing the children.

One night he came home late, pulled a gun, and shot at Susan. A neighbor called the police; he was handcuffed and arrested. Ted's father, who had previously been completely out of the picture, now came to Ted's aid by paying his bail. This became a regular routine. Each time Ted was out of jail, he would return home to drink and terrorize Susan and the children. After six months, Susan told Ted she wanted a divorce. He became enraged and threatened her. She persisted and engaged a lawyer.

Her intention was to return to the university to finish her education and continue with her plans to be a teacher. She had less than two years to go and was confident that with child support, income from a job, and financial aid, this plan was feasible. Until the divorce, Ted refused to leave the house. The boys suffered terribly, seeing their mother beaten and their father handcuffed and taken to jail in a police car.

Currently, the youngest child, Matthew, now 14, works part time while attending high school as a sophomore. He is doing poorly in school but is managing to pass his courses. He likes his job and the money he makes. He is able to help pay for some of the things the family needs. He no longer has plans for college and, indeed, intends to continue working at the pizza restaurant if and when he graduates from high school. Although Matthew's grades have recently dropped from As to Cs and Ds, Justin's grades have suffered the most. He is now failing all his classes and has developed severe behavioral and emotional problems. He skips school, refuses to do his homework, and "hangs out with the wrong crowd." He takes drugs at home and school and sells drugs to his classmates. Justin is extremely depressed and hostile. He carries a knife to school and threatens classmates with it.

During one incident, when the victim's parents pressed charges, Justin was suspended from school and referred to the juvenile correctional department. He was placed in a program for adolescents who are dependent on alcohol or drugs. School officials realize that Justin "has problems" but have offered Susan no guidance or support, taking action only when Justin's behavior is life threatening.

Justin received correctional treatment in a private residential hospital, but it took some time to get him into treatment since he was not covered by his father's insurance plan. He had been admitted on his father's insurance card, but two days later the company denied the claim. Susan discovered that she was not covered by Ted's insurance and he refused to add Justin to his policy (he did not tell Susan that he did not have an insurance policy). Susan applied to the state for insurance and was covered after a two-month wait. Justin then entered the hospital and began to improve. Unfortunately, the state coverage limited the stay Justin needed. He remained and Susan is now received bills totaling more than $80,000 that she is expected to pay. She knows she will soon have to admit to the hospital that she cannot pay.

Susan is in trouble financially. She receives free medical aid from the university student clinic. Last Christmas, a church she joined took up a collection for her and the children and bought them $200 worth of groceries. She requested one month of subsidized utilities from the local utilities company but is eligible for this assistance only one time. She is concerned that she will not be able to afford utilities this month. Ted pays child support only sporadically, and he moves from town to town. He pays just enough to satisfy state requirements, so Susan has little legal recourse.

Susan never knows where she can find him in case of an emergency and is not certain he would even help. Ted continues to have visitation rights since visitation is not linked to child support. Susan is furious about this privilege but keeps thinking he will eventually take more responsibility for his children. Constantly depressed because of her situation, Susan also fears that bill collectors will start to hound her and that, if an emergency occurs, she will not be able to handle it. She does not know what to do.

As you think about these clients' needs from the human service perspective, you quickly realize that $200 for groceries and one month of subsidized utilities solve only immediate problems. The larger problems that Susan, Ted, Justin, and Matthew face are much more complex and will require comprehensive, coordinated service delivery.

You have learned in this chapter that human service professionals use three primary models of service delivery. In taking charge of this case, you will function within the context of the human service model. To promote the well-being of the whole person and to provide the comprehensive services necessary to that end, you may rely on professionals whose service delivery is guided by the public health model or by the medical model. To minimize duplication of services and to promote coordinated service delivery, you need to maintain active links with other professionals who may work with the same clients as you do.

Now that you are familiar with the history of Susan, Ted, Matthew, and Justin, review the problem-solving process. Select one of the individuals in the case study as your client and ask yourself the following questions:

- What is the mindset of this client now?
- What problems and subproblems does the client face?
- What alternatives are possible to solve these problems?
- How would you as the helping professional use the human service model in this case?

- What services might be provided by professionals who practice the medical model, the public health model, or both?
- How can a human service professional facilitate the interaction of all three models in resolving client problems?

Using models is a helpful way of identifying the different approaches to clients' problems. The distinctions among the models are not arbitrary, for each has a separate history and has developed in response to different social needs. From the human service perspective, however, each model has a part in the problem-solving process. The worker is responsible for blending the models and the treatments or services they represent in response to client needs. Indeed, one strength of human services is the focus on clients' needs and the flexibility to use approaches from various models to meet those needs.

KEY TERMS

antianxiety drugs	electroshock therapy	neurosis	psychoanalytic method
antidepressant drugs	generic focus	patient	psychopharmacology
antipsychotic drugs	human service model	prevention	psychotropic drugs
client	medical model	problem solving	public health model
consumer	mood stabilizers	psychiatry	

THINGS TO REMEMBER

1. Three different models represent orientations in service delivery: the medical model, the public health model, and the human service model.

2. Underlying each of the three models is a set of philosophical assumptions that guide the delivery of services and shape beliefs about the causes of problems, their treatment, and the role of the professional in service delivery.

3. The medical model views the person coming for help as a *patient* whose problem is diagnosed as a disease or sickness and treated by a physician or service provider who prescribes a treatment or cure for the "disease."

4. At the turn of the 20th century, Mary Richmond, author of *Social Diagnosis,* used the medical model to describe social casework.

5. Until the end of the 19th century, insanity was socially defined, but when psychiatry emerged as a medical specialty, insanity became a medical label.

6. Psychotropic drugs are now among the most widely used treatments for mental disorders. Psychopharmacology, the study of the effects of drugs on mental health, is an area of interest to human service professionals.

7. The public health model, like the medical model, focuses on individuals and larger populations; it attempts to solve many of society's social problems.

8. Communicable diseases, poor sanitation, and lack of medical knowledge have been primary community health problems since ancient times. Laws such as the Massachusetts Poor Law of 1692 in North America and the

Public Health Act of 1848 in Britain initiated efforts to improve public health conditions.

9. The U.S. Sanitary Commission was the first major public health group in the United States. Its efforts were primarily preventive, alerting the public to the benefits of preventive sanitary measures.

10. A primary focus of the human service model is to provide services that help individuals solve their problems, including a consideration of client problems within the context of their environments.

11. Individuals are among the clients of the human service system, as are small groups, larger geographic populations, populations defined by lifestyle, and populations that have problems in common.

12. The primary method of treatment is problem solving, a process focused on the here and now that encompasses three phases: problem identification, decision making, and problem resolution.

13. The human service philosophy emphasizes both the responsibilities of society and the importance of working with the whole person.

14. Themes characteristic of human service delivery are its generic focus; accessible, integrated services; problem-solving approach; treatment of the whole person; and accountability to the consumer.

15. Using models is a helpful way to identify the different approaches to clients' problems.

ADDITIONAL READINGS: FOCUS ON MENTAL ILLNESS

Karp, D. (2002). *The burden of sympathy: How families cope with mental illness.* NY: Oxford University Press.
The experiences of family members of the mentally ill who have survived provide caregivers aid, guidance, and solace. The similarities of caregiver experiences, the challenge of finding and maintaining equilibrium, and a critical look at what it means to be a moral and caring person come from 60 extensive interviews.

Kotuiski T. (2006). *Saving Millie: A daughter's story of surviving her mother's schizophrenia.* Madelia, MN: Extraordinary Voices Press.
The author recounts her experiences with her mother to serve as a resource for families dealing with schizophrenia and a broken health care system.

Pederson, J. (2004). *The panic diaries: The frightful, sometimes hilarious truth about panic attacks.* Berkeley, CA: Ulysses Press.
The focus of this book is what panic is, how it is experienced, and how it is treated. Interviews with psychiatrists, psychologists, and other health professionals offer suggestions for treatments. Symptoms, treatments, advocacy, and resources add to its comprehensiveness.

Slater, L. (1999). *Prozac diary.* New York: Penguin Books.
Lauren Slater, patient, therapist, and author of *Welcome to My Country,* shares what it is like to be cured by America's preeminent selective serotonin reuptake inhibitor.

Torrey, E. F. (2005). *Surviving manic depression: A manual on bipolar disorder for patients, families, and providers.* NY: Basic Books. This book provides a guide to living with bipolar disorder—symptoms, treatments, and advocacy.

Whitaker, R., & Whitaker, B. (2001). Mad in America: Bad science, bad medicine, and the enduring mistreatment of the mentally ill. Boulder, CO: Perseus Publishing.
Why are the cure rates for schizophrenia so low in America, the most well-developed country in the world? This exposé surveys 300 years of mental health treatments and attitudes.

References

Afifi, A., & Breslow, L. (1994). The maturing paradigm of public health. *Annual Review of Public Health, 15,* 223–235.

Burger, W. R., & Youkeles, M. (2004). *Human services in contemporary America* (5th ed.). Pacific Grove, CA: Brooks/Cole/Thomson Learning.

Clear, T. R., Cole, G. F., Resig, M. D. (2005). *American corrections.* Belmont, CA: Wadsworth/Thomson.

Committee Study of the Future of Public Health Institute of Medicine. (1988). *The future of public health.* Washington, DC: National Academy Press.

Eriksen, K. (1981). *Human services today.* Reston, VA: Reston Publishing.

Hamlin, P. (1985). *Experiences in mental institutions: Case studies.* Unpublished manuscript.

Harris, H. S., Maloney, D. C., & Rother, F. M. (2004). *Human services: Contemporary issues and trends* (3rd ed.). Needham, MA: Allyn & Bacon.

Ingersoll, R. E., & Rak, C. F. (2006). *Psychopharmacology for helping professionals: An integral exploration.* Belmont, CA: Thomson Brooks/Cole.

Mehr, J., & Kanwischer, R. (2004). *Human services: Concepts and intervention strategies* (9th ed.). Boston: Allyn & Bacon.

National Center for Life Health Statistics. (2006). *Life expectancy.* Retrieved August 10, 2006, from http://www.cdc.gov/nchs/fastats/lifexpec.htm.

Okun, B. F. (2002). *Effective helping: Interviewing and counseling techniques* (6th ed.). Pacific Grove, CA: Brooks/Cole.

Pichot, P. (1985). Remedicalisation of psychiatry. *Psychiatrial Fennica, 16,* 9–17.

Reinhard, S. (1986). Financing long-term health care of the elderly: Dismantling the medical model. *Public Health Nursing, 3*(1), 3–22.

Richmond, M. (1917). *Social diagnosis.* New York: Sage.

Seligman, M. (2004). *Authentic happiness: Using the new positive psychology to realize your potential for lasting fulfillment.* New York: Free Press.

Shirreffs, J. H. (1982). *Community health: Contemporary perspectives.* Englewood Cliffs, NJ: Prentice Hall.

Spake, A. (2003, September 15). Public health. *U.S. News and World Report, 135*(8), 30.

Trattner, W. I. (1999). *From poor law to welfare state: A history of social welfare in America.* New York: Free Press.

Zimbalist, S. E. (1977). *Historic themes and landmarks in social welfare research.* New York: Harper & Row.

CLIENTS AND HELPERS IN HUMAN SERVICES

© John Birdsall/The Image Works

Questions to Consider

- What types of problems lead people to human services?
- How do people find help?
- What are helpers like? What are the different ways of categorizing professionals who deliver human services?
- How do human service professionals provide services to those who want or need them?

. . .

Part Two focuses on the people who are involved in the practice of human services, either as recipients or as service providers. Chapter 5 introduces the client or consumer—who may be an individual, a group, or a population—and gives examples of these different types. The chapter examines how they get help, barriers they encounter, and their perspectives on help.

Chapter 6 shifts to the human service professional, the provider of human services, with an examination of helpers' motivations, values, and characteristics. It also provides an overview of the categories of human service professionals and insights about them. The chapter concludes with a description of the roles and responsibilities of human service professionals.

The primary purpose of Part Two is to further refine the definition of human services by considering the individuals who are involved in service delivery. As you read the two chapters in this part, think about the Questions to Consider.

THE CLIENT

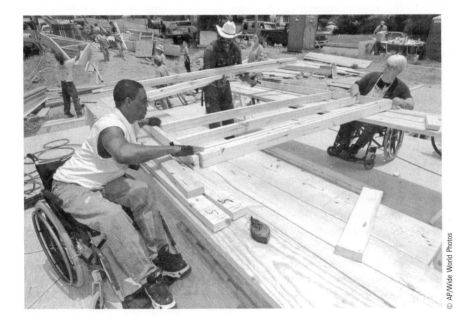

CHAPTER 5

© AP/Wide World Photos

After reading this chapter, you will be able to:

- Define "the whole person."
- Differentiate among four perspectives of client problems.
- Define "client(s)."
- List the ways people get help.
- Identify the barriers to getting help.
- Summarize the influence of client expectations on the helping process.

Self-assessment

- What are the strengths and limitations of the different ways to categorize problems?
- Explain the problems of homelessness based upon the developmental, situational, and human needs perspectives.
- What are the barriers to receiving services and how might a human service professional counter them?
- What are the possible sources of client reluctance?
- What expectations do clients have of human services?

The purpose of this chapter is to explore the recipient of human services. This individual may be called a *client*, a *consumer*, or a *customer*. Some consumer groups are concerned with the "client" label because of the stereotype it generates. The term *consumer* is used to emphasize the business nature of the delivery of services. The term *customer* connotes an individual who is actually purchasing the services and the need to be accountable to that individual. The term **client** describes the engagement of a professional in order to get advice and/or services. For this text, we have elected to use the term *client* since it is most often used in agency settings. Understanding the client is critical to any study of human services. Indeed, the client is the reason there are helpers and a helping process. Part One has already established that some people, in some circumstances, need assistance from others to survive and to develop the ability to help themselves.

In an effort to define the term *client* comprehensively, this chapter introduces several ways of thinking about the user of human services. One way of viewing the client is to study the meaning of the phrase "working with the whole person." This guiding principle in human services focuses on the many components that define an individual and the areas of support a helper must consider when providing assistance.

Describing the problems that clients experience is also an important consideration in defining the client. Problems can be considered in various ways. Several possible theories can be used to define the problems and difficulties that confront individuals. The developmental theory approaches problems from the life span perspective and defines them in terms of life crises or tasks that occur during a lifetime. The situational perspective describes problems that occur from accidents and other traumatic points in time. Meeting human needs, both physical and psychological, is another approach to explaining the problems that individuals encounter. One theory posits that **social change** has a primary effect on the problems individuals experience. Finally, culture may also be a critical factor in understanding the problems an individual or group experiences and may present challenges to the human service professional to consider its influence. Each of these perspectives is defined and its impact on the delivery of human services is described in this chapter.

The term *client* has many meanings. In some cases, clients are individuals; in others, the client may be a small group such as a family, or even a larger population such as the residents of a geographic area. In this chapter you will meet several individuals who are clients: Mary, who was hit by a car; two individuals who share first-person accounts as victims of random violence and nonphysical assault; Kisha, a homeless teenager; and a pregnant teenager who is involved in a gang. In the international arena, you will also read about countries in crisis. These accounts will illustrate the concepts introduced in this chapter.

Finally, in defining the client, we explore the experience of getting help from the client's perspective. Sometimes it is difficult for human service professionals who themselves have never been clients to understand thoroughly what it is like to ask for and receive services. We discuss the many ways of getting help, the barriers to be surmounted, clients' expectations, and their evaluation of services.

THE WHOLE PERSON

Clients enter the human service delivery system as individuals with multifaceted perspectives that include psychological, biological, cultural, social, financial, educational, vocational, and spiritual components. These components encompass life experiences such as family, friends, health, school, work, legal status, residence, safety and security, finances, play, well-being, and accomplishments. These perspectives are integrated within the individual to form the **whole person** that the human service professional encounters. During the helping process, the professional is continually aware that the client does not simply represent "a housing issue," "a food-stamp dilemma," or "a child-care consideration." Problems for clients are rarely single issues, and the human service professional should approach each client with the expectation of more than one problem. In fact, one problem can cause, influence, or at the very least be related to other difficulties.

The case of Mary is a good example of how problems in one area influence problems in other areas. The following is from the official record.

> The client, a 38-year-old white female, was involved in an accident while standing on the corner of a busy street in her hometown. She was hit by an automobile driven by a drunk driver. She sustained a severe head injury, a neck injury, and multiple orthopedic injuries at the scene of the accident. She was rushed to the hospital by ambulance and suffered cardiac arrest in route. Her recovery was slow and she was in the hospital for over three months. She was moved to a rehabilitation facility in a town 60 miles away. After three months in rehabilitation, the professionals involved in Mary's staffing indicated that she would need at least six additional months of rehabilitation. She was unable to speak, had limited daily living skills and limited ambulation, and could communicate slowly. The case manager, team leader of the human service professionals working with Mary, spent time on funding issues. At present, and projected for the future, Mary needed 24-hour support to sustain her activity and her safety. Her husband, Seth, worked in their hometown and visited each day.

The initial concerns for Mary were physical. She sustained multiple injuries and experienced cardiac arrest, so attention to her physical well-being was of primary importance. Once her physical condition stabilized, human service professionals involved with planning and providing her care—using the "whole person" perspective—established the following treatment plan that addressed other issues.

The Intervention. Client receives 0.5 hour of occupational therapy 2 days a week. Client receives physical therapy for 1.5 hours per day, 5 days per week or as tolerated. Client has been tested by speech therapist; the test indicated that she does not respond to interaction or treatment.

Mobility. Client is not mobile. This immobility places the client at risk.

Nutrition. Client's usual weight is approximately 130 lbs. Client eats poorly and current weighs 115 lbs.

Communication. Professionals report the client will not interact with others. The client does not make eye contact. The client does watch television.

Elimination and urination. Client is unable to eliminate and urinate without assistance.

Daily living. Client is able to help with bathing and dressing, but does not appear interested in expanding or improving skills. Client is uninterested in these activities.

Mental health assessment. Client is seen by a psychiatrist once a week. Medications have been used consistently for clinical depression.

Safety. Client needs to be supervised 24 hours, seven days a week.

Social history. Client is married and having difficulty with home visits. The client rejects help from spouse but cannot manage daily living skills. It is difficult for the spouse to visit during the day since he works in a neighboring town. The spouse indicates that there were marital problems before the accident.

This treatment plan illustrates a multiproblem client who is receiving help in the human service delivery system. Note that, in this case, severe physical problems affect other areas, such as psychological functioning, relationships with family, vocational limitations, and financial difficulties. Although the financial and vocational are not addressed specifically in the treatment plan, advocates for the client are currently trying to find financial resources for her as she does not have long-term care benefits or home-care benefits. Vocational needs are addressed by recognizing that the client will not be able to work and will need 24-hour supervision or care.

As a human service professional working with clients, the critical point to remember is that the client is an individual made up of psychological, social, economic, educational, vocational, and spiritual dimensions and possibly will have needs in many of those areas. Even if a client appears only to be looking for housing, the helper realizes that the client may possibly have other difficulties such as unemployment, illiteracy, or a lack of child care. If single problems are solved with little attention to the other difficulties the client is experiencing, then that person may not be able to become self-sufficient.

A majority of clients enter the human service delivery system because they are experiencing problems. Those problems can be defined in many ways.

PERCEPTIONS OF CLIENT PROBLEMS

Problems are a normal part of life. This concept is central to understanding who a client is and what problems the client encounters. As you recall from Chapter 1, the "problems in living" approach, which is basic to our definition of human services, has been a major factor in shaping the human service model (as described in Chapter 4).

DEFINING PROBLEMS

Thinking about problems is one way to understand the concept of "problems in living." Problems usually indicate something exists that is causing the client to experience trouble or discomfort. Usually the act of problem solving is an associated action, indicating the problems, whether short- or long-term, have solutions or that there are possible ways of addressing them. Problems in living, from the human service perspective, can have two components: a description of the problem and a course of action leading to its resolution. First, the problem is described as a situation, event, or condition that is troublesome for the client. It can be as simple as a pregnant 20-year-old married woman's request for information about prenatal care programs or as complex as an unmarried, pregnant 15-year-old's need for counseling. The second component occurs in several stages: The problem is identified and discussed, solutions are formulated and implemented, and the results are evaluated.

One complicating factor in identifying and resolving problems is the difficulty of predicting what an individual will experience as a problem. Factors such as the cultural values of the society and the developmental needs of the individual influence how problems are defined. For example, an increasingly common problem in this society is adult children caring for aging parents and relatives. The extended family that once cared for elderly relatives has been replaced by the smaller nuclear family, a unit whose living space and lifestyle are sometimes not suitable for the care of others. This new generation of caregivers is known as the "sandwich generation." Many of them are caring for children at home while assisting aging relatives with their needs.

How clients view their own situations and what they perceive to be problems are important factors in problem identification. It is possible that individuals either lack the resources or the skills, or both, to solve the problem. It is also possible that the client and the helper may disagree about the client's situation. For example, the helper may believe the client lacks resources or skills, while the client may perceive no problem at all. In the client's environment, unemployment, poor school attendance, and illiteracy may be normal conditions among neighbors and family members. The client experiences these conditions as a way of life, not as situations that must be corrected or problems that need to be solved. The helper, on the other hand, may view these conditions as problems that should be faced and resolved.

Even if clients recognize the existence of problems, there is no guarantee that they will seek assistance. If they do ask themselves whether help will alleviate the problems

TABLE 5.1 | SUMMARY POINTS: CLIENT PROBLEMS

- It is difficult to predict what an individual will experience as a problem.
- The individual perspective is part of the problem definition.
- A person often lacks resources or skills, or both, to solve problems.
- No guarantee exists that an individual will seek help.

they have, they may conclude that it will not. They may see the condition as something to be endured, or they may feel that having the difficulty is preferable to seeking assistance.

UNDERSTANDING CLIENT PROBLEMS

Despite the difficulties of identification, **problems** are still a useful way to address the identity and needs of the client. It is because individuals have unmet needs that they come in contact with the human service delivery system. The system uses a variety of conceptual frameworks to aid in identifying problems. This section introduces models to address four types of problems: developmental and situational problems, hierarchical needs, needs created by social change, and environmental influences.

A DEVELOPMENTAL PERSPECTIVE   According to developmental theorists, individuals engage in certain tasks or activities at different points in their lives. Describing the **developmental process,** experts in developmental psychology suggest that human development is a continuous process and that there are certain phases and stages that individuals experience during the life span (Trotter & Swartwood, 2007). The development begins at the point of conception and ends at the time of death. During the time between these two points, the individual experiences systemic changes. The change of dependent children into independent adults was studied by Erik H. Erikson, a psychoanalyst and expert in adult development, whose major contribution to the understanding of human development was his description of the "eight stages of man" (Erikson, 1963). Erikson's stage model is one of many perspectives on development. His stages, summarized in the list that follows, reflect the tasks through which individuals work during the different stages.

> *Basic trust versus basic mistrust.* Infants learn to trust in an environment that consistently provides for their needs—that is, one in which the caretaker is sensitive to the needs of the infant. A person who does not experience this warmth and caring in infancy will have difficulty trusting others in later years.

> *Autonomy versus shame and doubt.* In this stage, the toddler wishes to "let go" and try new things but does not know the alternatives and consequences of such actions. The child at this stage needs both urging to try new things and gentle protection from the consequences of his or her lack of experience. A toddler who does not experience such support may later be reluctant to try new things and may doubt his or her abilities.

Initiative versus guilt. The child who moves beyond the stage of autonomy is able to define a task and work to complete it. Initiative means cooperative effort, enthusiasm for new things, and acceptance of responsibility. When a person experiences success at this stage, he or she will generally become an adult who is willing to accept moral responsibility and takes pleasure in developing his or her abilities. A child who does not develop the ability to take initiative becomes an adult who is unable to take risks and meet new challenges.

Industry versus inferiority. In this period of growth, the child begins to experience life as a worker and provider. Receiving instruction and evaluation (in the culture, in school), the child learns to enjoy work and develops good work skills, such as the ability to concentrate and to manipulate the tools of the society. If the child does not develop a sense of being capable, he or she may later have a fear of inadequacy, resulting in poor performance, low expectations, or both.

Identity versus role confusion. In this stage, the adolescent begins to combine the identity formed in the previous stages with the work he or she must accomplish in the future. The stage is complicated by physical growth and sexual maturation. The adolescent rebels against those who previously provided support and relies on peers and heroes and heroines for guidance and care. During this stage, the individual struggles to make sense of an adult world in terms of childhood experiences.

Intimacy versus isolation. The young adult, having formed an identity during the previous stage, desires to establish intimate relationships that may include the components of mutual love, sexual intimacy, and parenting. An inability to establish intimacy with others may result in isolation.

Generativity versus stagnation. The adult assumes the responsibility for "parenting" the next generation, guided by the children's needs, as described for the previous stages. This parenting responsibility is required of all adults, not just those who are biological parents. During this stage, acceptance of this role helps the adult avoid stagnation and loss of purpose.

Ego integrity versus despair. The ego integrity that is possible at this stage represents the culmination of the successful development of identity through the previous seven stages. The older adult understands and accepts life as it has been experienced, assumes responsibility for that life, and accepts death as the final part of the life cycle.

Erikson's stages provide the foundation for thinking about human development, but other theorists have expanded what we know about the lifespan perspective for adults. For instance, Sheehy (1995) reported on mid-life transition periods for adults where the focus becomes reflection and evaluation of the past and the future. During this time, adults search for a sense of wholeness and meaning rather than perfection, they begin to see their lives within a cultural context and feel they belong to a community (Trotter & Swartwood, 2007). Levinson (1975) posited that during this time, individuals begin to build structures that would last the remainder of their lives. These new structures focus on the meaning of work, relationships, and spirituality.

BOX 5.1	WEB SOURCES
	Find Out More about Client Problems

http://www.ncadv.org/

The National Coalition Against Domestic Violence is dedicated to the empowerment of battered women and their children and therefore is committed to the elimination of personal and societal violence in the lives of battered women and their children. This site offers information about the problem, community response, public policy, and getting help.

http://www.unaids.org/

The Joint United Nations Program on HIV/AIDS is the main advocate for global action on the epidemic. This site provides information about events, geographical areas, partnerships, and other links.

http:www.nilc.org/

The National Immigration Law Center (NILC) is a national support center whose mission is to protect and promote the rights and opportunities of low-income immigrants and their family members. NILC has offices in Los Angeles, Oakland, and Washington, D.C. This site provides information about NILC, publications, immigrants, employment, and public benefits, and other links.

http://www.nami.org/

The National Alliance for the Mentally Ill is the nation's voice on mental illness. As such, this site offers up-to-date information on mental illness in the news, communities, annual meetings, legislation, and publications.

http://www.ojjdp.ncjrs.org/

The Office of Juvenile Justice and Delinquency Prevention's site offers information about the agency's organization, staff, and employment opportunities. It is also the place for the latest information from this agency on facts and figures, publications, programs, and events.

Developmental theorists view life as a *process* from birth until death, from the beginning to the end. Although everyone goes through the same developmental stages, individuals experience these stages in different ways. Development may be affected by the social context in which the individual lives—the home, family, community, culture, country, and sociopolitical climate. A person's characteristics, including traits, wishes, values, and childhood experiences, may also influence the way that person experiences each stage. Determining the stage on which the individual is working is sometimes difficult. Moving from task to task and from developmental stage to developmental stage are not activities as discrete as having a birthday or completing a list of jobs or chores. Sometimes an individual is deeply focused on the tasks of a certain developmental stage, but there are also times of transition between stages, when the tasks are being completed and the individual is only beginning to formulate the questions that will signal the next stage (Levinson, 1978; Shaffer, 2002; Trotter & Swartwood, 2007).

An individual deeply focused on a specific developmental stage experiences a time of intense questioning and exploring. A developmental stage begins when the tasks of that stage are of primary importance, and the stage ends when the individual's focus has changed. For example, a toddler who has learned to walk may want to explore every nook and cranny at one instant but be paralyzed by a new environment a moment later. When the child's focus changes from the independence of walking to the independence of exploring new environments, his or her developmental tasks have changed.

TABLE 5.2 | SUMMARY POINTS: ERIKSON'S DEVELOPMENTAL PERSPECTIVE

- Individuals engage in certain tasks or activities at different times during their life.
- Stages are experienced differently by each person.
- The social context affects movement through developmental stages.
- Traditional stages are changing as society changes.

There is a dimension of quality to the completion of developmental tasks. Even if a task is finished, it is not necessarily finished well. As mentioned earlier, developmental tasks are addressed within the individual's social context, and that context may not support individual development. In addition, how the individual has completed previous developmental tasks affects his or her work on the next stage. An individual may not reach the next stage with the necessary skills or confidence to continue developing.

In Western culture, the traditional ways children and adults develop are changing (Sheehy, 1995). Young females are maturing earlier, children are carrying weapons to school, women are marrying later, women are having children later, individuals are retiring earlier, and, at the same time, individuals are working in their 70s. Even the concept of "elderly" or "being old" is shifting as we see increasing longevity. These and other changes represent changes in the traditional life span development stages. When developmental theories are used to identify problems that individuals experience, an important point to remember is that these traditional stages are changing.

Using a developmental model to view problems may be helpful to the human service professional because it provides the helper with a basic understanding of the process of growth and change that individuals normally experience. Workers can use Erikson's stages to help describe problems in terms of current tasks that require the client's focus, as well as to determine whether the previous developmental tasks have been adequately completed.

Human service professionals can also use developmental models to provide a framework for identifying problems not regarded as normal. For example, certain problems associated with mental illness (such as hallucinations and delusions) and with criminal behavior (such as aggressive, violent behavior) are labeled deviant. In any attempt to account for this deviance, Erikson's developmental model is a starting point for identifying whether a problem can be categorized as a problem in living or as a departure from the expected. With clients who have very serious problems not classified as problems in living, it may be necessary to use several problem identification models.

A SITUATIONAL PERSPECTIVE   Another way of viewing problems in living is from the situational perspective. Problems resulting from accidents, violent crimes, natural disasters, and major changes in life—such as a move, job change, or divorce—are all defined as **situational problems.** The characteristics of these problems are very different from those of the developmental problems discussed in the preceding section. First, these problems usually occur because the individual is in a particular place at a particular time. It is difficult for individuals to "be in the world" without experiencing some situational problems. Such problems can occur even if the individual has not done anything to contribute to or cause them. In such cases, individual responsibility begins once the situation has occurred and is identified as a problem situation. Linking situational problems with a specific event may be difficult because the event might be only a marker of a more complex situation. For example, with divorce or a geographic move, there are obviously contributing factors that precede the event. However, the problem may still be characterized as situational because of the existence of the marker—a clear problem on which the client and the human service professional can focus.

Another characteristic of situational problems is that they can lead to short-term or long-term difficulties, or both. Most such problems require, at a minimum, immediate action. The complexity and quantity of assistance required depend on the severity of the problem and the state of the client when the situation occurs. Situational problems may require additional help after the short-term assistance has been provided. Yet another characteristic is that individuals experiencing situational problems are often viewed as victims—people who suffer injury from their own fault or that of others. One of the first responsibilities of the helper is to move the client from the role of victim to the status of taking responsibility for personal actions and thoughts.

> I first became involved with human services in January. As a victim of aggravated assault, attempted murder, and mayhem in a case of random violence, my situation was severe. As the result of the assault, I was blinded in my right eye and impaired in my left eye. The first person I saw was my physician, who gave me the prognosis and told me what medical treatment I would need, including surgery. The second person was a hospital administrator, who told me I had no major insurance that would cover my needs and the costs of surgery. The third person I talked to gave me hope. He was a case manager who worked with victims of violent crime. He talked with me for two hours about what legal processes were involved, how to apply for assistance, and whom to see in the different agencies. He told me to have faith in the system. And he told me that his job was to help link me to services that I need and then monitor progress.

Violent crime, such as the assault just described, is a situational problem experienced by Americans every day. Problems also include the unreported violence that occurs behind the doors of homes, workplaces, and institutions and the nonphysical assaults that go unreported. The emotional sufferings of these victims can be the most serious result. One explanation for this finding is the damage that occurs after the crime to previously psychologically healthy individuals. After the crime, even healthy individuals are likely to experience depression, anger, shame, and anxiety. They begin to question their previous sense of social order and to redefine their ideas of fairness and justice. Women in particular experience a sharp increase in physical and psychological stress after such victimization, feeling both powerless and helpless. The following account describes the fear and terror that accompanied a nonphysical assault.

> It was an ordinary day like any other, exceptionally cold and dreary. The walk to class was an ordinary walk, exceptionally quick in order to keep warm from the cold. Few walkers were walking so the pace and the tempo were the only interests keeping me alert. A hand, his hand, dipped to below his belt whereupon he unzipped his pants.

Odd, I thought. In order to keep warm, I kept walking. Not only was he unzipping his pants but he was showing me the most private part of his body. The only tempo I felt now was that of pounding beating inside my chest in sheer and utter panic. I was moved to another place, another time, another element. I panicked. I was terrified. What would he do from here? The ordinary day became a tangled net of confused thoughts, options. Where do I go? Where was he? Where did he go? Was he behind me? Watching me? Would he try to get me, touch me, hurt me? The numbers were all mixed up in my head. They were simple numbers. I know them. The police dispatch woman talked me through the incident quicker than it happened. Sirens, lights flashed, and uniformed men pounced. Safety. Was it safe? Am I safe? Can I move? Breathe? Walk? Think? Was it a dream? Did this just happen to me? The litany of questions confirmed my story as truth. The story was told again. And again. And yet again. The story will be told a fourth time on Tuesday to a judge and then again to an administrative hearing board for the university. My story. Will he be convicted? Will he go to jail? Will he be expelled from this university? He never touched me, yet he scarred me irreparably. The terror and the fear will never escape me. (Willis, 1999)

Differences in behavior, customs, or traditions that are cultural often cause situational problems for people. The behavior or custom in question may be considered normal in one culture but unacceptable in another.

A Danish woman, visiting from Copenhagen, left her 14-month daughter in a carriage outside a restaurant in New York City. While having dinner with the child's father, she was separated from the child by two tables and a window. Another customer, concerned about the child's safety, called 911. Police arrested both parents, charged them with child abuse, and placed the child in foster care. The mother and child were reunited five days later (Harpaz, 1997).

In Denmark the practice of leaving a young child outside in a carriage is normal and acceptable. Often parents stop in for a cup of coffee or a snack in a fast-food restaurant, leaving the baby outside, or leave the baby napping in a stroller in the back of a housing complex. Child kidnappings are rare in Denmark, so this practice is safer there than in New York City.

Another situation that creates problems is unemployment. Corporate downsizing, closing of mills and factories, and the high rate of small-business failures are factors that have made unemployment a situational crisis for many individuals. These new unemployed are finding it difficult to secure jobs comparable to the ones they lost. Many are now working in retail outlets and shopping malls. Their jobs are part time or temporary, the pay less than their previous jobs with fewer benefits and often less job satisfaction. Overall, the affected individuals feel ashamed and unappreciated. The situation also creates economic difficulty that the whole family faces as the chief breadwinner's ability to provide the basics such as food, clothing, and shelter is threatened.

MEETING HUMAN NEEDS   Another way of defining human problems is to identify basic human needs and ask, "Which of these are being met and which are not being met?" Abraham Maslow developed a **hierarchy of needs** that is helpful in the problem identification process. Maslow's hierarchy begins with the most basic of physical human needs and ends with the need of individuals to become self-actualized, to strive to develop their understanding of themselves and their environment (see Figure 5.1).

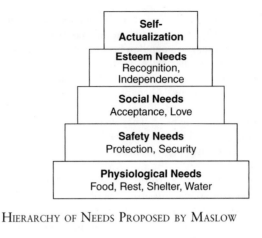

FIGURE 5.1 | HIERARCHY OF NEEDS PROPOSED BY MASLOW

According to Maslow, these needs exist in a hierarchy, which means that individuals cannot address higher-order needs until their most basic needs have been met. If an individual is hungry, cold, scared, or in a life-threatening situation, this person will have difficulty concentrating on love and belonging needs. Likewise, people who get little acceptance or respect from others will have difficulty involving themselves in activities that will lead to self-actualization. Brammer and MacDonald (2003) suggested that the needs can be divided into two categories: "D" needs (*deficiency* needs) and "B" needs (*being* needs). "D" needs comprise the first four levels, wherein an individual seeks to achieve calm and satisfaction. After these "D" needs are met, the individual seeks to achieve the "B" needs and concentrates on developing the self.

The importance of meeting basic needs is a primary consideration in the case of child abuse and neglect. An estimated 872,000 children were victims of abuse and neglect in 2004 (Department of Health and Human Services, 2006). When children are abused and neglected, many of their basic needs are threatened, including their physical, safety, social, and self-esteem needs. Even though experts agree on the needs that are not being met, they have not always agreed on the way to restore children to a supportive environment.

During the 1960s and 1970s, the emphasis was on removing the child from the home and placing the child in foster care. During the 1980s, the approach was to leave children in the home and provide services to parents that helped them better meet their

TABLE 5.3 | SUMMARY POINTS: SITUATIONAL PROBLEMS

- Such situations occur because an individual is in a particular place at a particular time.
- Problems can lead to short- or long-term difficulties or both.
- Experience results in a variety of feelings for the person.
- A person experiencing situational problems is often viewed as a victim.

children's needs. Today, the debate continues about whether foster care or family reunification is the best approach to meet the children's basic needs.

On a larger scale, natural disasters such as hurricanes, tornadoes, floods, and earthquakes may result in human needs by many people at the same time. Immediate needs may be physiological, safety, or both (e.g., food, clothing, shelter, and water). When these needs are met, concern shifts to higher-order needs. Moving from a shelter to more permanent housing, returning to school and jobs, and dealing with the longer-term emotional effects of a large-scale disaster will be the focus of many victims.

SOCIAL CHANGE AND ITS EFFECTS Axelson (1999) suggested another view of the problems of human existence. Human beings experience problems not just because of their needs as individuals but also as a result of rapid social changes, the breakdown of many traditional forms of society, and conflicts between old and new values. In this century, many changes have occurred rapidly in society—sometimes explosively. Rapid social change leaves individuals in unfamiliar situations. Often, people do not have the skills, self-confidence, and support from others to adjust to changing demands. You can imagine the alienation and isolation experienced by people who retain the "old" way or who are no longer part of the mainstream of society as a result of changing urban areas, population shifts to suburbia, or a move to another country. The homeless constitute one such group. Today that definition has expanded to include children, individuals with a dual diagnosis of mental illness and substance abuse, and those who live in the rural areas.

Homeless people have a variety of needs. This group can serve to illustrate the developmental and situational perspectives, as well as the approaches of Maslow and Axelson. Most people know there are homeless individuals, either from seeing coverage of their situation in the media or actually seeing homeless people in their community. In the discussion that follows, you will see that the homeless have multiple needs. Very basic survival needs come first; without a home, existence becomes a struggle to secure food, shelter, rest, and safety. However, homeless people also need recognition and acceptance by the community.

Few people choose to be homeless, yet many individuals find themselves in this situation as the result of rapid social change, unemployment, fire and flood disasters, or eviction. The homeless are single men and women and poor elderly who have lost their marginal housing, ex-offenders, single-parent households, runaway youths, youths abandoned by their families or victims of family abuse, young people who have moved out of foster care, women escaping from domestic violence, undocumented and legal immigrants, Native Americans leaving the reservation after federal cutbacks and unemployment, alcoholics and drug abusers, and ex-psychiatric patients. The so-called "new poor" who are victims of unemployment and changes in the job market may also become homeless.

Accurate statistics describing the homeless have been difficult to obtain; the very nature of the problem makes counting difficult. In many cases, **homelessness** is a temporary circumstance rather than a permanent condition. It is estimated that 760,000 people are homeless on any given night, and 1.2 to 2 million people experience homelessness during one year (National Alliance to End Homelessness, 2006).

BOX 5.2	INTERNATIONAL FOCUS
	Communities in Crisis—Reaching the Vulnerable

The following excerpt illustrates the effects of war, poverty, disasters, and violence on women and children throughout the world. As you read about UNICEF, consider the following questions:

1. What problems do people experience?
2. How are they related to Maslow's hierarchy of needs?
3. What do you think the impact is developmentally and situationally?

Countries in Crisis:

Reaching the Vulnerable

The devastation wrought by emergencies is particularly harsh for children and women. In the last decade alone, more than 2 million children have died as a direct result of armed conflict, and more than three times that number have been permanently disabled or seriously injured. An estimated 20 million children have been forced to flee their homes. More than 1 million children have been orphaned or separated from their families. HIV/AIDS, rampant in war-affected countries, has orphaned more than 13 million children. The majority of displaced persons and refugees are children and women.

UNICEF's mission is to provide special protection for the most disadvantaged children: victims of war, disasters, extreme poverty, all forms of violence and exploitation, and those with disabilities. The human dignity of children and their families is often the first casualty of a crisis. During an emergency UNICEF focuses on meeting the basic needs of women and children as well as protecting their fundamental rights.

Reaching the most vulnerable during humanitarian crises is our greatest challenge. During many emergencies, safe access to vulnerable populations is often delayed because of armed combat, nonexistent roads and bridges, land mines or weather conditions. Sometimes access is simply denied by those in control. The consequences are usually devastating, leaving entire communities deprived of the most basic assistance and protection. Most of those who die in wartime, for instance, do not die as a direct result of violence but from the loss of basic health services, food, safe water, or adequate sanitation. This is especially true for children. The countries with the highest rates of preventable deaths among children are countries which have experienced protracted periods of armed conflict: India, Nigeria, China, Pakistan, Democratic Republic of Congo, and Ethiopia.

Discrimination based on ethnicity, gender, health status, or age keeps people from having a voice in decision making. Vulnerability is often exacerbated when war or natural disasters cut people off geographically. These factors—isolation, lack of voice, discrimination—make it imperative that we reach affected children as quickly as possible. Not only must we meet their basic needs, we must also protect their fundamental human rights and take the necessary steps to restore their dignity.

Source: http://www.unicef.org/emerg/index.html

People are homeless for any number of reasons. One is that the technological society in which we live has eliminated many unskilled and semiskilled jobs; downsizing, the closing of factories, and the outsourcing of the production of goods to countries with cheaper labor have been the direct cause of job loss. In fact, employment-related problems such as unemployment and low wages represent the primary reason why individuals become homeless. A second reason is urban renewal or **gentrification,** which many municipal governments promote as a way to revitalize the downtown areas of cities. This movement has brought a decrease in low-cost housing, displacing individuals without providing any alternative affordable homes. The changing structure of the American family has also contributed to the growth of this population. Because the nuclear family is more isolated than in previous generations, such events as divorce and the death of a spouse have forced individuals (and in some cases, whole families) to adapt to a lower level of survival. Finally, deinstitutionalization, which many blame for most of the homeless population, in fact accounts for only 20 or 30% of this group (Nooe, 2001).

Families with young children are among the fastest-growing segments of homeless. Although some are without family and friends, many have relatives or other social ties, but they believe those in their support network would not "take them in" for more than a day or two. Urban schools are struggling to provide educational opportunities for homeless children. The schools are faced with the challenge to educate during a time when children do not have a stable home and do not know where they will be living from day to day. There is also a growing number of teens who are homeless and not living with a parent or older adult.

Children in homeless situations are vulnerable. These children live in poverty and have a higher percentage of risk for domestic abuse, live with one or more parents with a substance abuse problems, have developmental delays, and experience mental health problems such as anxiety and depression. They also face barriers to attending school because they may lack transportation, records from previous school, immunization records, and clothing (National Coalition for the Homeless, n.d.). The following story illustrates one teen's experience. Kisha became homeless when her parents threw her out of the house with only the clothes on her back.

> Kisha lived in four different places from January until March of last year. Over the years she has lived in a variety of housing that includes a VW bus, a tent, an apartment, in a temporary housing shelter, under a bridge in a sleeping bag, and in a cardboard box in an alley. She has lived alone, with her mom, with her grandmother, with friends, and with a couple of other teens that she met on the streets. She is tired of moving from place to place, but she can't find anyone who will be able to help her for a long period of time. People don't mind helping her out for a while, but then she gets embarrassed that she is staying there and taking charity and sometimes they get tired of her living with them. She has attended three schools in the past four months and she wants a stable home so that she can go to school. She does not want the other kids to know that she has no home.

To improve your understanding of how human service workers understand this complex client group—the homeless—think of some homeless people in your community. As this group becomes more numerous and more visible, you may see them sleeping beside buildings or rummaging through garbage cans. Think of an individual you have seen, and describe his or her physical appearance. How old do you think this person is? How do you imagine this person spends an average day? Where in your community does this person stay at night? How might this individual fit into the categories of the homeless as described? Identify five problems that your homeless individual has. Which problems are represented in Maslow's hierarchy? Which problems are associated with rapid social change?

ENVIRONMENTAL INFLUENCES   The homeless population also emphasizes the importance of an individual's **environment** on one's history, living situation, and current problems. Understanding the influences of the environment in which clients exist is another helpful way to understand them. One type of environmental influence could be the results of rapid social change described earlier. Other environmental influences could include specific locations in which a client lives, friends and family that influence

TABLE 5.4 | SUMMARY POINTS: HOMELESSNESS

- Basic survival, security and safety, and recognition and acceptance are needs.
- Homelessness results for a variety of reasons.
- The very nature of homelessness makes a count of the numbers of homeless difficult to obtain.
- Families with young children, dually diagnosed individuals, and teenagers comprise large groups of homeless.

the client, groups to which the client belongs, and activities in which the client engages. These dimensions are part of the environment that influences a client's life.

Studying the impact of influences on the client allows the helper to better understand the reality of a situation. With an improved knowledge of the environment, the helper also can assist clients with adaptation to or alteration of their environments. Several theorists have contributed to the understanding of how the environment affects the individual.

Bronfenbrenner (1979) first presented his ideas concerning influence to explain how children grow and develop. Later he and others used his theory to explain difficult environmental situations such as child abuse and violence.

One way to consider a client's environment is to think of it in layers. The further the distance the factors are from the individual, the less influence they have. In other words, those factors or individuals closest to the client are considered primary influences, or have a stronger impact than those that are not so close.

The most immediate and earliest influences on individuals, as children, are family (those who interact with the child), school peers and teachers, daycare or child-care workers, and social and sports organizations. Family influence includes parent interactions, child-care situation, presence of or absence of the mother or father or both, and age and gender of siblings. These are key variables that determine the world of the child. At times, primary influences are complicated by divorce or blended families. Physical characteristics of the environment also contribute a direct influence and can include living space and television, computers, and reading materials.

A middle layer of influences, or secondary influences, is represented by the neighborhood, social organizations, and faith-based organizations in which the individual is involved. The beliefs, common roles, and norms of the community also exert an influence. For example, the neighborhood may play a significant role in the individual's life, including location (rural, suburban, urban), playmates, sense of community (involved, friendly, or isolated), traffic patterns (quiet or busy streets), and play areas. The interactions within the secondary environment are also influences. For example, a child who lives at home and attends school is influenced by both. A child who is home-schooled experiences different influences.

The factors with the least influence in the life of a child are those such as international, regional, or global changes. For example, children in the 1950s grew up with threats of nuclear holocaust, spending time in school practicing civil defense drills and stocking community bomb shelters with food and water. Children of the 1960s became part of a well-known rebellious generation, the baby boomers, who both protested and fought in the Vietnam War. Certain factors in this increasingly global environment will help define the children of this new millennium and shape what they believe. Such factors include increased violence in homes, schools, and the workplace; unemployment; migration to the cities; fear of substance abuse and AIDS; and the threat of terrorism.

CASE STUDY

Another way to understand these influences is to see how a human service provider would consider them.

SUE ELLEN DRAPER

Don Regalis has worked with Sue Ellen Draper, a welfare client, for the past nine years. Sue Ellen has four girls: Sharon, age 10; Suzie, age 8; and twins, Sarah and Sindy, age 5. Sue Ellen has always lived in this sparsely populated rural county. Welfare has been part of her family history. Her mother, Sarah McCall, raised Sue Ellen and her five brothers, Darin, Donnie, David, Drew, and Doug, on welfare. Sarah depended on both welfare and food stamps to feed and clothe the children. For years, with few services available for welfare clients in this small community, Sarah pieced together a living that combined taking in washing, using church donations, and accepting government help to provide for her children.

Don Regalis has known Sue Ellen since birth, but his first encounter with her as a client occurred when she became pregnant at the age of 16. She was married and her husband, Phil, could not find work. Don's involvement with Sarah McCall and her family, and now Sue Ellen and her family, has spanned his own career with the Department of Human Services. It has been a continuous relationship filled with successes and challenges. He is a consistent presence for this family.

Throughout the years, Don has considered environmental factors as important to an understanding of his clients. The following example illustrates how Don thinks about Sue Ellen and her environment.

SUE ELLEN DRAPER

- Sue Ellen is of childbearing age, slender, and attractive.
- She is a confident homemaker.
- She lacks assurance to work outside the home.
- She is able to think through difficult issues.
- She excels at accounting tasks.
- She is willing to share her skills.
- She has mechanical aptitude and ability.
- She lives in poverty.

According to Don Regalis, Sue Ellen's primary environment includes her family, neighborhood, school, and her physical environment.

SUE ELLEN DRAPER: THE PRIMARY INFLUENCES

- Sue Ellen was the youngest in the family and the only girl.
- Sue Ellen's mother focused on her to the exclusion of her brothers.
- She grew up without a father.

- She learned from her family that school was not important.
- She learned that the role of mother and homemaker was important.
- The home she lived in was small.

The larger environment in which Sue Ellen lived also affected her development. Don Regalis believes that the culture of her rural environment has had its influence.

SUE ELLEN DRAPER: THE SECONDARY INFLUENCES

- There were strong influences of neighborhood and school, which is where Sue Ellen spent a majority of her time.
- Sarah McCall's work (washing) and gregarious nature established interactions with many of the neighbors.
- Sarah McCall had multiple interactions with her neighbors, since she both worked for and socialized with them.
- Sue Ellen had an active interaction within her neighborhood, helping with her mother's small business, drinking coffee with neighbors in their kitchen, providing meals and recreation space for neighborhood children, and participating in large-group summer play.
- School had the "feel" of the neighborhood.
- Teachers continually associated Sue Ellen with her five older brothers.
- Many were also acquainted with her mother.
- One math teacher, in particular, was especially encouraging to Sue Ellen and two of her brothers.

As he works with her, Don Regalis continues to gain information about Sue Ellen's environment. This information helps him think about the problems she faces and the needs she has.

DEFINING STRENGTHS   Defining the strengths of clients is an important consideration and is included in assessing the nature of problems. In human services, client strengths refer to the positive characteristics, abilities, and experiences of the client. It is important to understand the nature of the strengths that clients have. This information, paired with an identification of problems they are experiencing, provides the helper with information that can help the client grow and change. The concept of building on strengths can help clients approach their problem areas by using their past successes.

Clients come to the helper with strengths. These represent the activities, characteristics, and achievements of the individuals, families, or communities who need help and support. Usually it takes the professional time to help clients identify past successful behaviors and situations; once identified, the clients can be more hopeful about solving their current problems.

Another positive focus of identifying strengths is asking the clients to take a new perspective on their difficulties. Although it is important to ask, "What brings you here today?" or "Tell me about your current situation," the conversation expands as clients have the opportunity to recall how they have solved problems in the past and what successes they have had at home, at school, in relationships, and at work. Helping clients set an agenda that builds on successes establishes a positive tone to the helping relationship and the work to be done.

If you review the notes of Don Regalis, he has begun to identify several strengths of Sue Ellen Draper and her family. Note that she is described as a confident homemaker, is able to think through difficult situations, excels at accounting tasks, is willing to share her skills, and has mechanical aptitude and ability. One strength that she learned from her family is that homemaking is important. Her neighborhood environment provided her with social opportunities; she has good relationships with her neighbors; and her math teacher has been supportive. Sue Ellen can probably provide Don Regalis with additional information about her strengths. He can help her assess her emotional make-up, behavior, life skills, and other areas of functioning to assess the strengths upon which they can build during problem solving.

CLIENTS AS INDIVIDUALS, GROUPS, AND POPULATIONS

This chapter has presented approaches to identifying problems through understanding human needs. This section examines three ways to think about the term *client,* using a brief client history to illustrate different perspectives about client identity.

In many cases, the client will be an individual. In fact, most of us will think about each of our clients as one person. This means working one-on-one to define problems, assess possible interventions, and provide services. In the following case history, you will read one person's account of her life. Think about her as your client. As you read, make note of the facts you learn about her and her situation. What are her problems? Using the models discussed in the previous section, apply what you have learned to help you understand her situation.

When I was 12 years old, my mother and her boyfriend left me with my grandmother and never returned. Momma told me they would be gone for the weekend and would pick me up on Monday. That was four years ago. My grandmother tried to do right by me, but she is old and can't get around very well. After Momma left, I was angry, hurt, and sad. How can a mother leave her child and never want to see her again? I managed to finish the school year, but my grades were down and I was absent a lot. The guidance counselor at my school talked to me about the importance of staying in school and working hard. That might be important to kids who have a family, but I was alone. School was just a place for other kids to make fun of me and call my mother names. When kids laughed at me, I wanted to die. I couldn't take it. I started fighting back. I was suspended from school for "consistent and persistent, disruptive behavior." It wasn't my fault that I had to fight. I only went off when kids picked on me or laughed at me. Why am I the one getting suspended?

Over the summer vacation, I met Victor. He was really nice to me. He was in a gang. He told me the gang would protect me from anyone who tried to mess with me. The school couldn't make that promise. Me and Victor started off as friends, but we got closer. I had sex with Victor on my 13th birthday. He said it would be really special. It wasn't. It hurt like hell. Not only that, but I got pregnant. Victor said not to worry, the gang family would be the baby's family. I really didn't want to get involved with the gang, but I felt like I didn't have any choice now with the baby coming. Victor was right about being protected. Once I joined the gang, nobody bothered me or laughed at me anymore. I moved out of my grandmother's house and lived with Victor. I guess Granny didn't care because she never came after me.

Things were good for a while. Soon after I got pregnant, Victor changed. He was distant and not around at night anymore. Even though I was Victor's girlfriend, I had to have sex with all the guys in the gang. Having sex with all the gang bangers in one night is called "pulling a train." They "pulled trains" on me until I got big with the baby. Victor stopped having sex with me, but he said he still loved me and wanted to be with me and the baby. I didn't believe him. I knew he was sleeping with a lot of other girls.

I wanted to go home to Granny's but Victor went crazy when I talked about leaving. We had a huge fight. Victor covered my mouth with his hand while he held a knife to my stomach. He cut a "V" on my arm with a knife and said if I left he would do more than "scratch me on the arm" next time.

I didn't have to go to school because I was pregnant. The school sent a teacher to our apartment once a week to help me keep up. I told her she was wasting her time. I didn't want to go back to school, but she came every week. She also made arrangements for me to see a doctor for prenatal care check-ups at the health department. They gave me free food vouchers there to buy cereal, cheese, and milk. Victor liked it when I came home with the food vouchers. He used them to get weed. That was OK with me cause I liked to smoke pot. I was getting high as often as I could. When I was stoned, I could forget about all the shit in my life.

One night I was with Victor at a party. His fellas were getting too wild. They wanted Victor to be the shooter at a drive-by. He didn't have to do it, but I could tell he was not going to back down from a challenge. Victor didn't even say goodbye to me. I somehow knew I would never see him again. None of those guys came back. They shot up the wrong 'hood. The boys they wanted to pop found out they were planning a drive-by and were waiting for them. Victor shot up the crack house but when they tried to drive away, their car crashed into the curb. Before they could turn around, the other guys started shooting up the car. They shot Victor. I don't know how many times. Then they pulled Victor and his crew out of the car and crushed their faces with baseball bats. The police came too late. Victor was dead. I guess I should have been more upset. It really seemed more like a dream.

That was four years ago. I had my baby, but he was very small and sick when he was born. I named him Victor and call him Little Vic. We live in a group home for single teen mothers. I get a lot of help from the houseparents. They take good care of me and my little boy. I go to school here and want to get my GED. Little Vic has something called "developmental delays" and goes to a special school for special needs children. My life is not great but it's getting better.

If we think about clients as individuals, then there are several clients in this situation. The young woman who is sharing her story is a client and is, in fact, currently receiving services to help her with her education, housing, and parenting. Her son, little Victor, is also a client with special needs that may be both physical and mental. He is attending a special school. At some point, Victor, the father, may have been a client, but he is now dead. In any case, these individuals have needs and problems that they are unable to address alone. If they became our clients, we would use the concept of the whole person introduced earlier in this chapter to assess their needs and problems, think about the four models that would help us understand their situations, and consider ways to access the services that are needed.

Another way to think about this case is to consider a broader definition of client—groups as clients. Examples of such groups may be a couple, a family, or several individuals who share a similar situation or problem. In this case history, we might think of Granny, little Victor, and his mother as a family unit that might be a client. It is also possible to think about Victor's **gang** as a client group who needs human services. If we focus on the gang as a potential client group, then we would need to understand the gang culture, which might include the structure of gangs, the ways of identifying gang members, and why and how kids join gangs.

We can also think of larger groups as clients—neighborhoods, cities or counties, problem populations, or geographic regions. In this case history, we might consider

BOX 5.3	WEB SOURCES

Find Out More about Gangs

www.streetgangs.com

This site provides access to reports by the *Los Angeles Times* related to gangs in Los Angeles, California.

www.lib.msu.edu/harris23/crimjust/gangs.htm

This site, sponsored by the University of Michigan, provides a definition of the term *gangs* and links visitors to reviews of literature that focus on gang issues.

www.iir.com/nygc/maininfo.htm

The National Youth Gang Center is one of five major components of a comprehensive,

coordinated response to the gang problem by the Office of Juvenile Justice and Delinquency Prevention. Its purpose is to expand and maintain the body of critical knowledge about gangs and effective responses to them. Topics include frequently asked questions, legislation, community gang problems, and federal gang programs.

www.lunaweb.com/memgang.htm

This site is an example of a community's response to the gang problem. The Memphis Police Department promotes gang awareness by providing answers to often-asked questions, suggestions for public participation, and a list of resources.

gangs as a client group that is a community or a national or societal problem. For example, the United States has seen rapid proliferation of youth gangs since 1980. Their presence is felt in communities in several ways, including their dress, language, colors, and music. Perhaps of greatest concern though is the increase in violence and crime. Assaults and batteries, drug-related crimes, auto thefts, home invasions, drive-by shootings, graffiti, and an increase in truancy and school dropouts are associated with gangs. One response to community needs is the National Youth Gang Center, which is funded by the U.S. Department of Justice's Office of Juvenile Justice and Delinquency Prevention. The center assists state and local jurisdictions in the collection, analysis, and exchange of information on gang-related demographics, legislation, literature, research, and promising program strategies. Its website (http://ojjdp.ncjrs.org/) provides current information. See Box 5.3 for more information.

Please note as you think about your role as a human service professional that your work with clients is not restricted to individuals, families, and groups. It may also include others such as your employers and society at large. Human service professionals are employed within a social service delivery system and work for a specific organization or agency. Chapter 8 introduces this work environment and helps you understand your place in it. Society as a client emerges from human service professionals' explicit and implicit commitment to bettering the lives of others on a social scale. For example, a commitment to educate all children or eradicate poverty may guide your work in advocacy, outreach, and mobilizing, roles that are introduced in Chapter 6.

GETTING HELP

Having discussed *what* problems clients face and *who* the clients are, we now address the question of *how* clients get help. The answer is not simply that clients experience problems and then find the appropriate human service agency, because people do not always use the services they need.

Questions that are often raised about the help-seeking process are "Why don't people use available services? Why don't they ask for what they need if it is not available?" These are questions we continue to ask today. A discussion of the conditions under which clients enter the human service system, the barriers clients experience as they enter the system, and clients' perspectives on human services immediately before and after receiving assistance will provide answers to these questions.

WAYS OF GETTING HELP

As stated, people do not experience problems and automatically go directly to the appropriate human service agency. Individuals can become involved with the human service delivery system in several ways, including self-referral and referral by other professionals. Clients can also be forced to receive services or can receive services inadvertently as members of a larger population. The Internet has made it possible for clients to find services on their own using search engines and internet service directories.

REFERRAL   **Referral,** a common method of getting help, includes self-referral and referral by others. Those individuals who initiate help themselves may experience a more productive helping relationship than individuals who are forced into a helping situation. Individuals may voluntarily seek assistance from human service agencies because they are desperate and confused. They have experienced a traumatic event or are in a situation so intolerable that they can no longer ignore it. Self-referral typically occurs when clients have tried every way they know to cope, to no avail, and have no other ideas about how to address their problems. Some potential clients have heard about services from their friends and neighbors or through television, radio, or billboard advertising and know exactly what their problem is and where to go. Others in desperate condition stop at the first agency available, regardless of its function, hoping that someone will be able to refer them to the right service.

Another type of referral is from another professional to a human service agency. Ministers, physicians, mental health workers, and other helping professionals often see an individual who needs assistance for problems beyond their expertise. The referring professional first assesses the client's complex situation and then refers this person to one or more additional human service agencies. For such a referral to be successful, the referring professional must help the potential client clarify problems and begin to provide some alternative solutions. (Referral may be one of those solutions.) This action may preempt the next professional's work, but it assures the client that the referring professional is not just "passing the buck." The referring professional should also provide the potential client with as much information as possible about the agency to which the referral has been made. If the client is somewhat reluctant to go to another professional for help, more assistance from the referring professional will increase the probability that the referral will be successful.

INVOLUNTARY PLACEMENT IN THE SYSTEM   Another way of getting into the human service system is to be placed in the system by others. **Involuntary clients**—referred by schools, prisons, courts, marriage counselors, protective services, and the juvenile justice system—are potentially difficult to work with because they have not chosen to

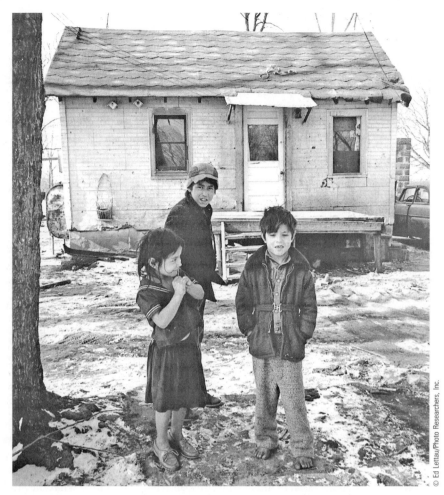

© Ed Lettau/Photo Researchers, Inc.

receive services. The service to which they are referred usually offers only part of the treatment they are to receive. Their cooperation and participation in that service is often monitored, and decisions about subsequent treatment (including release from treatment) are partially based on their observed attitudes and progress. This creates some pressure on the clients to treat the referral seriously.

One example of the use of involuntary referral of clients is the case of child abuse. The decision to allow a child to remain in or return to a home may be contingent on agreement by one or both parents to receive counseling services. For another example, the juvenile court may order involuntary services for first offenders. Depending on the crime and the circumstances, judges often sentence juveniles to receive counseling, to perform tasks in the social services, or to assume other responsibilities related to their crimes. A third example involves individuals incarcerated for crimes. Much of their time in prison is programmed by others, and they have little say over their treatment.

| BOX 5.4 | GETTING HELP: *LOCATE SERVICES* |

If unsure where to go for help, talk to someone you trust who has experience in mental health—for example, a doctor, nurse, social worker, or religious counselor. Ask their advice on where to seek treatment. If there is a university nearby, its departments of psychiatry or psychology may offer private and/or sliding-scale fee clinic treatment options. Otherwise, check the Yellow Pages under "mental health," "health," "social services," "suicide prevention," "crisis intervention services," "hotlines," "hospitals," or "physicians" for phone numbers and addresses. In times of crisis, the emergency room doctor at a hospital may be able to provide temporary help for a mental health problem, and will be able to tell you where and how to get further help. Listed below are the types of people and places that will make a referral to, or provide, diagnostic and treatment services.

- Family doctors
- Mental health specialists, such as psychiatrists, psychologists, social workers, or mental health counselors
- Religious leaders/counselors
- Health maintenance organizations
- Community mental health centers
- Hospital psychiatry departments and outpatient clinics
- University- or medical school-affiliated programs
- State hospital outpatient clinics
- Social service agencies
- Private clinics and facilities
- Employee assistance programs
- Local medical and/or psychiatric societies

Source: The National Institute of Mental Health, September 30, 2005. Getting help: Locate services. Retrieved October 20, 2006, from http://www.nimh.nih.gov/healthinformation/gettinghelp.cfm

Involuntary clients and voluntary clients may feel very differently about human services. Someone else has decided that the involuntary clients need assistance; they have not admitted that they need help and probably would not have chosen the human services they are receiving if they had decided to seek help on their own. They are often embarrassed or angry that someone else has decided what they need and has sent them to receive the services in question. Because they have not chosen the assistance, they may also feel trapped. Their alternatives are much more limited than those of voluntary clients. If they do not like the treatment or the helper, they may have little ability to change the helping situation.

INADVERTENT SERVICES Another way of entering the human service system is to be part of a larger population that is targeted for services. In this situation, receipt of services does not depend on the individual's need or ability to qualify for the services, and the client does not have to ask for them. Although inadvertent services can often help the client, they also have their limitations. Ideally, before services are provided to a large population, the consumers using the services are consulted. However, some of the clients receiving the services may not have had any input about the type of service provided or the manner in which it is delivered. In such cases, the services provided may seem useless to the client. Services that clients receive inadvertently include the redevelopment of low-cost housing; neighborhood crime-watch programs; shelters for the homeless, AIDS victims, or the elderly; and emergency help for disaster areas.

Many clients who need help do not receive the services they need, nor do they seek them for a variety of reasons. **Barriers** that clients experience are discussed next, including how they view the problem, the cost of the resources, and the reluctance to use friends as helpers. Reading a description of these barriers may be frustrating, because the problems are presented from the client's point of view, without any discussion of how helpers can overcome such client barriers. We have chosen to separate client barriers from helper responses to retain the focus on the client. Subsequent chapters will provide a human service response to such barriers.

Barriers to Seeking Help

In discussing barriers, one of the first factors to consider is how the client views the problem. If the client considers the problem too difficult to solve, too overwhelming to consider, or too embarrassing to admit, then the person is less likely to seek help. Clients who perceive the problem in these ways may consider the process of seeking help a burden or a waste of time. From the client's perspective, the problem cannot be solved even by experts.

If the client is embarrassed at having the problem, seeking help means admitting to others that there is a problem. The very nature of many problems in living involves a reluctance to admit to having problems. Spouses in troubled marriages may be reluctant to talk about their difficulties because parents and significant others have warned them about the trouble this could cause them. Abused children, spouses, and parents keep the abuse quiet because making an accusation would cause great disruption and because they, the abused, feel that the situation is ultimately their fault. Men in this society are less likely to seek help than women experiencing similar problems because men are socialized to solve problems on their own.

Another barrier is the individual's perception of the human service professional. Such helpers are viewed as strangers and experts—two categories that establish immediate barriers for those in need. The helping process requires the individual in need to talk about personal issues and concerns with someone unknown. For many individuals in our society, the "stranger" evokes distrust and suspicion. The expert commands respect but also fear. The client initially sees the expert as an "accomplished" person who has little in common with individuals who have overwhelming problems. Fears of the stranger and the expert are barriers that prevent individual clients from seeking services and from trusting workers in the initial stages of the helping process.

Cultural factors sometimes prohibit seeking help. In some ethnic groups and in some areas of the country, there is a strong prohibition against sharing problems or concerns with people outside the family. In Appalachia, for example, problems remain within the family, or in some instances, the extended family. For an individual to seek help means embarrassment, ostracism, or both to the individual and the family. For Asian cultures the concept of losing face is important; many individuals do not seek help because they do not want to bring shame to the family. In many cultures the help that is offered is not the help that they need. For example, within the African American culture, religion and spirituality is an important source of help. Often traditional Western ways of helping do not embrace the cultural support of the client.

Three barriers are directly related to available client resources: money to pay for the services, transportation to reach the place of service delivery, and the time and distance involved in traveling to receive the services. For the disabled, architectural barriers may present additional problems. Many clients may be ready and willing to seek assistance but cannot determine a way to surmount the problems of paying for services or of finding time and transportation to receive them. One solution to the inability to pay is to provide services to poorer clients on a realistic sliding scale. Transportation is a difficult problem for rural clients who live miles from the nearest population center. Equally vulnerable are clients who live in smaller cities without mass transportation or in larger cities with expensive mass transportation. Other clients cannot use services because they work long hours or are caring for children or an elderly parent. Unless service hours are extended and family care relief is provided, services may be inaccessible (from the client's perspective) even if they are affordable and nearby. What makes these barriers particularly frustrating for the clients is that they add one more set of problems to an already troubled situation.

The psychological costs of seeking help are also serious barriers. Some clients view help as effecting an immediate loss of their freedom; they fear that helpers will demand changes in their behavior, lifestyle, and work habits. They do not want to lose what little freedom they have. Clients also fear that they will ultimately have to assume responsibility for their problems, and this may frighten them. When clients admit that they need help and seek assistance, they are also afraid that they will be considered inadequate. When a person seeks help, it is a signal to others that the individual cannot solve problems alone and that his or her efforts have failed. To admit such "failure" is very difficult. Sometimes there is considerable pressure from peers not to seek help, especially if the peers see themselves as having a similar problem. Finally, clients resist seeking help because they fear being indebted to a human service worker or agency. Asking for and receiving help means giving the worker the power of a caregiver. Clients feel pressed to live up to the worker's expectations, and they fear disappointing the worker if little or no change takes place in their lives.

BARRIERS TO FRIENDS AS HELPERS   The barriers are very real to individuals who are experiencing problems in living and choose not to seek help. Besides being reluctant to seek the help of professional workers, such individuals often hesitate to seek out informal help from family and friends. This reluctance stems from their own fears and fear of the reactions of others. Some of the barriers to seeking help from significant others are similar to the barriers to seeking professional services. Telling friends about their problems may cause a loss of face; reputations and good appearances may suffer if others know about the problems. People want others to think well of them. It is a common worry that once others know about their problems, then they will lose friendships or respect. People also fear that the disclosure will be a burden to those who have been told—that the problems might upset the listener or place him or her in an uncomfortable situation. To impose on friends might violate the "rules" of the friendship.

Another reason individuals do not ask their friends for help is that they do not find them helpful. Many friends do not know how to respond appropriately, offering only

TABLE 5.5	SUMMARY POINTS: BARRIERS TO HELP

- Client's perspective of the situation
- Embarrassment
- Reluctance to admit to having a problem
- Perceptions of the helper
- Cultural factors
- Cost of services
- Transportation
- Time
- Fear

advice, authoritarian "shoulds," and cliches. Many friends also cannot be trusted. What the individual experiencing problems considers confidential may be considered public information by the friend. Most potential clients do not want their problems to be common knowledge in their own environment.

THE RELUCTANT CLIENT   **Reluctance,** in its many forms, may have its positive characteristics, although many experienced helpers believe that establishing a bond with a client is easier if the client wants and seeks help. Client reluctance is to be respected. Reluctance is often self-protective, designed to maintain personal integrity. Part of the helping process requires clients to admit there is a problem, to share information about themselves and their environment, and to engage with the helper to change their behaviors and then evaluate the change. This process requires an inner strength that potential clients may lack at the beginning of the process.

THE CLIENT'S PERSPECTIVE

People often decide to use the human service system with preconceived ideas or expectations about what will happen. Sometimes their expectations are confirmed; other times, they lead to misunderstandings. One reason client expectations are important is the emphasis many agencies and helping professionals place on client satisfaction.

CLIENT EXPECTATIONS

To understand clients, we must know what each expects from both the human service system and the service professional and how each person perceives that same system after receiving help. Today's clients are focusing more than ever on the quality of care they will receive. The following discussion of client perceptions before and after receiving services is based on the results of several studies of client perception of the juvenile justice system, family services, protective services, and services to unmarried mothers. Although the information was collected from clients requiring different services, the results are surprisingly similar.

BOX 5.5	GETTING HELP
	One Client's Perspective

I needed help, and I had mixed feelings. I felt guilty needing help. It probably had something to do with the way I was raised. If you're strong enough, you shouldn't be having emotional problems. The barriers to getting help were mostly internal. I didn't feel like it was okay to be as angry or depressed as I was. I felt I should just snap out of it. There's a family history of breakdowns. I really don't know if it's hereditary. Some people thought that was an excuse.

I had one doctor who put me on so many medications; I gained weight until I weighed over 200 pounds, which was just making me more depressed. I had to go for a physical, and the doctor said one of those medications shouldn't even be mixed with the others. That added to the depression, so I took myself off everything and I lay down to die. And my husband would have allowed it. It seemed like the depression was in cycles, too. I'd be depressed and I'd want to die, and then I'd get angry. When I got angry the last time, I was the one who called the doctor and said I needed help.

First, many clients imagine that the helper will have an unbiased attitude toward them and will have experience in working with the problems they are experiencing. The helper will understand the problems because he or she will have the client's point of view. Clients might also expect the helper to listen, help them decide what to do, and help them do whatever needs to be done. Clients also expect the helper to assist them in dealing directly with the environment.

Clients may also have clear expectations about the helper's behavior. For example, a client may expect the helper to tell him or her what to do. Helping professionals should be able to understand what clients say, provide them with necessary information, and offer an opinion of their own if it differs from the clients' opinions. In other words, the helper is expected to take a very active role in the helping process.

Clients also have ideas about what they expect from the helping process. First, clients want to resolve the problem they are facing, and they may expect quick solutions. Often, results are defined as change—either in themselves or in other people, and these changes are described in concrete terms. For example, a client may identify lack of resources and the need for tangible goods and services as the problems. Clients may also be reluctant to define something as a problem if they think it cannot be resolved.

CLIENT EVALUATIONS OF SERVICES

Clients today are much more sophisticated in the area of client satisfaction. They are acquainted with issues of access and quality of services, and many of them provide feedback to agencies and service providers by filling out satisfaction surveys and questionnaires after they have received services. Because of the current climate of accountability, clients are more vocal about what they expect and what will satisfy them.

Clients' views of services after the process are often consistent with their prior expectations. The most positive outcomes are the practical improvements in their lives, such as better living conditions, food, and clothing, as well as intangible improvements, such as increased self-confidence, assumption of new roles, acquisition of new skills, and solution of their problems in living. Helper activities that may be helpful are the ones that go beyond talking.

BOX 5.6	A CLIENT SPEAKS

About Being a Client

When I chose to be a client, I didn't think there was any hope for me as far as my disease of alcoholism was concerned. I thought that I didn't have a choice, that I would end up one day dying as an alcoholic. And I didn't know anything about AA or about treatment centers. One day I stumbled on this information from another alcoholic who was still practicing his disease, and he told me they had a treatment program for veterans. At that point, I was in school, I was trying to get some education to better myself, and I was sick and tired of trying to fight this disease on my own. I wasn't getting anywhere with it. I might go two or three days, but then the next thing I know I'm back out there again.

When exams came around, I got test anxiety, and just to relieve that pressure I would take a drink, saying to myself, "I'm just gonna take a couple of drinks." But I would drink until I'd get sick. So I called the hospital and they set up an appointment. I really didn't know what to expect when I got there. I was kind of fearful. I thought it was a place where you go to dry out and get back on your feet and then they send you back out. But it was not that way. They educated us about the disease of alcoholism and that people were beginning to accept it as a disease, and that there was hope for the alcoholic. I started to feel a little better, because until then I didn't think there was any hope for me. And I found out that I had a choice. I had a choice to drink, or to go to AA meetings to get help.

About Barriers to Getting Help

I think the biggest barrier was myself. I don't think it's anything out there, because wherever I go, there I am, and I still have those same problems. The world is not gonna change; you can't change other people, places, and things.

About Human Service Workers

The majority of the workers are compassionate people and are very understanding. The ones that I find are not understanding are the ones that have not experienced this disease. They don't know what alcoholism is all about. People who have been through alcoholism understand, and they can see through all your cunning, manipulative ways.

About Getting Help

I think the biggest thing for any person seeking help, or anyone who is in an institution, is to break out of the denial stage. I think that is the biggest downfall for everybody, for any client. That was my biggest problem for years. I knew I had a problem, but I would not admit it. I always said, "No, it was just circumstances, I was at the wrong place at the wrong time," or "I just had one beer too many." The key is awareness; today I'm aware of what my downfalls are, and what I need to do to make life better. If you really and truly want to do something about your problem, you have to be totally honest with yourself, because you can't be honest with other people until you start being honest with yourself. In my case, I needed to stop being passive and start being assertive and not letting people control my feelings.

Clients often want workers who will help them get something, take them somewhere, talk with someone for them, see someone with them, and refer them. Many clients consider the outcomes of the helping experience to be very positive, view workers as helpful and fair, and believe that things will be better for them after the service than before. Many also will perceive at least some improvement or the potential for improvement in their situations.

Factors linked to client satisfaction and client dissatisfaction follow.

SATISFACTION

1. Client satisfaction is linked to the client's perceptions of the helper. Specifically, clients are more satisfied with the services they receive if they perceive the worker as having similar values, if the helper accurately

perceives their needs, and if they perceive the worker as an expert with experience in the problem area.

2. Clients also want to have a good relationship with their human service professional. For them that means that the helper spends time with them, listens to their problems, and provides emotional support. This includes being called prior to appointments and receiving follow-up contacts.

3. Clients want to participate in the process of helping, especially if they are long-term clients. They want to have input into the decisions about their treatment. They also base their satisfaction on the amount and accuracy of the information that they receive.

4. Satisfaction is also linked to the helper's ability to solve problems and the amount of change that clients think occurs during the helping process.

5. A supportive environment also makes a positive difference.

Conversely, clients who are dissatisfied can be described as follows:

DISSATISFACTION

1. Dissatisfaction arises when clients want material assistance from the helper, but the helper wants to focus on personal and interpersonal problems. This may lead to a clash between the helper's and the clients' expectations.

2. Receiving unwanted help and advice may lead to dissatisfaction.

3. Clients may experience dissatisfaction when there is a lack of clarity about the problem and what the intervention or plan will be to resolve it.

KEY TERMS

barriers	gang	involuntary clients	situational problems
client	gentrification	problems	social change
developmental process	hierarchy of needs	referral	whole person
environment	homelessness	reluctance	

THINGS TO REMEMBER

1. The term *client* may refer to an individual, a small group such as a family, or a larger population such as the residents of a geographic area.

2. The definitions of problem suggest that "problems in living" can have two components: a description of the problem and a course of action for resolving the problem.

3. A way of defining human problems is Abraham Maslow's hierarchy of needs, which begins with the most basic of physical human needs and ends with the need of individuals to become self-actualized.

4. Human beings experience similar problems, not just because of their individual needs but also as a result of rapid social changes, the breakdown of many traditional forms of society, and conflicts between old and new values.

5. Learning about environmental influences is one way to examine client needs.

6. Individuals can become involved with the human service delivery system in several ways, including self-referral, referral by other professionals, or involuntary placement.

7. Self-referral occurs when individuals have tried every way they know to cope, to no avail, and have no other ideas about how to address their problems.

8. Ministers, physicians, mental health workers, and other helping professionals often see an individual who needs assistance for problems beyond their expertise, and after assessing the client's situation, refer the client to one or more additional human services agencies.

9. Client expectations fall into three categories: to find a cure or straighten out a situation, to define results as change in themselves and change in others, and to describe what changes should occur as concrete rather than general or abstract.

10. From the clients' perspective, positive outcomes were the practical improvements in their lives, such as better living conditions, food and clothing, and intangible improvements, including increased self-confidence, assumption of new roles, acquisition of new skills, and solution of their problems in living.

11. Clients' satisfaction is linked to their perceptions of the helping professional and of the relationship, the helper's ability to solve problems, and the amount of change the clients thought occurred during the helping process.

12. Conversely, clients who expressed dissatisfaction did so because they wanted material assistance from the helper or they received unwanted advice and help.

ADDITIONAL READINGS: FOCUS ON CLIENTS

Currie, E. (2004). *The road to whatever: Middle-class culture and the crisis of adolescence.* NY: Metropolitan Books.
Adolescent crime is now an issue of the suburban middle class and author-sociologist. Currie suggests why teens from ideal homes are engaging in irresponsible and criminal behavior.

Harrison, K. (2003). *Another place at the table.* NY: Tarcher/Penguin.
This book is Harrison's personal account of foster parenting needy children and emergency care "hot line" foster children. In addition to abandoned infants, runaway teens, disabled preschoolers, and children with psychiatric problems, Harrison also deals with lawyers, social service providers, and therapists who are involved in the lives of foster children.

Lahiri, J. (2003). *The namesake: A novel.* Boston: Houghton Mifflin.
This novel is the story of Gogol, a second-generation immigrant who can never quite find his place in the world. His family leaves their tradition-bound life in Calcutta to be transformed into Americans, and Gogol is raised as an American boy.

Morales, A. T., Sheafor, V. W., & Scott, M. E. (2007). *Social work: A profession of many faces.* Boston: Allyn & Bacon.
The focus of this book is the various groups of people who need help, including children, older adults, women, disabled people, and members of minority racial and ethnic groups.

Shakur, S., & Scott, M. K. (2004). *Monster: Autobiography of an L. A. gang member.* NY: Grove Press.
"Monster" Kody, today known as Sanyika Shakur, spent 16 years as a "gangbanger" in South Central Los Angeles. His story begins with his induction into the Crips at age 11 and ends with a 7-year prison term for beating a crack dealer.

REFERENCES

Axelson, J. A. (1999). *Counseling and development in a multicultural society* (3rd ed.). Pacific Grove, CA: Brooks/Cole.

Brammer, L. M., & MacDonald, G. (2003). *The helping relationship: Process and skills*. Boston: Allyn & Bacon.

Bronfenbrenner, U. (1979). *The ecology of human development*. Cambridge, MA: Harvard University Press.

Erikson, E. (1963). *Childhood and society*. New York: Norton.

Harpaz, B. J. (1997, May 15). NYC case highlights a culture clash. *USA Today*, 9A.

Levinson, D. (1978). *The seasons of a man's life*. New York: Ballantine.

National Alliance to End Homelessness. (2006). *Policy book 2006*. Retrieved October 22, 2006, from http://www. endhomelessness.org/content/article/detail/586.

National Coalition for the Homeless. (n.d.). *Research on homelessness from the National Coalition for the Homeless*. Retrieved October 22, 2006, from http://www.nwrel.org/cfc/frc/pdf/Handout2.PDF.

Nooe, R. (2001). Mental illness and homelessness. In T. McClam & M. Woodside (Eds.), *Human services in the 21st century* (pp. 205–214). New York: Council for Standards in Human Service Education.

Shaffer, D. R. (2002). *Developmental psychology* (6th ed.). Pacific Grove, CA: Wadsworth/Thomson.

Sheehy, G. (1995). *New passages*. New York: Ballantine.

Trotter, K. H., & Swartwood, M. (2007). *Life span: A multimedia introduction to human development CE-ROM 2.0*. Pacific Grove, CA: Wadsworth/Thomson.

U. S. Department of Health and Human Services. (2006). *Summary. Child maltreatment: 2004*. Retrieved October 22, 2006, from http://www.acf. hhs.gov/programs/cb/pubs/cm04/summary.htm.

Willis, R. (1999, November). Looking for sense in a senseless crime. *Counseling Today*, 16.

THE HUMAN SERVICE PROFESSIONAL

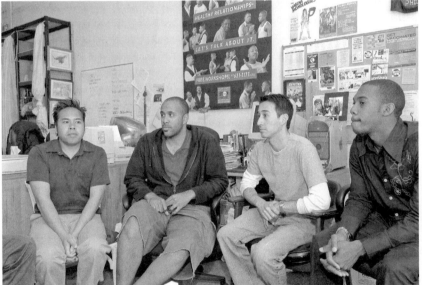

CHAPTER 6

© Rachel Epstein/Photo Edit

After reading this chapter, you will be able to:

- Write a description of the five commonly accepted human service values.
- List four characteristics or qualities of helpers that are identified by a number of studies.
- Distinguish the three categories of helpers.
- Identify the other helping professionals with whom a human service professional may interact.
- List the three areas of job responsibilities for human service professionals.
- Provide examples of the roles included in each of the three areas of professional responsibilities.

Self-assessment

- Describe the motivations for choosing a helping profession.
- How do values and a philosophy of helping relate to motivations for choosing a helping profession?
- List the helper characteristics that are important for the human service professional.
- What are the similarities and differences among human service professionals, physicians, psychologists, social workers, and counselors?
- How does the *Occupational Outlook Handbook*'s entry on human service workers help you define them?
- What are the three primary areas of job responsibilities for human service professionals?

Helping means assisting other people to understand, overcome, or cope with problems. The *helper* is the person who offers this assistance. This chapter's discussion of the motivations for choosing a helping profession, the values and philosophies of helpers, and the special characteristics and traits helpers have will assist in establishing an identity for the helper. We also define workers as human service professionals, as well as introduce other professionals with whom they may interact. An important key to understanding human service professionals is an awareness of the many roles they engage in as they work with their clients and with other professionals.

In this chapter you will meet two human service professionals, Beth Bruce and Carmen Rodriguez. Beth is a case manager at a mental health center and has previous experience working with the elderly and adolescents. Carmen is a vocational evaluator for a state agency. She has varied responsibilities related to preparing clients for and finding gainful employment.

WHO IS THE HELPER?

In human services, the helper is an individual who assists others. This very broad definition includes professional helpers with extensive training, such as psychiatrists and psychologists, as well as those who have little or not training, such as volunteers and other nonprofessional helpers. Regardless of the length or intensity of the helper's training, his or her basic focus is to assist clients with external or internal problems and help clients help themselves (Brammer & MacDonald, 2003; Okun, 2002).

The human service professional is a helper who can be described in many different ways. For example, effective helpers are people whose thinking, emotions, and behaviors are integrated (Cochran & Cochran, 2006). Such a helper, believing that each client is a unique individual different from all other clients, will greet each one by name, with a handshake and a smile. Others view a helping person as an individual whose life experiences most closely match those of the person to be helped. The recovering alcoholic working with substance abusers is an example of this perspective. Still another view of the helper, and the one with which you are most familiar from your reading of this text, is the generalist human service professional who brings together knowledge and skills from a variety of disciplines to work with the client as a whole person.

Your understanding of the human service worker as a professional helper will become clearer as this section examines the reasons why individuals choose this type of work, the traits and characteristics they share, and the different categories of their actual job functions.

Motivations for Choosing a Helping Profession

Work is an important part of life in the United States. It is a valued activity that provides many individuals with a sense of identity as well as a livelihood. It is also a means for individuals to experience satisfying relationships with others, under agreeable conditions.

Understanding vocational choice is as complex and difficult a process as actually choosing a vocation. Factors that have been found to influence career choice include individuals' needs, their aptitudes and interests, and their self-concepts. Special personal or social experiences also influence the choice of a career. There have been attempts to establish a relationship between vocational choice and certain factors such as interests, values, and attitudes, but it is generally agreed that no one factor can explain or predict a person's vocational choice. Donald Super, a leader in vocational development theory, believes that the vocational development process is one of implementing a self-concept. This occurs through the interaction of social and individual factors, the opportunity to try various roles, and the perceived amount of approval from peers and supervisors for the roles assumed. There are many other views of this process, but most theorists agree that vocational choice is a developmental process.

How do people choose helping professions as careers? Research in this area tells us that the choice is influenced by direct work experience, college courses and instructors, and the involvement of friends, acquaintances, or relatives in helping professions. Money or salary is a small concern compared with the goals and functions of the work itself. In other words, for individuals who choose helping as their life's work, the kind of work they will do is more important than the pay they will receive (Brown, 2007).

There are several reasons why people choose the helping professions. It is important to be aware of these motivations because each may have positive and negative aspects. One primary reason why individuals choose helping professions (and the reason that most will admit) is the desire to help others. To feel worthwhile as a result of contributing to another's growth is exciting; however, helpers must also ask themselves the following questions: To what extent am I meeting my own needs? Even more important, do my needs to feel worthwhile and to be a caring person take precedence over the client's needs?

Related to this primary motivation is the desire for self-exploration. The wish to find out more about themselves as thinking, feeling individuals leads some people to major in psychology, sociology, or human services. This is a positive factor, because these people will most likely be concerned with gaining insights into their own behaviors and improving their knowledge and skills. After employment, it may become a negative factor if the helper's needs for self-exploration or self-development take precedence over the clients' needs. When this happens, either the helper becomes the client and the client the helper, or there are two clients, neither of whose needs are met. This situation can be avoided when the helper is aware that self-exploration is a personal motivation and can be fulfilled more appropriately outside the helping relationship.

Another strong motivation for pursuing a career in helping is the desire to exert control. For those who admit to this motivation, administrative or managerial positions in helping professions are the goal. This desire may become a problem, however, if helpers seek to control or dominate clients, with the intent of making them dependent or having them conform to an external standard.

For many people, the experience of being helped provides a strong demonstration of the value of helping. Such people often wish to be like those who helped them when they were clients. This appears to be especially true for the fields of teaching and medicine. Unfortunately, this noble motivation may create unrealistic expectations of what being a helper will be like. For example, unsuccessful clients do not become helpers; rather, those who have had a positive helping experience are the ones who will choose this type of profession. Because they were cooperative and motivated clients, they may expect all clients to be like they were, and they may also expect all helpers to be as competent and caring as their helpers were. Such expectations of both the helper and client are unrealistic and may leave the helper frustrated and angry.

VALUES AND HELPING

Values are important to the practice of human services because they are the criteria by which helpers and clients make choices. Every individual has a set of values. Both human service professionals and clients have sets of values. Sometimes they are similar, but often they differ; in some situations, they conflict. Human service professionals should know something about values and how they influence the relationship between the helper and the client.

Where do our values originate? Culture helps establish some values and standards of behavior (Schmidt, 2006). As we grow and learn through our different experiences, general guides to behavior emerge. These guides are **values,** and they give direction to our behavior. Because different experiences lead to different values, individuals do not have the same value systems. Also, as individuals experience more, their values may change. What exactly are values? Values are statements of what is desirable—of the way we would like the world to be. They are not statements of fact.

TABLE 6.1	SUMMARY POINTS: WHY INDIVIDUALS CHOOSE TO WORK IN HELPING PROFESSIONS
Help others	Contribute to another's growth
Self-exploration	Discover more about self
Exert control	Good in administration organization
Positive role models	Inspired by help from others

Values provide a basis for choice. It is important for human service professionals to know what their own values are and how they influence relationships with coworkers and the delivery of services to clients. For example, professionals who value truth will give the client as much feedback as possible from the results of an employment check or a home visitation report. Because human service delivery is a team effort in many agencies and communities, there have to be some common values that will assist helpers in working together effectively. The following are the most commonly held values in human services: acceptance, tolerance, individuality, self-determination, and confidentiality.

The next paragraph introduces Beth Bruce, a human service professional with a variety of experiences. In this section, her experiences are used to illustrate the values that are important to the human service profession.

> Beth Bruce is a human service professional at the Estes Mental Health Center, a comprehensive center serving seven counties. She has been a case manager at Estes for the past eight months and has really enjoyed her first year's work in mental health. Her first job was as a social service provider in a local nursing home, where she worked for two years. She then worked with adolescents as a teacher/counselor at a local mental health institution before joining the Estes staff.

Let's see how human service values relate to Beth's experience as a human service professional.

Acceptance is the ability of the helper to be receptive to the client regardless of the way a client is dressed or what the client may have done. Professionals act on the value of acceptance when they are able to maintain an attitude of goodwill toward clients and to refrain from judging them by factors such as the way they live or whether they have likable personalities. Being accepting also means learning to appreciate the client's culture and family background.

> One of the most important values that Beth holds is accepting her clients for who they are. She has worked with the elderly, teenagers, and now people with mental illness. These populations are different, but they retain one important quality for her: They are all human beings. Her acceptance of all clients has been put to the test. She had a male client in the nursing home who had once been tried for murder and found guilty. Because Beth believed that no circumstance justifies the killing of another, she had difficulty accepting that man as a worthwhile human being.

The second value of human service work is **tolerance**: the helper's ability to be patient and fair toward each client rather than judging, blaming, or punishing the client for prior behavior. A helper who embodies this value will work with the

BOX 6.1 | MY WORK AS A HUMAN SERVICE PROFESSIONAL

Thomoa Pressa, a case manager at a community health agency, describes his work and the skills necessary to be effective.

In my job, I am working hard to help children. That means that I listen to them and then I have to sell to others the idea of helping them. When children are remanded to custody of the state, then I have quite a lot of work to do. I have to conduct several assessments, and once those are complete, then I have to develop a plan for the child. This includes what services the child will receive. My work includes working with the child and, of course, the family. But I also have involvement with members of the court and members of other social service agencies.

My job is really important when I get ready to place a child. I have to know and understand what the child needs but I also have to know what services the child will need. I have to make an assessment about how to match the child with the service. Not everyone in the community agency system can work with these children. I have to find the right place for the child and get the child to the placement at the right time.

It is a challenge sometimes to facilitate communication. I am working with lots of individuals who don't have very good communication skills—in fact, this is one of the reasons that these children are having difficulties. And sometimes I just have to tell people what to do and what their responsibilities are. I will need for everyone to understand the role each plays in helping this child. And all participants in a staffing have to agree with this plan that I have drawn up. In fact, I am telling parents what they need to do if they want to have their children living with them again. And finally, I have to talk to the child about what is happening to him or her and why we are taking the steps that we are taking. This is difficult at times. This is where the selling comes in—selling to the child.

A lot of what I do feels like crisis intervention. And the pace is fast. No day is the same. There are lots of interruptions and then crises involving the children and their families. And we are making critical decisions about these children and the care they need. Two important decisions are deciding what level of care the child needs and who is going to have custody of the child. Then in my job I spend time talking with review boards about the child's case and I have to make reports to the courts.

One thing that has held me in good favor is that I have great professionals on my team and we support each other. And I always strive for the work/life balance and take good care of myself and my own needs.

client to plan for the future, rather than continually focusing on the client's past mistakes.

Beth works with a friend and coworker who is not very tolerant of people with mental illness. Several times, this coworker's intolerance of client behavior has caused problems for the client. Just yesterday, a problem arose with Ms. Mendoza, a 26-year-old woman with schizophrenia who is currently receiving day treatment and lives in a group home. She refused to see her parents when they came to see her at the day treatment center. Mr. Martin, Beth's coworker, forced Ms. Mendoza to see them because he believes that family is very important and that parents have a right to see their children. Now the parents are upset because Ms. Mendoza threw a chair at them. Ms. Mendoza is upset with Mr. Martin for making her see her parents, and Mr. Martin is angry with his client because he feels he was right to insist that she see them.

Individuality is expressed in the qualities or characteristics that make each person unique, distinctive from all other people. Lifestyle, assets, problems, previous life experiences, and feelings are some areas that make this person different. Recognizing and treating each person individually rather than stereotypically is how helpers put this value into practice.

> When Beth first started working with the elderly, she had had little contact with older individuals. What she knew about them she had learned from her grandparents. She thought of the elderly as lively and quick-witted like her grandmother or quiet and shy, living in the past, like her grandfather. During her first months at the nursing home, the clients she encountered continually surprised her. They represented a broad range of human attitudes, behaviors, and experiences. She learned to distinguish between the generalizations she had made about the elderly and the information she now possessed based on her experiences at the nursing home.

Deciding for oneself on a course of action or the resolution to a problem is **self-determination.** The helper allows clients to make up their own minds regarding a decision to be made or an action to be taken. The helper facilitates this action by objectively assisting clients to investigate alternatives and by remembering that the decision is theirs. In some cases, clients are limited by their situations or their choices. For example, a prison inmate may have restricted alternatives from which to choose recreational activities; however, it is the inmate's right to choose from the available alternatives.

> When Beth worked with teenagers, she was constantly aware that although these clients were not of legal age, they needed to believe they had some control over their own lives. She often helped them sort out alternatives, but she constantly resisted when they asked her to give advice or to make their choices for them. In most situations she believed they should assume some responsibility.

The last human service value is **confidentiality.** This is the helper's assurance to clients that the helper will not discuss their cases with other people—that what they discuss between them will not be the subject of conversation with the helper's friends, family, or other clients. The exception to this is the sharing of information with supervisors or in staff meetings where the client's best interests are being served.

> A speech that Beth learned early when she was working with the elderly still applies in her work with clients in community mental health. When clients ask if she will keep information confidential, she responds, "Most information that you give me I will keep to myself. I do keep records about my discussions with you to share with other colleagues who need the information. But at any time, if you tell me of your plans to hurt yourself or others, I will need to tell the appropriate people." This speech reminds Beth of the practical application of this important value.

You should consider the following questions as you think about the meaning of these values in your own life and practice.

- What kinds of client behaviors would be the most difficult for you to accept? How would you meet the challenge of working with these clients?
- When was the last time you felt uncomfortable sharing information about another person? How did you resolve the situation?

As you think about these five values in relation to yourself as a future human service professional, consider the possibility of working with many different clients. As you think about the clients listed here, place a check beside those clients who would be difficult for *you* to work with. Which values might present problems or conflicts for you? Try to respond honestly, not what you think would be socially or professionally desirable.

_____ a man with religious beliefs that cause him to refuse treatment for a life-threatening illness

_____ a same-sex couple who wants to resolve some conflicts they are having in their relationship

_____ a man who wants to leave his wife and two children in order to have sexual adventures with other women

_____ a young woman who wants an abortion but is seeking your help in making the decision

_____ a person who has severe burn scars on the face, shoulders, arms, and hands

_____ a man or woman from a culture where the male is dominant and the female submissive

_____ a person who does not want to work

_____ a man who strongly believes the only way to bring up his children is by punishing them severely

_____ a woman who wants to leave her husband and children in order to have a career and independence but is afraid to do it

_____ a person who is so physically attractive that you cannot concentrate on what the person is saying

_____ a person who speaks no English and makes no effort to do so

Values are the groundwork for creating a philosophy of helping, which in turn provides a basis for working with people. A philosophy of helping embodies beliefs about human nature, the nature of change, and the process of helping. As individuals grow and develop and as their values change, their helping philosophy and style also develop. An example is the way Beth's values translate into her philosophy of helping, which influences her human service practice.

> Beth believes that all human beings are good and that all behavior is directed to the good. She thinks that violence to others, cruelty, and self-abuse are all behaviors that the perpetrators consider to be positive ways to meet their personal needs. She also believes that people have the capacity to change, if only they believe they can change. Hence, the helper's responsibility is to develop clients' belief in themselves and help provide alternatives for change, practical assistance, and support. Because of these views, Beth has high hopes for her clients, and she believes that her major responsibility is to educate and motivate them. She is frustrated when she works with clients who have tried to hurt others, and she is puzzled when those clients do not want to change. In spite of her frustration, she has maintained her belief in the goodness of human beings.

CHARACTERISTICS OF THE HELPER

To be an effective helper demands the use of the helper's whole self, not just a professional segment of it. This requirement creates difficulty when one tries to generalize about the values and characteristics that helpers ought to have. Ideas differ widely about what helpers should be like and what they bring to their work with others. In this section, you will read about some of these ideas. You will also be

| BOX 6.2 | MASLOW'S VIEW OF HELPING |

Abraham Maslow, a man of vision, described life by taking into account "its highest aspirations." He was dedicated to encouraging development of human potential. This enthusiasm led Maslow to make statements on how people can help each other more effectively. The following written statement demonstrates his creativity and his sensitivity toward helping.

Helping? Well, I have a label for it (labels are good, they are useful for me), I call it the Bodhisattvic Version (Path)....There are two Buddhistic legends. In one the Buddha sat under a tree and had the great revelation he saw the truth. It's very Socratic. He saw the truth, the truth was revealed to him, and then he ascended to heaven, so to speak, to Nirvana. In another version, the Bodhisattvic Version, the Buddha sat under the tree, had a great illumination, saw the truth, ascended to the gates of heaven, and there, out of compassion for mankind, could not bear to selfishly enter heaven and came back to earth to help—on the assumption that nobody could go to heaven unless we all go to heaven.

So this is a beautiful legend, and what it means for us, I think, is to recognize that helping in the first place is a very, very hard job and the helper can be a clumsy fool—the helper can be a hurter....To know when to be available and when not is to think of the helper as being available, being the consultant, rather than being the manipulator, controller, interferer, giving orders and telling people what to do....

This is a very hard thing to do—that is, to know when to keep your hands off and when you help and when to be available and so on—especially with our young children, where frequently we do have to interfere. What is implied, therefore, is that one of the paths to being a helper is to become a better and better person, in the psychotherapeutic sense, in the sense of maturing, evolving, becoming more fully human, and so on. If you want to help others best, improve yourself. Cure yourself.

Source: Excerpt from *Abraham H. Maslow: A Memorial Volume, an International Study Project*, pp. 39–42. Copyright © 1972 by Wadsworth Publishing.

encouraged to think about the qualities you possess that might be important to your work as a helping professional, as well as qualities you may want to develop more fully to increase your effectiveness. Box 6.2 outlines how Abraham Maslow thinks about helping and the helping process.

Individuals learn attitudes and behaviors as they respond to their circumstances (Cochran & Cochran, 2006). Some responses may even be unconscious. Through the learning process, a person internalizes these attitudes and behaviors and they become a pattern in his or her life. A major influence on how an individual reacts to these needs is culture. Families, schools, and peers are among the agents who communicate ways of behaving and help determine what an individual considers to be acceptable and unacceptable behavior in different situations. An increasing body of research supports

TABLE 6.2	SUMMARY POINTS: VALUES THAT GUIDE PRACTICE
Acceptance	Maintain goodwill and refrain from judging
Tolerance	Be patient and fair
Respect for individuality	Respect differences, avoid stereotypes
Self-determination	Help clients make decisions
Confidentiality	Will not disclose client information

the concept that the personal characteristics of helpers are largely responsible for the success or failure of their helping (Brown & Srebalus, 2003). In fact, numerous studies concluded that these personal characteristics are as significant in helping as the methods helpers use (Brammer & MacDonald, 2003).

A number of researchers have examined these characteristics, and we studied this work to identify the traits that seem to be universal in effective helpers. The helping person should be able to hear the client and then use his or her knowledge, skills, values, and experience to provide help. To do this, the helper should be self-aware, objective, professionally competent, and actively involved in the enabling process (Okun, 2002). In a review of a number of research studies, Okun (2002) concluded that certain qualities, behaviors, and knowledge on the part of the helper most influence the behaviors, attitudes, and feelings of clients. Self-awareness, honesty, congruence, the ability to communicate, knowledge, and ethical integrity are also included on her list.

Effective helpers have definite traits (Brown & Srebalus, 2003). One way to discuss what these are is to use a framework that suggests two sets of attitudes: one related to self and the other to how one treats another person (Brammer & MacDonald, 2003). Personal congruence, empathy, cultural sensitivity, genuineness, respect, and communication are considered important traits.

All the characteristics mentioned are important ones for helpers. Many other perspectives can be studied, but this brief discussion shows that certain characteristics tend to be common to most studies. In preparing this text, we have reviewed a number of perspectives. Our guiding question was "What characteristics are important for the beginning human service professional?" We identified the following qualities as important: self-awareness, the ability to communicate, empathy, professional commitment, and flexibility. Each of these is discussed in depth to help you understand what the quality is and why it is important for entry-level practice.

SELF-AWARENESS   Most authorities in the helping professions agree that helpers must know who they are because this self-knowledge affects what they do. Developing **self-awareness** is a lifelong process of learning about oneself by continually examining one's beliefs, attitudes, values, and behaviors. Recognizing stereotypes, biases, and cultural and gender differences are part of the self-awareness process. So is our desire for acceptance and client success; "needing" our clients to like us and to do well may be a sign of trouble, however. Self-awareness, then, is a particularly critical process for helpers because it assists them in understanding and changing their attitudes and feelings that may hinder helping. The importance of self-acceptance is underscored by the helper's use of self in the helping process.

Beth Bruce's awareness of self expanded greatly when she began to work in the field full time. As she began to learn about the culture and beliefs of others, she developed a keener sense of who she was. It seemed that, as she developed the patience to work with her first clients—who were mentally ill clients—she also became more patient with herself.

ABILITY TO COMMUNICATE   Helpers' effectiveness depends in part on their ability to communicate to the client an understanding of the client's feelings and behaviors (Okun, 2002). Listening, a critical helping skill, is the beginning of helping and is necessary for establishing trust, building rapport, and identifying the problem.

TABLE 6.3	SUMMARY POINTS: CHARACTERISTICS OF EFFECTIVE HELPERS
Self-awareness	Helper understands self
Ability to communicate	Being "tuned in" to client's message
Empathy	Understand experience from client perspective
Responsibility/commitment	Devoted to well-being of others

Careful listening means being "tuned in" to all the nuances of the client's message, including verbal and nonverbal aspects of what is said as well as what is not said. Such focused listening enables the helper to respond with thoughts and feelings to the client's whole message.

Beth Bruce's ability to communicate was challenged when she began her work with adolescents at the hospital. These young people were aggressive, belligerent, and violent. She worked hard to listen, gain their trust, and provide them honest, constructive feedback. One of the most important skills Beth learned was to listen to the client's entire statement before formulating a response.

EMPATHY **Empathy** is acceptance of another person. This quality allows the helper to see a situation or experience a feeling from the client's perspective. This may be easier for helpers who have had experiences similar to those of their clients. For example, this may explain the understanding that recovering alcoholics have for other alcoholics, widows for the recently bereaved, and parolees for the incarcerated. It does not mean, however, that helpers whose experiences are different cannot express the unconditional acceptance of the client that is a characteristic of empathy.

When Beth worked with her elderly clients, they used to tell her "you will not really understand until you are older." Beth used her communication skills to reflect feelings and content of her clients in order to demonstrate her understanding of their plight.

RESPONSIBILITY/COMMITMENT Feeling a responsibility or commitment to improve the well-being of others is an important attribute of human service professionals. This includes attending to the needs of clients first and foremost. It also means a commitment to delivering high-quality services. In other words, human service professionals act in the best interests of clients and do so to the best of their ability. One way that workers do this is by following a code of ethics or a set of ethical standards that guide professional behavior or conduct. Among other things, codes of ethics in the helping professions spell out what the client has a right to expect from the helper. Honesty may be one expectation of the client—a belief that the professional will be honest in answering questions or in practicing only what he or she is trained to do.

Beth has been troubled by ethical dilemmas throughout her work experience. Fortunately her values have guided her practice and her supervisors have praised her responsible actions. Several examples of ethical codes and standards are presented in Chapter 9.

FLEXIBILITY **Flexibiity** is a multifaceted trait that allows human service professionals to shift their perspectives on the nature of helping, their view of the client and the client's problems, and their preferred interventions. Professionals are willing to reconsider, modify, or abandon their approaches to helping when they encounter difficult or unusual situations. Continually seeking new ways of understanding or other options for providing support to the client, helpers who are flexible understand the complexities of human service work. Sometimes it is challenging for new professionals to be flexible in their approaches to work responsibilities because of their limited experience and inability to consider alternatives. Flexibility is an increasingly important characteristic as human service professionals work with individuals representing different ethnic and cultural groups.

Just as self-awareness helped Beth Bruce be more aware of herself, as she worked with others from different cultures, she has increased her knowledge and understanding of other cultural norms. Her work with African Americans, Cubans, Haitians, and a new wave of Russian émigrés continually expands her perspectives on family, gender roles, the role of spirituality in individual health and development, and the meaning of work. She keeps an open mind in each encounter as she listens for cultural values that differ from her own.

TYPOLOGY OF HUMAN SERVICE PROFESSIONALS

Besides understanding who the human service professional is in terms of characteristics and values, the student of human services should also know the professional categories that describe such workers. The human service profession includes several levels of workers, which may be classified in a variety of ways. Two considerations present in most categorizations are educational preparation or training, and competence. The next subsection discusses categories of professional work developed by two professional educators.

CATEGORIES OF WORKERS

One way to categorize helpers is to divide them into two classes (Brammer & MacDonald, 2003). The first, the nonprofessional, includes helpers who offer unstructured assistance through friendships, family relations, and community and general human concern. The second category, the professional who provides structured helping, is the one in which we are interested. It is further divided into three categories of workers: *professional helpers, paraprofessionals,* and *volunteers* and *peers.* Professional helpers are characterized by certification from professional groups, licenses by governing bodies, and degrees from educational institutions. Examples of professionals in this category are social workers, nurses, ministers, and counselors. The second group consists of **paraprofessional helpers** who perform some of the traditional counseling functions but also engage in broader roles, such as those of advocate and mobilizer. Peers and volunteers are a third broad group that encompasses those with little or not training as well as those with extensive training. Often training and orientation is offered to prepare these workers for their responsibilities working with clients and providing indirect administrative services.

What distinguishes each group is the amount of formal training its members have had, their level of responsibility, and their degree of participation in policy formation. In addition, members of the professional group possess research skills, a wider theoretical background, and clinical judgment, a result of their clinical training and supervision. Tension may occur between paraprofessionals and professionals, in part because of increasing evidence that each group may be as effective as the other in delivering services.

A second way to categorize helpers, similar to Brammer and MacDonald's (2003) system, is one proposed by Okun (2002), who categorizes workers as *professional helpers, generalist human service workers,* and *nonprofessional helpers.* Workers who are trained specialists with graduate-level training in helping theory and skills and who often have supervised clinical experience are classified as professional helpers, even though their training and credentials may vary. These professional helpers may work with generalist human service workers as part of a team, as supervisors, or as consultants. Generalist human service workers have education and training at the undergraduate level and job titles such as psychiatric technicians or aides, youth street workers, day care staff, probation officers, and church workers. Okun's third category, **nonprofessional helpers,** includes workers with some training in helping and little agency responsibility. They use communication skills to develop helping relationships with those people they are assisting. Included here are volunteers who work for no pay and peer helpers who may be similar in age and experience to the clients.

THE HUMAN SERVICE PROFESSIONAL

As a result of an unmet need for trained, educated workers in human services, the 1992–1993 edition of the *Occupational Outlook Handbook (OOH)* included an entry on the human service worker. The latest edition of the handbook divides careers into several categories, including one for community and service occupations such as counselors, probation officers and correctional treatment specialists, social and human service assistants, and social workers. According to the descriptions of these occupations, probation officers and correctional treatment specialists, social and human service assistants, and social workers fit within the definition of those performing human service work (Bureau of Labor Statistics, 2006).

According to the *OOH,* those who work in the field of corrections usually have a bachelor's degree in social work, criminal justice, or a related field. The primary job responsibilities include working in probation, in parole, or at correctional institutions. When describing the field of social and human service assistants, the *OOH* states, "Social and human service assistant is a generic term for people with a wide array of job titles, including human service worker, case management aide, social work assistant, community support worker, mental health aide, community outreach worker, life skill counselor, or gerontology aide" (Bureau of Labor Statistics, 2006). The *Handbook* suggests that these professionals work under the supervision of other helping professionals such as nurses, physical therapists, psychologists, and others. The jobs vary, as do the responsibilities and type of supervision. Job opportunities in these two categories are growing rapidly.

The category titled "social workers" also describes opportunities for both social workers and human service professionals, especially those graduating from four-year human service programs. The nature of the work is described "for those with a strong desire to help improve people's lives . . . help people function the best way they can in

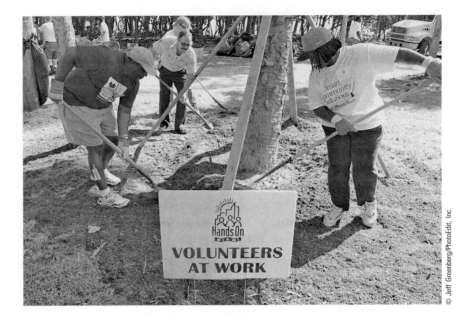

their environment, deal with their relationships, and solve personal and family problems . . . see clients who face a life threatening disease or social problem" (Bureau of Labor Statistics, 2006). The various areas of responsibility include counseling, child welfare, family services, child or adult protective services, mental health, substance abuse, criminal justice, occupational counseling, and work with the aging. Job opportunities for social workers and professionals from related fields will increase through the next decade.

OTHER PROFESSIONAL HELPERS

As a human service professional, you will be working with a variety of other professional helpers. This section, adapted from the 2006–2007 *Occupational Outlook Handbook,* identifies the nature of the work and the training of these individuals so that you will be familiar with them.

PHYSICIANS **Physicians** perform medical examinations, diagnose illnesses, treat injured or diseased people, and advise patients on maintaining good health. They may be general practitioners or specialists in a particular field of medicine. Physicians are required by all states to be licensed. It usually takes about 11 years to become a physician: 4 years of undergraduate school, 4 years of medical school, and 3 years of residency. Those who choose to specialize usually spend 3 to 5 years in training and another 2 years in preparation for practice in a specialty area.

One example of a specialist with whom you will likely be in contact is a **psychiatrist.** Concerned with the diagnosis, treatment, and prevention of mental illness, psychiatrists may be found in private offices and institutional settings, courtrooms, community-centered care facilities, and specialized medical areas such as coronary and intensive care units. They frequently act as consultants to other agencies. Psychiatrists are medical doctors who have an additional five years or more of psychiatric training and experience and are qualified to use the full range of medical techniques in treating clients. These include drugs, shock therapy, and surgery, in addition to counseling and behavior modification techniques.

PSYCHOLOGISTS   Although their training and the kinds of treatment they use are different, **psychologists** are sometimes confused with psychiatrists. Psychologists study human behavior and mental processes to understand and explain people's actions. An individual may specialize in any of several areas within psychology, including clinical, counseling, developmental, industrial organizational, school, and social psychology. Each specialty focuses on a different aspect of human behavior. For example, the developmental psychologist is concerned with the behavioral changes people experience as they progress through life. Clinical psychologists, on the other hand, may work in hospitals, clinics, or private practice to help individuals who are mentally or emotionally disturbed adjust to life, and to help medical and surgical patients deal with their illnesses and injuries. They may use interviews, diagnostic tests, and psychotherapy in their work.

Psychologists may practice with a master's degree or a doctoral degree. A master's degree prepares the person to administer and interpret tests, conduct research, and counsel patients. The doctoral degree usually requires five to seven years of graduate study and is often required for employment as a psychologist. A doctorate in psychology and two years of professional experience are generally required for licensure or certification; although requirements may vary from state to state, certification is necessary for private practice.

SOCIAL WORKERS   The focus of **social workers** is helping individuals, families, and groups cope with a wide variety of problems. The nature of the problem and the time and resources available determine the methods used, which may include counseling, advocacy, and referral. Social workers also function at the community level to combat social problems. For example, they may coordinate existing programs, organize fund-raising, and develop new community services. Social workers may also specialize in various areas. Medical social workers are trained to help patients and their families cope with problems that accompany illness or rehabilitation. Those who specialize in family services counsel individuals to strengthen personal and family relationships. Corrections and child welfare are other popular areas of study and employment.

Preparation for the field of social work occurs at two levels. The baccalaureate level (BSW) is the minimum requirement, followed by the master's degree in social work (MSW), which is usually required for positions in mental health and for administrative or research positions. Training generally includes courses of study focusing on social work practice, social welfare policies, human behavior, and the social environment. Supervised field experiences are also necessary.

The National Association of Social Workers (NASW) awards certification in the form of the title ACSW, which stands for the Academy of Certified Social Workers. Licensing or registration laws have also been passed by many states to regulate social work practice.

COUNSELORS One of the largest categories of professional helpers is **counselors.** Although their exact duties depend on the individuals or groups with whom they work and the agencies or settings in which they are employed, counselors help people deal with a variety of problems, including personal, social, educational, and career concerns. Examples of the different types of counselors are school and college counselors, rehabilitation counselors, employment counselors, and mental health counselors. Two with whom you may interact as a human service professional are mental health counselors and rehabilitation counselors.

The *mental health counselor* works with individuals who are dealing with problems such as drug and alcohol abuse, family conflicts, suicidal thoughts and feelings, stress management, problems with self-esteem, issues associated with aging, job and career concerns, educational decisions, and issues of mental and emotional health. Their work is not limited to individuals, however; it may involve the family of the individual. These counselors often work closely with other specialists such as psychiatrists, psychologists, clinical social workers, and psychiatric nurses.

The *rehabilitation counselor* helps people deal with the personal, social, and vocational effects of their disabilities. Disabilities may be social, mental, emotional, or physical, calling for the services of counseling, evaluation, medical care, occupational training, and job placement. Rehabilitation counselors also work with the family of the individual when necessary and frequently with other professionals such as physicians, psychologists, and occupational therapists.

Positions as a counselor usually require a master's degree in a counseling discipline or a related area. This preparation frequently includes a year or two of graduate study and a supervised counseling experience. Licensure and certification are available; requirements vary, depending on the specialty. The National Board for Certified Counselors (NBCC) and the Commission on Rehabilitation Counselor Certification (CRCC) are two national certifying bodies. There are also certifying boards in each of the 50 states.

Human service professionals could assume the responsibilities of social workers or counselors, or be given this title, even though they might not be specifically certified as such. The variation in the needs of agencies and the competencies of individual workers makes it difficult to establish rigid categories for function or title. However, having the title or performing the job of a mental health counselor is definitely not the same as being nationally certified. Some states and agencies will only hire workers with national certification, whereas other sites have more flexible hiring categories.

TABLE 6.4 | SUMMARY POINTS: OTHER PROFESSIONAL HELPERS

Physicians	Licensed medical professionals who provide general medical services or specialty services
Psychologists	Study human behavior to understand individual thoughts and actions
Social Workers	Help individuals, families, and groups cope with problems
Counselors	Help people deal with a variety of problems

HUMAN SERVICE ROLES

At this point in Chapter 6, you have some idea about the identity of the human service professional and the relationship of this individual with other helping professionals. An examination of their roles further defines the human service professional.

The many human service roles to be introduced provide the framework for the helping process. In performing the various roles, the human service professional is continuously focused on the client; this client focus provides the common thread to connect the roles.

Although the roles of human service professionals are constantly evolving, the helper remains a "Jack or Jill of all trades," or, in human service terms, a generalist. The generalist knows a wide range of skills, strategies, and client groups and is able to work effectively in a number of different settings. Engaging in a variety of roles enables the human service professional to meet many client needs. What exactly do these helpers do?

Many professionals have attempted to answer this question. The Southern Regional Education Board (SREB) conducted a study in the late 1960s to define the roles and functions of human service professionals. As a result of this analysis, SREB identified 13 roles that human service workers could engage in to meet the needs of their clients, agencies, or communities (Southern Regional Education Board, 1969). These 13 roles include administrator, advocate, assistant to specialist, behavior changer, broker, caregiver, community planner, consultant, data manager, evaluator, mobilizer, outreach worker, and teacher/educator.

In a more recent study, the U.S. Department of Education funded the Community Support Skills Standards Project to define the skills that human service personnel need to work in the field. The result of the work was a set of 12 broad, functional themes of work in human services. These emerged from a job analysis and are reflected in the project's report as competency areas. The areas are as follows: participant empowerment; communication; assessment; community and service networking; facilitation of services; community living skills and supports; education, training, and self-development; advocacy; vocational, educational, and career support; crisis intervention; organizational participation; and documentation (Community Support Skill Standards Project, 2006).

The National Organization for Human Services in concert with the Council for Standards in Human Service Education also define the human service professional and summarize the work that these helpers do. In a document that defines the human service worker, commitment to others in need is emphasized. The document states:

> "Human services worker" is a generic term for people who hold professional and paraprofessional jobs in such diverse settings as group homes and halfway houses; correctional, mental retardation, and community mental health centers; family, child, and youth service agencies; and programs concerned with alcoholism, drug abuse, family violence, and aging. Depending on the employment setting and the kinds of clients served there, job titles and duties vary a great deal. The primary purpose of the human service worker is to assist individuals and communities to function as effectively as possible in the major domains of living (National Organization for Human Services, 2006).

To better understand the varied roles that are assumed by the human service professional, we used the results of these studies to categorize three areas of responsibility:

TABLE 6.5 | HUMAN SERVICE ROLES

Providing Direct Service	Performing Administrative Work	Working with the Community
Behavior changer	Broker	Advocate
Caregiver	Data manager	Community and service networker
Communicator	Evaluator	Community planner
Crisis intervener	Facilitator of services	Consultant
Participant empowerer	Planner	Mobilizer
Teacher/educator	Report writer	Outreach worker
	Resource allocator	

providing direct service, performing administrative work, and working with the community. Next we examine these three categories and the roles that represent each area of responsibility. (See Table 6.5.)

PROVIDING DIRECT SERVICE

Providing direct service to clients is a responsibility with which many beginning professionals are familiar. This work represents the development of the helping relationship and the work that helpers do in their face-to-face encounters with their clients. Many roles, such as behavior changer, caregiver, communicator, crisis intervener, participant empowerer, and teacher/educator, are included in the category of direct services. The following illustrate many of these roles and how human service professionals perform them.

Behavior changer—carries out a range of activities planned primarily to change clients' behavior, ranging from coaching and counseling to casework, psychotherapy, and behavior therapy.

> Sun Lee Kim is a substance abuse counselor at a drug and alcohol inpatient clinic at a local hospital. Sun Lee, one of the staff group leaders, facilitates a reality therapy group each day. The purpose of this group is to encourage participants to change their communication behavior, first in the group and later in the wider context of the facility. Peer support and pressure are used to facilitate this behavior change.

Caregiver—provides services for people who need ongoing support of some kind, such as financial assistance, day care, social support, and 24-hour care.

> Jim Gray works in foster care. His major responsibility is to provide support to families with foster children. One of his favorite activities is to visit foster homes to determine the success of the foster care situation and provide emotional and practical assistance to the families.

Communicator—is able to express and exchange ideas and establish relationships with a variety of individuals and groups, including clients, families, colleagues, administrators, and the public.

> Dal Lam works with AIDS patients in a self-help center established by a regional hospital in a rural desert area. His responsibilities require him to communicate with different populations that include individuals who are testing HIV positive, individuals with AIDS, medical staff, insurance providers, families, and community groups. He spends much of his time in prevention work that takes him to the elementary schools, local high schools, civic meetings, and churches. His approach is always the same: clear, articulate, compassionate, and confident.

Crisis intervener—provides services for individuals, families, and communities who are experiencing a disruption in their lives with which they cannot cope. This intervention is short term, focused, and concrete.

> Christy Holston works in a sexual assault crisis center and is a victim advocate. She receives four or five new clients a week, mostly women, who are dealing with issues of sexual assault, attempted rape, or rape. Some of her clients call through the hotline immediately after being assaulted, others are referred through the emergency room at the hospital, and others call to ask for help many years after the crisis.

Participant empowerer—shares with clients the responsibility for the helping relationship and the development and implementation of a plan of action. This helper ultimately encourages clients to care for themselves.

> Judy Collins is a case manager for young adults who are developmentally disabled. In the program, First Steps, she works with clients to move from group home living to apartment living. She coordinates daily living training, vocational assessment and training, and first employment. Her clients participate fully in the case management process and are called "co-case managers." There is a graduation ceremony when these clients become their own "case managers."

Teacher/educator— performs a range of instructional activities, from simple coaching to teaching highly technical content, directed at individuals or groups.

> Dr. Washington Lee, a physician, and Ned Wanek, a human service professional, work in a family planning clinic. They spend two mornings a week teaching classes to women and men about the reproductive system and alternative methods of family planning. In addition, they counsel individuals, provide physical exams, plan educational media, and talk to schools and community groups about family planning.

PERFORMING ADMINISTRATIVE WORK

Performing administrative work is another important responsibility for many human service professionals. In addition to providing direct services to clients, many helpers are involved in managerial activities as they supervise or oversee processes or projects. As they work with clients, they assume administrative responsibilities such as planning, linking clients to services, allocating resources, and evaluating. The specific administrative roles are broker, data manager, evaluator, facilitator of services, planner, report (documentation) writer, and resource allocator.

Broker—helps people get to the existing services and helps make the services more accessible to clients.

> Maria Giovanni's caseload at the Office for Student Services consists primarily of students with physical disabilities. One of her functions is to make sure these students have their classes scheduled in accessible buildings on campus and are able to get around campus to their classes and school events. To achieve this goal, Maria may have to help students reschedule classes or arrange for parking. She is also "on call" to assist these students in getting other services they might need.

Data manager—gathers, tabulates, analyzes, and synthesizes data and evaluates programs and plans.

> Roosevelt Thompson is part of the staff of a local day care center. Although he assists the child-care staff when needed, his actual responsibilities are business oriented. The day care center is privately owned but partially funded by the city. Its clients include children referred to the center from the courts for temporary care as well as children of working parents. His concern is to see that the center maintains an appropriate balance between referred and regular paying clients to maintain its financial stability. He continually gathers information and projects the financial needs of the day care center.

Evaluator—assesses client or community needs and problems, whether medical, psychiatric, social, or educational.

> Karen Tubbs leads a community planning organization established to assess the community's needs in the event of a national disaster. In her coastal region, disaster means the threat of damaging winds, rain, and numerous hurricanes. Its meetings are part of a complex process of planning for and developing resources to begin providing human services should a hurricane strike their region.

Facilitator of services—brokers (links the client to services) and then monitors the progress the client makes with the various helping professionals. This helper also uses the problem-solving process when services are deficient or inappropriate.

> Louisa Gonzales works in a group home for young children who need a short-term safe haven. During the time the children are in the home, Louisa spends many hours coordinating their care with schools, child-care agencies, the health department, and the welfare department. Many times, without her services, these children would get lost in the system and would receive substandard care.

Planner—engages in making plans with both short-term and long-term clients in order to define accurately their problems and needs, develops strategies to meet the needs, and monitors the helping process. Planners also help develop programs and services to meet client needs.

> Ruth Strauss works with families who are planning for the long-term care of aging parents. This requires careful attention to the needs and priorities of all involved. She has better luck with her families when she uses a very structured planning and decision-making model. With this model, everyone in the family has a clear understanding of the problems and the goals and can monitor the success of the plan. She also serves on a program development team that creates new programs for families.

Report (documentation) writer—records the activities of the agency work. This can include intake interview reports, social histories, detailed treatment plans, daily entries into case notes, requests for resources, rationale and justification for treatment for managed care, and periodic reports for managed care.

> Lisa Wilhiem is a social worker in a local hospital emergency room. She is the intermediary for clients who will potentially need longer-term care. It is her responsibility to coordinate the initial requests for services to the managed care organizations or insurance companies. Although she spends several hours of her day with patients and the medical care staff, a majority of her time is spent documenting how the patient entered the health care system and what the current needs of the patient are.

Resource allocator—makes recommendations on how resources are to be spent to support the needs of the client. These recommendations are made once priorities are set and prices for services are determined.

> Hoover Center, a psychiatric facility for adolescents, is developing a new program that will individualize the treatment of its clients. In the past, there was a standard treatment for all clients regardless of their problems. Because of the pressures from managed care and the limited resources available for the center, the decision has been made to ask each client's case manager to establish priorities and determine how the resources per client are to be spent. The case manager will submit a plan that will be approved by the supervisor and then submitted to the managed care organization for review and final approval.

WORKING WITH THE COMMUNITY

Many professionals are also very involved with their community as they develop collegial networks and work on behalf of their clients to create and improve services within the local area and beyond. The roles of advocate, community and service networker, community planner, consultant, mobilizer, and outreach worker are those which the helper assumes responsibility in the community context.

Advocate—pleads and fights for services, policies, rules, regulations, and laws on behalf of clients.

> Jose Cervantes is a lawyer for a legal aid clinic in an urban area. His clients, referred by the courts, are individuals who need legal services but cannot pay for them. Most of his cases involve marital separation, divorce, custody of children, and spouse and child support. Besides handling individual cases, Jose works with politicians, judges, and other lawyers to develop a legal system that is sensitive to the needs of his clients.

Community and service networker—works actively to connect with other helpers and agencies to plan for providing better services to the community and to clients, share information, support education and training efforts, and facilitate linking clients to the services they need.

> Ian DeBusk has been working for the public schools for the past 20 years. Early in his career he worked with in-school suspension programs and today he supervises school counselors in 15 high schools, 12 middle schools, and 32 elementary schools. One of his responsibilities is to help his counselors find the services their students need. Ian has colleagues within the criminal justice system, child welfare services, health department, and vocational rehabilitation agency, to name just a few. Each day he spends

time on the phone and on the road helping those in his network and also asking them to help his counselors and their students.

Community planner—works with community boards and committees to ensure that community services promote mental health and self-actualization, or at least minimize emotional stress on people.

> Hector Gomez is director of the local department of human services. As director, part of his responsibility is to provide leadership in human services to the city and county. He spends many evenings attending board meetings with other members of the community discussing funding and future planning for human services.

Consultant—works with other professionals and agencies regarding their handling of problems, needs, and programs.

> Three members of a pediatric language lab serving young children with communication disorders have formed a consulting service as part of their job responsibilities with the lab. The focus of the service is to educate teachers and day care staff about communication disorders and help them work with children in their own facilities. The consulting activity will enable the lab to expand the impact of its services.

Mobilizer/Community organizer—helps to get new resources for clients and communities.

> Just last week James Shabbaz, a psychiatric social worker at the research hospital, discovered that the funding for the newly formed hospice service was not being renewed. The support services provided to family members of dying patients will be difficult to replace. James has decided to schedule a meeting with hospital staff and members of local churches to assist him in thinking about alternative support for these family members.

Outreach worker—reaches out to identify people with problems, refer them to appropriate services, and follow up to make sure they continue to their maximum rehabilitation.

> Greg Jones from the local mental health center travels into rural sections of a three-county area to follow up on patients who have been released from the regional mental health facility. His primary responsibilities are to provide supportive counseling, assess current progress, and make appropriate referrals.

Each job in the human service field represents a unique combination of roles and responsibilities. The following list shows the way in which roles and responsibilities can be configured.

HOME HEALTH CARE COORDINATOR
- Broker
- Data manager
- Evaluator
- Facilitator of services
- Report writer (documentation)

PAROLE OFFICER
- Broker
- Data manager

- Planner
- Report (documentation) writer

MENTAL HEALTH CASE MANAGER
- Behavior changer
- Caregiver
- Crisis intervener
- Data manager
- Evaluator
- Facilitator of services
- Report (documentation) writer
- Resource allocator

CHILD CARE PROFESSIONAL
- Advocate
- Behavior changer
- Communicator
- Report (documentation) writer
- Teacher/educator

FOOD BANK ORGANIZER
- Communicator
- Community and service networker
- Community planner
- Mobilizer
- Outreach worker

As you learn more about human services and meet human service professionals, try to determine the roles they are performing and the responsibilities they assume as they work with clients, their colleagues, and the community.

FRONTLINE HELPER OR ADMINISTRATOR

Helpers may generally be categorized as having either frontline or administrative responsibilities. Using only these two categories may oversimplify the actual responsibilities of a given helper, but the categorization is useful when you are visualizing what human service professionals actually do. The schedules that follow outline the typical day of a **frontline helper** and an **administrator.**

FRONTLINE HELPER: WOMEN'S CASE COORDINATOR (SHELTER FOR BATTERED WOMEN AND THEIR CHILDREN)

8:00 A.M. Use this time to finish what needs to be completed from the previous day if planned activities were interrupted by an emergency with a client. Read the progress notes in the case files. See clients at about 8:30—set up the appointments a day in advance. See each client two or three times each week, depending on their schedules. Be prepared for a crisis and a new client.

10:00 A.M. Go to court for orders of protection. This can last all day, depending on how many cases are on the docket. Go to court with a client for her hearing or to file for an order of protection.

11:00 A.M. If back from court, see clients or do paperwork. Return phone calls and e-mails.

12:00 noon Go to the dining room to eat with clients.

1:00 P.M. Run errands with clients; go to their homes for clothing or important documents. Get a police escort for entering the home.

3:00 P.M. Attend staff meetings once a week (usually lasting a couple of hours). During these meetings, discuss each case and service issues.

5:00 P.M. Update case notes. Set up appointments for the next day. Make phone calls and check e-mails.

ADMINISTRATOR: DIRECTOR, SOCIAL SERVICES

8:00 A.M. Attend morning meetings to coordinate staff activities. Prioritize week's projects.

9:00 A.M. Check client vacancies; plan for number of admissions. Make phone calls. Check e-mails. Gather information, review referrals, and schedule meetings and follow-up activities.

10:00 A.M. Meet with families, phone hospitals for possible admissions, meet with clients.

11:00 A.M. Meet with head administrator. Make plans, revise schedule for afternoon. Check phone calls and emails.

12:00 noon Eat at desk or with clients. Catch up on mail, read reports, write letters.

1:00 P.M. Discharge planning for clients. Meet with part-time staff. Reprioritize based on morning's activities.

2:00 P.M. Meet with other professionals, such as bookkeepers and nurses; contact services outside agency for information, planning, and referrals.

3:00 P.M. Complete referral book and complaint log. Make sure all tasks and written correspondence are completed. Be available to see clients and families. Follow up on a crisis encounters by a case manager. Client is in jail.

4:00 P.M. Answer phone calls. Check e-mails. Finish reports due that day. Visit with clients and families.

5:00 P.M. Complete paperwork. Plan for the next day. Answer phone calls, call people at home. Check e-mails.

7:00 P.M. Evening visit with family or client in hospital, read mail, work on big projects to improve services, attend professional meetings.

As you can see by reading these examples, both professionals perform more than one role. Although frontline helpers and administrators sometimes have similar responsibilities, each has a different focus. The frontline helper focuses on caring for the client; the administrator's primary focus is on planning and organizing

BOX 6.3	WEB SOURCES

Find Out More about Helper Roles

http://www.caregiver.com/

This site provides help to those providing 24-hour services to individuals who cannot care for themselves. It provides online discussions and resources for those providing this care. Sometimes the human service professional is the caregiver; other times the professional is supporting the "at-home" 24-hour caregiver.

www.apa.org

This website of the American Psychological Association provides information for students who are interested in pursuing careers in psychology. It also offers an opportunity for users to search more specific topics such as roles.

www.acsu.buffalo.edu/~drstall/hndbk0.html

This site is a handbook for the caregiver of the elderly. It contains in-depth discussion of issues that caregivers (both professional and lay) face and provides suggestions for help and support. It is comprehensive and covers topics such as legal and ethical issues.

www.crisishotline.org/

This website is the crisis hotline in Houston, Texas. Many helping professionals are involved in crisis intervention. This site describes the services provided, including a hotline and crisis counseling.

services. Both have valuable responsibilities in human service delivery and share the ultimate goal of helping clients.

CASE STUDY

The following case study provides an example of a human service professional who is involved with many of the issues helpers encounter. As you read the case study, consider the helper's roles, values, and characteristics. Are there any potential sources of frustration for the helper? What are her expectations?

Carmen Rodriguez has worked as a vocational evaluator for a state agency in the southwestern United States for the past four years. She considers herself a human service professional; with most of her clients, the focus of her work is much broader than just vocational counseling. She describes her job as follows.

MEET CARMEN RODRIGUEZ

I have been a work evaluator for the past four years. In my position, I work with clients to assist them in preparing for and finding gainful employment. One of the requirements for eligibility for services at my agency is that the individual must have a mental, physical, or emotional disability that is a handicap to employment. There must also be a reasonable expectation that the person can be gainfully employed after receiving services.

One of the aspects of my work that I like a lot is the variety of clients I encounter. They are of different ages and from varied backgrounds. I work with many Mexican Americans and Native Americans. My clients are both males and females and, as I said, they have various disabilities. Usually I work with a client every day for a period of six to eight weeks. Because of this close contact, I feel that I get to know my clients well.

Clients come first with me. I constantly think about what I can do for them, and I want to help them in any way I can. Sometimes their circumstances seem so poor, but I know that if I work hard enough I can make their lives better.

Another rewarding part of my job is working with other professionals. We are all committed to meeting client needs, although at times we are limited by the purposes of our various agencies. We've found that we are much more successful working together. In fact, ten of us from different agencies meet monthly for lunch to talk about our work and find out about other services that may be available. It's also a good time to find out about new legislation and regulations and the ways agencies are dealing with funding problems or new grants.

Another part of my work that I find particularly challenging is consulting with a variety of specialists, including psychologists, psychiatrists, and other medical specialists. It's important that I be able to speak their language to a certain extent so that I can tell them what we want them to evaluate and the kinds of information they can provide to assist us in our evaluation of the client. It's also helpful to know some of the terminology so that I can understand their reports. It does make me nervous to talk to these professionals, because their training is different from mine. It is easier now than when I first began working here.

I guess it's pretty obvious how I feel about my work. It's rewarding and challenging, and I feel as if I learn something new each day. It may seem as if it's the perfect job, but it really isn't. There are some negative aspects to it, and probably the most frustrating is that in a bureaucracy things never seem to move as quickly as I want them to. For example, there is quite a bit of paperwork. To receive an authorization for services, I have to go through several channels. This sometimes takes days, and since I work with the client on a daily basis, I get as impatient as the client.

The other aspect of my job that I sometimes find frustrating is that clients often do not do what I would like them to do. When you work with people, it's important to realize that you don't tell them what to do. Actually, we try to teach them to take responsibility for their actions, and this involves making decisions for themselves. When they make a decision that is not in their best interest or may lead to problems or failure, it's very difficult for me not to intervene. I want so much for my clients to succeed, but I've learned that they are independent individuals who must live their own lives. In spite of the frustrations, I hope to keep this job for several years. It offers many opportunities for professional growth and gives me a chance to make a difference.

Apply what you have read in this chapter by answering the following questions about Carmen Rodriguez.

- What motivates Carmen in her work?
- What do you think Carmen's philosophy is? What are her values?
- Identify the professionals with whom Carmen works.
- What human services roles does Carmen play?

Key Terms

acceptance	flexibility	paraprofessional helpers	self-awareness
administrator	frontline helper		self-determination
confidentiality	individuality	physicians	social workers
counselors	nonprofessional helpers	psychiatrists	tolerance
empathy		psychologists	values

THINGS TO REMEMBER

1. Helping means assisting people to understand, overcome, or cope with problems. A helper is one who offers such assistance.

2. The primary reason why individuals choose helping professions (and the reason most will admit) is the desire to help others. Related to this is the desire for self-exploration.

3. Values are important to the practice of human services, because they are the criteria by which human service professionals and clients make choices.

4. Acceptance, tolerance, individuality, self-determination, and confidentiality are important values for human service professionals.

5. Characteristics that are important for the entry-level human service professional are self-awareness, the ability to communicate, empathy, professional commitment, and flexibility.

6. One way of categorizing helping professionals is a three-level system: professional helpers, entry-level professionals, and nonprofessionals.

7. Human service professionals work with other professionals, including physicians, psychologists, social workers, and counselors.

8. The broad range of job titles, duties, client groups, and employment settings in human services supports the generic focus of the profession.

9. Roles and responsibilities of human service professionals can be grouped into three categories: providing direct service, performing administrative work, and working with the community.

10. Frontline helpers and administrators are two more categories of human service professionals that describe the complexities of their roles.

ADDITIONAL READINGS: FOCUS ON HELPERS

Balfour, S. (2005). *Nursing America: One year behind the nursing stations of an inner-city hospital.* NY: Tarcher/Penguin.

The author follows eight nurses in a regional hospital in Memphis, Tennessee, as they work in trauma, burn, and adult special care units. Their daily routines are comprised of the challenges of constant emergencies, job uncertainty, and anonymity.

Blumberg, T. A. (2004). *No time for lunch: Memoirs of an inner city psychologist.* NY: Devora Publishing.

As a school psychologist for the Baltimore City Public Schools for almost 25 years, the author has worked with a cross-section of children—those who endured physical abuse, who chose elective mutism, who lived in fear, and who created fear.

Grobman, L. M. (2004). *Days in the lives of social workers: 54 professionals tell "real-life" stories from social work practice.* Harrisburg, PA: White Hat Communications.

Fifty-four different settings are represented in these accounts of social work practice by social workers themselves. They provide a firsthand, close-up look at their work.

Jacob, J. (2007). *Our school: The inspiring story of two teachers, one big idea, and the charter school that beat the odds.* NY: Palgrave Mac-Millan.

The account of an inner city school in San Jose, California, that adopted a new approach to charter school education. The book captures the struggles, inspiration, and gutsy determination of teachers, students, and parents.

Kidder, T. (2003). *Mountains beyond mountains: The quest of Dr. Paul Farmer, a man who would cure the world.* New York: Random House.

An account of the life of Dr. Paul Farmer, an infectious disease specialist who travels the world diagnosing and curing these diseases.

Parent, M. (1998). *Turning stones: My days and nights with children at risk.* New York: Harcourt Brace & Co.

The author, a caseworker for Emergency Children's Services in New York, has written this memoir about some of the abused children he has helped—or failed.

References

Brammer, L. M., & MacDonald, G. (2003). *The helping relationship: Process and skills.* Boston: Allyn & Bacon.

Brown, D. (2007). *Career information, career counseling, and career development* (9th ed.). Boston: Allyn & Bacon.

Brown, D., & Srebalus, D. J. (2003). *An introduction to the counseling profession* (2nd ed.). Boston: Allyn & Bacon.

Bureau of Labor Statistics. (2006). *2006–2007 Occupational outlook handbook.* Retrieved October 29, 2006, from http://www.bls.gov/oco/oco1002.htm.

Cochran, J. L., & Cochran, N. (2006). *The heart of counseling: A guide to developing therapeutic relationships.* Pacific Grove, CA: Brooks/Cole/Thomson.

Community Support Skill Standards Project. (2006). *About the CSSS Project.* Retrieved October 29, 2006 from http://www.hsri.org/ddworkforce/csss/aboutcsss.html.

National Organization for Human Services. (2006). *The human service worker: A generic job description.* Retrieved October 29, 2006, http://www.nationalhumanservices.org/hsworker.html.

Okun, B. F. (2002). *Effective helping: Interviewing and counseling techniques* (6th ed.). Pacific Grove, CA: Brooks/Cole.

Schmidt, J. J. (2006). *Social and cultural foundations of counseling and human services: Multiple influences on self-concept development.* Boston: Allyn & Bacon.

Southern Regional Education Board. (1969). *Roles and functions for different levels of mental health workers.* Atlanta, GA: Author.

The Practice of
Human Services

PART | III

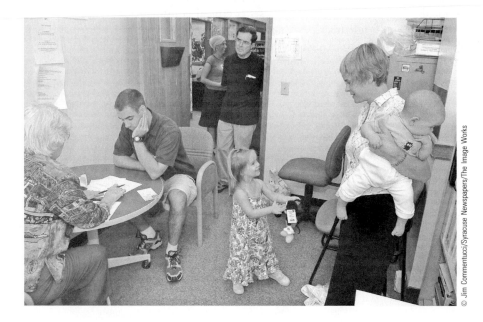

© Jim Commentucci/Syracuse Newspapers/The Image Works

Questions to Consider

- What is the nature of the helping process?
- What communication skills facilitate the process?
- How can knowledge of the working environment be useful in understanding human service delivery?
- What important ethical and professional issues must human service workers be prepared to face?

• • •

Part Three focuses on the practice of human services and the context in which helping occurs. Chapter 7 explores the helping process, introducing the skills helpers need to do their jobs well. The chapter concludes with a section on brief therapy and crisis intervention. Chapter 8 addresses the environment of the human service system. It begins with an examination of components such as mission and goals that help define the nature of the organization. The chapter then covers the referral process, challenges human service professionals face in their day-to-day work, and ways of using the system to assist clients and the community at large. As community organizers, human service professionals are able to extend their work to meet the needs of a wider audience and to serve as advocates for those in need. Part Three concludes with Chapter 9, Professional Concerns. This chapter presents ethical considerations for the human service professional and describes practical applications of ethical principles. The purpose of Part Three is to refine the definition of human services (developed in Parts One and Two) by examining the helping process in actual practice. As you read the three chapters in this section, think about the questions to consider.

THE HELPING PROCESS

CHAPTER 7

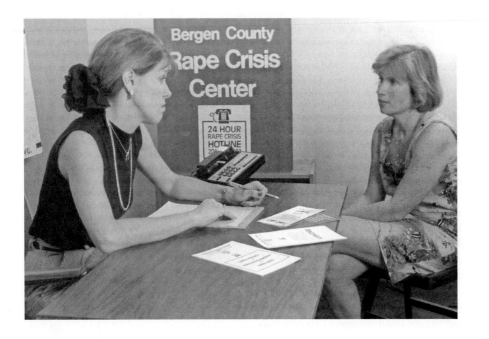

After reading this chapter, you will be able to:

- Distinguish helping relationships from other relationships.
- Recognize the skills essential for the development of a helping relationship.
- Demonstrate how a helper listens and responds to a client.
- Describe challenging clients.
- Identify the phases of a crisis and the skills necessary for crisis intervention.
- List the four stages of resolution-focused brief therapy.

Self-assessment

- What distinguishes the helping relationship from other relationships?
- Explain the purposes of each of the five stages of the helping process. What special attitudes, skills, and values do helpers need for each of the five stages?
- What special knowledge do helpers need to understand nonverbal messages? How can this understanding aid in the helping process?
- Why are verbal messages important? How does an understanding of verbal messages help when working with culturally different clients? Reluctant/resistant clients?
- Describe how the helper might best listen and respond to the client.
- What special understanding do helpers need to work with culturally different clients and reluctant/resistant clients?
- Why is a crisis different from other helping situations?

Helping can take many forms, such as gathering information from the client and other sources, looking for assistance, deciding how to solve a problem, and talking about feelings. Yet it is always guided by two questions: (1) What is helpful? (2) How can the needs of the client be met? In human services, assistance to the client occurs through the *helping process*. As they engage in this process, human service professionals must remember that clients are responsible for themselves and make their own decisions. Giving advice or telling someone what to do does not encourage responsibility or promote self-help, which are goals of the helping process.

The effectiveness of the helping process depends greatly on the skills of the helper, which is the focus of this chapter. The helper's ability to communicate an understanding of the client's feelings, clarify what the problem is, and provide appropriate assistance to resolve the problem contributes to the effectiveness of the process. The nature of the helping relationship, the skills of helping, group work, and the challenges of difficult clients will be investigated in this chapter. A look at special human service methodologies such as crisis intervention and resolution-focused brief therapy will provide an overview of the helping process.

To illustrate some of the important concepts in this chapter, you will read about three individuals. We first renew our acquaintance with Carmen Rodriguez, the rehabilitation professional you met in Chapter 6. Then, Michiko, an international student from Japan, struggles with living in a new environment. Finally, Joan, a wife abandoned by her husband, needs support and assistance during this crisis and help after the crisis event has been resolved.

THE NATURE OF THE HELPING PROCESS

The helping process occurs in both formal and informal settings. In this chapter we will explore the helping that occurs in formal settings, for example, offices, institutions, agencies, street corners, and any other setting where human service workers deliver services to clients. As noted in Chapter 5, the term *client* can refer to an individual, a small group such as a family or a street gang, or a larger group such as a neighborhood or a geographic area.

The Helping Relationship

The cornerstone of helping, the medium through which help is offered, is the **helping relationship.** The helping process takes place within the context of a relationship that differs from others in that one person sets aside personal needs to focus on the needs of the other (or others), refraining from expressing opinions or giving advice.

Each participant brings to the relationship different perspectives and experiences. (See Figure 7.1) Both the client and the helper bring attitudes, values, feelings, and experiences, which may be similar or may be very different. In addition, the client brings needs, problems, and expectations about what will happen, as well as personal and environmental strengths. The helper comes with knowledge, training, and skills to assist with the problems of the client. Matching clients with helpers is often random, but there is considerable evidence that compatibility between the two is important for an effective helping relationship.

Because the helper has the knowledge and expertise that the client is seeking, much of the initial responsibility for establishing the relationship rests with the helper. The importance of the characteristics and values of the helper are discussed in Chapter 6. A growing body of research shows their importance in establishing and maintaining the helping relationship. The following questions (adapted from Rogers, 1958) may help you increase your self-awareness in relation to your own helping skills:

Can I be perceived as trustworthy, dependable, and consistent?

Can I express myself well enough that the client understands what I am saying?

Can I experience attitudes of warmth, caring, liking, interest, and respect for the client?

Can I separate my needs from those of the client?

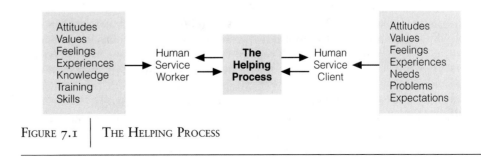

FIGURE 7.1 | THE HELPING PROCESS

Am I secure enough myself to allow the client to be separate and independent from me?

Am I able to see the world as the client does?

Can I accept the client as he or she is?

Can I help the client see his or her strengths?

As you begin to grasp the concept of the helping relationship and its importance to human service delivery, you may be asking yourself how it differs from other relationships. Several characteristics help make it unique (Perlman, 1983). First, helping relationships are formed for a recognized and agreed-upon purpose; they are goal oriented. Second, a helping relationship is time bound, which means it usually occurs over several sessions (depending, of course, on the nature of the problem); the relationship ends when the purpose has been accomplished. Third, the helping relationship carries authority. In this sense, the word *authority* has a very different meaning from the one with which you are probably familiar. The helper's authority consists of the knowledge and skills that enable him or her to work with the client toward resolving the problem. Finally, this relationship is for the client. The focus is always on the client's problems and concerns within the context of client strengths and the client's cultural context.

Among the most poignant illustrations of helping and the helping relationship is the work of Mother Teresa and the Missionaries of Charity. As you read about Mother Teresa in Box 7.1, think about how the characteristics of the helping relationship apply.

STAGES OF THE HELPING PROCESS

Usually the agency or organization with which a helper works shapes the focus, the services, and the duration of the helping process. For example, vocational rehabilitation agencies are concerned with the work histories of clients, any disabilities that may prevent them from being employed, and their vocational capabilities and aspirations. Finding low-income housing, arranging adoptions, and processing applications for food stamps are not part of their services. Regardless of the focus of an agency and its services, you will find that the stages of the helping process are similar. They will include components of the problem-solving process such as identifying the problem, setting goals to resolve the problem, and determining and applying strategies designed to help the client reach those goals.

PREPARATION   Before the client arrives, the helper will want to attend to several matters. One is the physical setting. Are there any barriers that will prevent or make it difficult to establish a relationship with the client? For example, many clients will perceive a desk as a symbol of authority, which may seem a barrier to them when the helper sits behind it. It may also be unwise to seat the client facing a window. Activities outside may distract clients and prevent them from focusing on what is happening in the office. Does the physical setting ensure confidentiality? Promising the client that all matters discussed will remain between the two of you means nothing if the setting is such that any discussion may be overheard by others.

BOX 7.1	INTERNATIONAL FOCUS

Mother Teresa and the Missionaries of Charity

Mother Teresa received God's call to serve the poorest of the poor in 1946. Her work began in Calcutta in a small way by caring for one sick and dying person she found on the streets there. Until March 1997, she was head of the Missionaries of Charity, a religious order she formed with the Vatican's blessing in 1950. The numbers of sisters and brothers in this order now total more than 4,000 worldwide.

They live what they teach, not owning more than the poor they serve. Mother Teresa won many awards, including the Nobel Peace Prize, Pope John XXIII Peace Prize, and India's Jawaharlal Nehru Award for International Understanding.

She founded hundreds of homes throughout the world, including four in Calcutta: Shishu Bhavan (the children's home); Prem Nivas (the center for leprosy patients in Titagarh); Nirmal Hriday (the home for the dying and destitute); and Prem Dam (the home for TB sufferers and patients with mental disabilities). As late as 1995, Mother Teresa was expanding her list of concerns. She was working with AIDS patients and fighting against abortion and prostitution, and for battered women. She traveled worldwide to advocate for the less fortunate and to enlist the support of others in the causes that she championed (Negri & Kramer, 1995).

Mother Teresa died on September 5, 1997. The Catholic Church is considering her for sainthood.

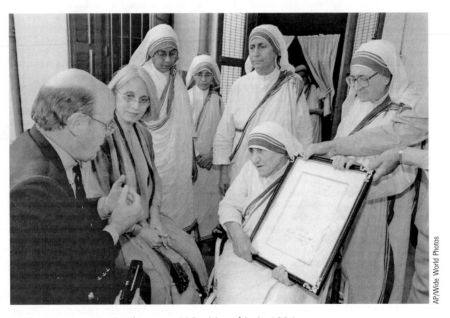

Mother Teresa accepting honorary U.S. citizenship in 1996.

Most agencies require extensive paperwork on clients. How will you handle note taking, filling out forms, and recording information? These decisions are best made before the client arrives. They can be handled in several ways; each helper must choose his or her own best method. For example, some helpers prefer taking notes while interviewing the client because it enables them to get all the facts while the client is present. Others say that taking notes while the client is talking is too difficult for them. They find that they miss important gestures and facial expressions.

The same is true of filling out forms. Some agencies require forms to be completed before the client sees a human service professional. In such cases, the helper may have little choice. If there is no such policy, the worker may choose to have the client complete necessary forms before their meeting, or the helper may wish to assist the client in completing the forms, using this opportunity to establish rapport with the client and begin developing a helping relationship.

Finally, before the client arrives, the worker reviews the information about the client that is already accessible. What records are available? Is additional information needed? Based on the information available, what is the best way to approach the client? Has the helper made arrangements to have uninterrupted time with the client?

What follows is one client's description of an initial visit to a Social Security office. As you read it, pay attention to the physical setting, the workers, and the climate. What messages do those seeking services receive?

> The first thing I noticed when I entered the double glass doors of the Social Security office was the back of everyone's head. I mean that there were rows of people sitting in metal folding chairs facing a blank white wall that had a door in the middle of it. All kinds of people were there—young, old, white, black, a couple of mothers with babies, some disabled. On the left side of the room was a counter with a glass partition. Three women were behind the counter. I watched the person who entered in front of me. He approached the counter and one woman told him, in a rather loud voice I thought, to take a number and sit down to wait his turn. I took number 38 before she could yell at me. As I sat there facing the blank white wall, I had a chance to observe how the agency operated. As each worker was ready for a client, she simply yelled out the number. The person then approached the counter, and there was an exchange of information, which I could plainly hear. In some cases, the individual then approached the door in the middle of the blank white wall. A buzzer sounded, unlocking the door, and the person entered. I suppose there were other workers behind the door, but I only made it to the counter. When number 38 was called, I found out I needed to write a letter to the regional office. The local office could not help me with my problem.

THE CLIENT ARRIVES   When the client enters the office, a climate of respect and acceptance is established if the client is greeted with a smile, a handshake, and an introduction. Remember that clients come with problems, feeling vulnerable and sometimes in pain or discomfort. A helper who takes charge of the initial meeting will help the client feel at ease by giving the client time to adjust to the new situation. The use of "ice breakers" or "door openers" allows the client to become accustomed to the setting and the helper: "Did you have any trouble finding the office?" or "Parking is sometimes a problem here. I hope it wasn't for you."

Since the helping relationship is time bound and goal oriented, the helper will at some point need to inquire about the client's problem. Many clients will be eager to share their problems. Others will be reticent about discussing problems that are personal and painful; they may test the helper by sharing less important problems first. The helper can initiate problem identification in a number of ways: "Let's talk about why you're here," "Tell me what's going on," "I'm wondering what's on your mind." In addition, the helper works with the client to identify personal and environmental

| BOX 7.2 | CARL ROGERS AND CLIENT-CENTERED THERAPY |

Carl Rogers, American psychologist and educator, was born on January 8, 1902, in Oak Park, Illinois. He attended the University of Wisconsin and graduated in 1924 with a degree in history. He then attended Union Theological Seminary in New York City and began to study for the ministry. He soon became influenced by a number of psychologists affiliated with Columbia University and transferred there to receive both his master's and doctoral degrees.

Rogers was initially concerned with environmental and institutional solutions to the problems of children, which he described in *The Clinical Treatment of the Problem Child* (1939). Later, he became interested in the psychotherapeutic process and gradually formulated the approach associated with his name—client-centered therapy. Client-centered therapy, or nondirective counseling, had a controversial beginning but proved to be a successful psychotherapeutic model. In *Counseling and Psychotherapy* (1942), Rogers maintained that the client knows better than anyone else what the problem is; with the help of a permissive, caring counselor, the client can find a solution to the problem. In client-centered therapy, the helper does not direct, give advice, or offer solutions and interpretations. The primary technique is "reflection of feelings." When the client speaks or acts, the helper responds by communicating perceptions of what the client means and feels. Through this "mirroring," the client can think more clearly about problems and feelings.

Source: From Taylor (1985).

strengths. "Tell me about a time when you solved this type of problem successfully." "What do you consider your best characteristic?" These are relatively nonthreatening ways of focusing on the client and the problem. Another way to do this is to have focused dialogue. After greeting the client, the helper and client can fill out the intake form together. This is a humanizing way to complete the form, and it does not require asking so many questions. Some forms include questions that build on strengths, such as "What do you enjoy?" "What do you do well?" "Who do you go to for help?" "What have you learned from your family and friends?"

During this initial stage, the helper can provide the client with information about the agency. For example, the client may want to know exactly what services the agency can provide. Other questions might concern the cost of the services, the criteria for eligibility to receive services, and the responsibilities of clients. In turn, the helper will probably have additional questions for the client. Does the client have any insurance? How did the client hear about the agency? Did someone refer the client here? What expectations does the client have for the agency and the helper?

EXPLORING THE PROBLEM   Chapter 5 discussed different perspectives on client problems. As the helper and the client begin to explore the problem, the helper should keep those perspectives in mind. The human service concepts of the whole person and the multidimensionality of problems will also guide this phase of the helping process (see Box 7.2). Once the problems are identified, it is time to move to the next stage.

INTERVENTION STRATEGIES   During this stage, the helper and the client set goals and determine how those goals will be reached to resolve the problem. This means addressing the current status of the problem, the client's aspirations and desires, and the client's personal and social resources. Should the helper find that the client's problem calls for expertise or experience that the helper does not have, the helper should refer the client to another professional who has the necessary knowledge and skills. Another reason for

TABLE 7.1	SUMMARY POINTS: HELPING STAGES

- Physical setting, paperwork, and review of information occur before the client arrives.
- When the client arrives, the helper greets the client, inquires about the problem, and provides information about the agency.
- Concepts of the whole person and the multidimensionality guide problem exploration.
- Intervention may involve referral, service provision, or both.
- Termination that is positive occurs when the needed services are provided and the objectives obtained.

referral at this point arises if, once the problem has been identified, the helper has such strong feelings or biases about the situation that he or she is unable to work objectively with the client. Referral will be discussed in detail in Chapter 8.

Depending on the problem, strategies may be as simple as providing a one-time service such as pregnancy testing or as complex as working with a client who has been injured in a car wreck and is permanently disabled. In the latter case, problems may include the client's loss of ability to work a previous job, difficulties of the client and the family in adjusting to the client's disability, and barriers in the home to the client's mobility. These issues must be addressed if the client is to adjust to his or her new reality. Each strategy used supports client strengths and helps the client negotiate his or her own environment.

The final stage of the helping process is **termination**. The relationship between the helper and the client may end in several ways. The most positive conclusion is when the services needed are provided and both participants are satisfied that the objectives have been reached. Unfortunately, not all terminations are so positive; services may be interrupted by either the helper or the client before the objectives have been reached. For example, the client moves from the area; the helper is transferred, promoted, or leaves the agency; or the client refuses to return for services.

In the case study that follows we visit Carmen Rodriguez, whom we met in Chapter 6. Here she discusses how she deals with many of the concepts discussed in this section.

One aspect of my work that makes it challenging is that I perform a variety of functions. For example, I always begin my work with a client with an interview. During this initial contact with the client, I try to establish rapport. I explain what we will be doing together for the next six weeks and what the schedule is like at our facility. It also helps clients to know what is expected of them. One of the best ways I've found to get this relationship off on the right foot is to talk to the client as someone I really want to get to know. I do have some background information on the client (usually an intake form, a medical evaluation, and a financial statement), and I briefly skim it before I see the client. When I meet with the client the first time, I always stand up and invite him or her in with a handshake and a smile. I leave the folder in a drawer, because I can concentrate on the client totally if I'm not distracted by reports.

After the initial meeting, I read the client's folder carefully. At that point, I usually ask myself the following questions: What do I know about this client? Does this client have a documented disability that is a handicap to employment? What evaluative information do I need to determine whether there is a reasonable expectation that this client can eventually be gainfully employed? Has this client been evaluated previously? Finally, what additional information would be helpful to best serve this client?

During the period of time that I work with the client on a daily basis, the goal is to determine what types of work the client would like to perform and what types the client is capable of performing. I always focus on the client's strengths as a way of boosting confidence and building on past successes. Staff members administer vocational tests, do some vocational counseling, and arrange for the client to try working as an employee in two or three different job settings. In most cases, I find myself going beyond these tasks. For example, many of the clients do not know about personal hygiene, so it is up to staff members to teach them about taking showers and using deodorant. Also, they may not know about proper work behavior. To succeed at a job, they must learn appropriate work habits such as being at work on time, taking limited breaks, dealing with conflicts, and getting along with other workers.

For the protection of the client, the agency, and the human service professional, it is necessary to maintain written case notes and documentation of services. This can be very time-consuming. I've noticed that each worker handles this task differently. What works for me is reserving the last 30 minutes of the day for updating files. I realize that these notes are important—the client may be transferred, I may change jobs, or I may be out sick—but some days it's a real chore to pull all the files and condense what's necessary into two or three sentences.

I hope to continue in my job for several more years, but eventually I would like to go back to school for further training. I want to develop my counseling skills to work with clients as individuals or groups in a more specialized way. My position as a case manager gives me practical experience and allows me to explore my career options by filling a variety of roles and working with other professionals.

AN INTRODUCTION TO HELPING SKILLS

Communication is the foundation for all interpersonal relationships. Exchanging messages to understand another's perceptions, ideas, and experiences is especially important in helping relationships. Helping others will be difficult if we do not understand their problems or concerns.

In this section we introduce basic helping skills. We begin by focusing on the client's message, which means perceiving both the verbal and the nonverbal messages of the client. Next, we focus on the helper's communication by identifying the skills necessary for effective listening and responding. Finally, we discuss what the helper needs to know about cultural differences.

One person sending a message to another person with the conscious intent of affecting the receiver's behavior is *communication* (Weiten & Lloyd, 2003). This process is illustrated in Figure 7.2. When the receiver interprets the message the way

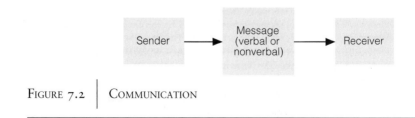

FIGURE 7.2 | COMMUNICATION

the sender intended, **effective communication** has taken place. When one person interprets the message differently from the way it was intended, the result is communication failure, the most common source of misunderstandings in interpersonal relationships.

The message that a person sends can be verbal or nonverbal. Both of these messages occur within a cultural context, and a message within one culture is not necessarily the same message in another culture. The most common example of a **verbal message** is the spoken word: "Hello, how are you today?" The smile and handshake or hug accompanying that verbal greeting are **nonverbal messages.** The skillful helper is able to "hear" the client's behavior (the nonverbal message), as well as what is actually said (the verbal message), and is able to respond verbally and nonverbally to these messages (Okun, 2002). It sounds complicated, and it takes practice to communicate effectively. A good beginning is through an introduction to each component of the communication process.

NONVERBAL MESSAGES

Nonverbal behaviors (body language) include a person's posture, tone of voice, gestures, eye contact, and touch. Everyone communicates nonverbally within the context of their own cultural environment. Each of us engages in some nonverbal behavior that we are aware of and perform intentionally. For example, when meeting someone for the first time, most of us want to make a positive first impression, so we deliberately greet that person with a smile or some other pleasant facial expression. However, we also communicate unconsciously in a nonverbal fashion. You may recall a time when you visited the doctor's office for shots and afterward wondered at the soreness in your muscles. The tension, fear, or hurt you experienced during the visit caused you to tense your muscles.

In a normal two-person conversation, more than 65% of the meaning is carried nonverbally. This fact emphasizes the importance of nonverbal communication in a helping situation. Frequently, you may find that a client's nonverbal message will provide you with valuable clues about what the client is thinking or feeling— important ideas that the client is unable to verbalize. Table 7.2 lists some common nonverbal cues and their meanings.

Another area in which nonverbal cues are important is the expression of feelings. Feelings are most often communicated nonverbally, particularly by facial expressions and tone of voice. One difficulty with "hearing" the nonverbal expression of feelings is the ambiguity of the nonverbal message. A nonverbal behavior such as crying could be interpreted in various ways; one cannot determine just from the tears on a person's face whether the person is sad, hurt, or disappointed. In fact, the person may be scared or even very happy.

Thus, we may think that nonverbal communication is a fairly straightforward process of sending and receiving messages, but it is actually a complicated mode of communication. Although they provide us with important clues about the person with whom we are conversing, nonverbal messages should be interpreted with caution.

Try this exercise: At some point today, select two people who are communicating with each other. (You may be in the library, a food-service area, or anywhere

TABLE 7.2 | NONVERBAL CUES AND THEIR POSSIBLE MEANINGS

Cue	Meaning
Lifting an eyebrow	Disbelief
Lowering eyebrows	Uneasiness, suspicion
Lifting both eyebrows	Surprise
Eye contact	Interest, confidence
Winking an eye	Intimacy
Slapping forehead	Forgetfulness
Rubbing the nose	Puzzlement
Turning up corners of mouth	Happiness
Cocking head to one side	Friendly, human
Little or no head and/or hand movements	Cool, no emotion
Raised shoulders	Fear
Retracted shoulders	Suppressed anger
Square shoulders	Responsibility
Bowed shoulders	Carrying a burden
Shrugging shoulders	Indifference
Sitting with arms and legs crossed	Withdrawal, resistance
Clasping arms	Protection
Tapping fingers	Impatience
Fondling and touching inanimate objects	Loneliness
Leaning forward in a chair	Interest
Leaning back, arms uncrossed	Open to suggestion
Leaning back, arms crossed	Not open to suggestion
Postural change—facing away	Finished with interaction

you choose.) For 10 minutes, observe the nonverbal communication of one of the participants. What behaviors do you observe? What possible interpretations can you make about the meanings of the behaviors?

VERBAL MESSAGES

Verbal messages consist of words spoken by a person, again within a cultural context. Such messages can be divided into a cognitive component and an affective component. The cognitive component consists of the facts of a message and reflects the person's thinking processes. This is the realm in which we are most comfortable. A cognitive message addresses such matters as who, what, where, when, and why. Consider the following statements and try to pick out the cognitive messages.

> I left work at 5:00 P.M. today. The last client I saw was Raphael Santini, and I just can't seem to get him off my mind. He is making such an effort to find a job, but he's had no luck. I couldn't believe it when he showed up today. I hardly recognized him, and I guess he could tell I was surprised, because I couldn't think of anything to say for a moment. He looked great. His hair was clean and neatly combed, and his clothes were new. He was so proud of himself, and I was proud of him too. I told him I was so pleased with the changes. I also felt good about myself, because some of my hard work with this client has paid off. I'm going to make some phone calls first thing in the morning to see what assistance I can find to help him locate a job. There's just got to be help for a motivated client like Raphael.

Some of the cognitive messages you probably identified were the speaker's leaving work at 5:00 P.M.; the appointment with Raphael Santini, who is trying to find a job; and the description of his neat, clean appearance. In the cognitive realm, facts are the focus.

The affective component, the feeling part of the message, may be expressed directly or indirectly. Many clients who are unsure about what they are feeling, or who are simply uncomfortable talking about feelings, may choose to express their feelings indirectly. This means that the individual may not name the feeling at all ("Stop driving so fast!"), or may describe it by telling what he or she feels like doing ("I feel like punching him in the nose"). One of the helper's main tasks may be to encourage the client to become aware of feelings and to learn to express feelings appropriately and directly: "I'm scared when you drive so fast," or "I'm angry at you for spoiling the surprise."

Review the statements about Raphael Santini. What feelings are expressed directly? In fact, there are very few, but they do include feeling "proud," "surprised," and "good." These feelings are named, and the reader clearly understands how the helper feels. Read the excerpt again, and consider the feelings that are being expressed indirectly. (It might be helpful to read it aloud.) You might identify such feelings as discouragement at Raphael's lack of success, exasperation at the job situation, disbelief at his appearance, and determination to find some type of assistance for Raphael. Determining exactly what the client (or, in this case, the helper) is feeling may be more difficult when feelings are expressed indirectly.

Listening and Responding

The way we listen and respond to the client is crucial in building a helping relationship. The first thing a helper must do before making any response to the client is to listen carefully to what the client is expressing, both verbally and nonverbally. Even though listening takes up more of a person's waking hours than any other activity and many people consider themselves good listeners, few of us actually are. This section will introduce listening behaviors and some helper responses that promote effective helping (see Table 7.3).

THE HELPER LISTENS   The kind of listening that helpers engage in is called **responsive listening** or **active listening**. These terms describe the behaviors of helpers as they

TABLE 7.3 | HELPFUL BEHAVIORS IN COMMUNICATING

Verbal	Nonverbal
Mirroring feelings	Making eye contact
Clarifying	Listening
Showing a sense of humor	Smiling
Providing support	Nodding one's head
Providing information that client needs	Leaning forward
Explaining helper's role	Maintaining a relaxed posture
Sharing information about oneself	Facing the client
Being nonjudgmental	Displaying facial expression
Asking few questions	Being punctual
Occasionally making appropriate use of gestures and touching	Maintaining a moderate rate of speech

attend to both the verbal and the nonverbal communication of the client. What makes this type of listening special or different from other listening behaviors is that helpers also attend to what is not said, that is, to the underlying thoughts and feelings of the client, which are not expressed in words. Two ways of considering responsive or active listening as helping behaviors are presented here.

Egan (2007, pp. 76–77) suggested several things helpers can do to communicate to clients that they are listening. These five behaviors are presented as a set of guidelines that helpers can follow to let their clients know they are physically present and actively involved in the helping relationship. You can easily remember the behaviors by thinking of the acronym SOLER.

- **S** Face the client *squarely*. This is a posture of involvement. To face away from the client or even at an angle lessens the degree of involvement.
- **O** Adopt an *open posture*. This is usually perceived as nondefensive. Crossing arms or legs may not communicate openness or availability.
- **L** *Lean toward* the other person. A natural sign of involvement, this posture is a slight forward inclination. Moving forward or backward can frighten a client or communicate lessened involvement.
- **E** Maintain *eye contact*. This is normal behavior for two individuals who are involved in conversation. It is different from staring.
- **R** Try to be *relaxed*. This means avoiding nervous habits such as fidgeting or tapping a pencil. Behaviors such as these can distract the client.

Remember that these are only guidelines. A helper's physical behavior may vary in accordance with the cultural identity of the client or what is comfortable for that particular helper.

Ivey and Ivey (2006) described **attending behavior** as another way to let the client know the helper is listening. The goal of attending behavior is to encourage the client to talk about and examine issues, problems, or concerns. Attending behavior has four dimensions: three nonverbal components and one verbal component.

1. *Visual/eye contact.* If you are going to talk to people, look at them.
2. *Vocal qualities.* Your vocal tone and speech rate indicate clearly how you feel about another person. Think of how many ways you can say "I am really interested in what you say" just by altering your vocal tone and speech rate.
3. *Verbal tracking.* The client has come to you with a topic of concern. Do not change the subject; stick with the client's subject matter.
4. *Attentive and authentic body language.* Clients know you are interested if you face them squarely and lean slightly forward, have an expressive face, and use facilitative, encouraging gestures. In short, allow yourself to be yourself; authenticity in attending is essential (p. 37).

Engaging in these behaviors encourages the client to talk, reducing the amount of talk from the helper. Benefits include communicating interest and concern to the client and increasing the worker's awareness of the client's ability to pay attention. Attending behaviors also allow the helper to modify helping behaviors to work effectively with clients who may be racially, culturally, or sexually different.

THE HELPER'S RESPONSE   Once the helper has heard the verbal and nonverbal messages of the client, it is time for the helper to speak. Remember that helpers' responses must be purposeful. Think about the characteristics of the helping relationship. This is not a casual conversation between two people, but a goal-directed exchange. Therefore, the helper must know his or her intent before speaking.

The helper has several options at this point. For example, did the helper understand what the client said? Was the message clear? Does the helper need further information to grasp the message correctly? Questions such as these will assist the helper in determining the intent of his or her response. Let us examine some of these options.

First, suppose the helper does understand the client's message and decides that the most helpful response would be one that lets the client know this. To communicate that intent, the helper may choose to **paraphrase,** to make a statement that is interchangeable with the client's own words.

CLIENT: I've been able to complete five tasks today that were on my list.

HELPER: You've had a productive day today.

The helper may determine that more than a simple paraphrase is needed to help the client become aware of or clarify feelings. In this case, a helper statement that reflects both the feeling (or affective component) and the facts (or cognitive component) is helpful. For example:

HELPER: You're really pleased that you were able to accomplish what you set out to do today.

If the helper is confused about what the client said, perhaps because the client was relating a complicated incident, the helper should ask the client for clarification. To attempt a response that will make little sense to the client and will let the client know that the helper did not understand what was said is not helpful. Responses such as "I'm not sure I understand . . ." or "I'm confused about . . ." are appropriate at this point. They also let the client know that the helper is interested enough to want to get the story right in order to be able to help.

Beginning helpers sometimes encounter situations in which clients are asking questions or seeking information that the helper does not know. Many helpers believe they should know everything and may feel embarrassed about being asked something they do not know. Unfortunately, they may attempt to answer off the tops of their heads or give an answer they believe may be correct. A better response in situations like this would be, "I do not have that information, but I do know where we can find it; let me check on that for you," or "I'm not sure about the eligibility requirements for that type of assistance, but I can refer you to someone who knows." Helpers are not supposed to have all the answers. The effective helper who wants to maintain a relationship with the client will enrich that relationship by being honest with the client.

ASKING QUESTIONS   Another technique that beginning helpers should be wary of is **questioning.** Most of us consider ourselves skilled at asking questions and find it a natural form of communication in everyday life—particularly questions that begin with the words *who, what, where, why,* and *when.* For the beginning helper, the question is the most common method of eliciting information from the client, and many helpers find themselves resorting to questions frequently. Unfortunately, one question seems to lead to another, and too many questions can interfere with the helping relationship, causing the client to feel like a witness. An overreliance on questioning, and neglecting other kinds of responses, hinders the helping process. It also creates a dependent client who has no role other than answering questions. Most questions can be rephrased as statements that elicit the same information. For example, the question "What was the last grade completed in school?" can be rephrased as "Tell me about your school experiences." In addition to discovering the final grade completed, the helper may learn how the client felt about school, whether the client enjoyed learning, and what circumstances surrounded the end of the client's educational experience.

Now that you have been alerted to the pitfalls of questioning, let us explore the time when asking questions is appropriate and how one asks good questions. There are several situations in which a question is helpful. You can begin the interview with a question: "How would you like to begin?" or "Could you tell me a little about yourself?" A second situation occurs when specific information is needed. Asking for information to clarify ("How long have you been ill?") or to elicit examples of specific behavior ("How does that make you feel?") can provide the additional information necessary for complete understanding. Finally, questions can be useful to focus the client's attention. For example, a client who is digressing or rambling on about several problems may need the helper's assistance to focus. Such assistance can be provided by statements such as the following:

> You've mentioned several concerns that you have about your daughter. You're afraid she is using drugs, and you suspect she is not doing well in school. I guess I hear you expressing the most concern, though, about your inability to talk with her. Let's focus on that. What happens when you do try to talk with her?

TABLE 7.4 | SUMMARY POINTS: WHEN TO ASK QUESTIONS

- To begin the interview
- To obtain specific information
- To seek clarification
- To elicit examples of specific behavior
- To focus the client's attention

Thus, there are times in a helping relationship when asking questions is appropriate and beneficial. How does one ask good questions? Egan (2007) suggested that the helper might first want to consider how the question will relate to and promote the helping relationship. Having specific objectives in mind before asking the question will help in formulating a good question.

Both closed and open questions can facilitate the development of the helping relationship when the helper has specific intentions. *Closed* questions are those that elicit facts necessary to facilitate the helping process. "How old were you when your father died?" and "How many brothers and sisters do you have?" may provide important information regarding the client's family situation if the client is having difficulties at home. Closed questions that require a "yes" or "no" answer should usually be avoided, because they lead the beginning helper to ask more and more questions.

Open questions, on the other hand, are broader, allowing the client to express thoughts, feelings, or ideas. They contribute to building rapport with the client and also assist him or her in exploring a situation, a problem, or an interaction. For example, "How did you feel after talking it over with your parents?" asks for the client's view. On the other hand, "Did you feel better after talking with your parents?" can be answered with a simple "yes" or "no," which does not enhance the helping process.

In summary, questions can be useful tools in the helping process. As with other types of responses, the key to effective questioning is knowing the intent of the question before posing it to the client. Are you seeking factual information or asking the client to offer thoughts or opinions about the topic of discussion? Considering how the question will promote the helping relationship will assist the helper in determining the appropriate strategy.

This section has been a brief introduction to helping skills. As you pursue your education and training in preparation for work in the human services, you will increase your knowledge about these skills and refine your use of them so that you become an effective helper. One area that requires a mastery of communications skills is working with groups of individuals. By the end of the 1980s, groups were recognized as viable means of helping individuals in a variety of settings. Group work flourished during the 1990s and will continue to be a major strategy in the 21st century to provide direct service to clients as well as to collaborate with colleagues and community groups. An introduction to basic group concepts and the role of communication in group work follows.

WORKING WITH GROUPS

Groups are natural. Since the beginning of time, individuals have banded together for survival, security, tasks, and problem solving, thus making groups a critical mode for accomplishing what needs to be done. Think about your own life—your living situation, your work, and even your leisure time. Most of these activities take place in groups. In human services, individuals also band together to accomplish tasks. Membership may be voluntary. For example, individuals with similar problems or experiences, such as victims of incest or suicide survivors or children of alcoholics, may work together on their problems. Involuntary membership occurs when participating in a group is mandated by some authority. Joining a group for abusive parents or one for substance abusers may be a condition for probation. In this section we will define groups, explore the skills necessary to work with a group, and consider the trends that will affect group work in the 21st century.

A **group** is a number of individuals who interact with each other. According to Brill and Levine (2004), groups have several characteristics. An important characteristic is the interaction that occurs among group members. This means that they participate in group meetings and discussions, share resources, give and receive help, and influence each other. Sharing common goals and values is a second characteristic. The group may be formed for an agreed-upon purpose or the group may establish its own goals once members meet. The group also develops its own values, identifying what is important to the group and translating it into behavior for individuals as members of the group and for the group as a whole. Groups also have a social structure. Roles define the formal structure of the group and influence how individuals act in the group. Different group members play different roles. Examples of roles include leadership, which may be a designated person or a shared role among members; the maintenance role, which sees to the well-being of the group by encouraging and compromising; the facilitative/building role, which helps everyone feel part of the group by initiating, seeking information and opinions, coordinating, and evaluating; and blocking, a role that is aggressive, dominating, and anti-group. A final characteristic of a group is cohesiveness among members. Members perceive that they belong to a group, they are interdependent in some way, and they work together to keep the group going as well as focus on common goals.

Groups have their own dynamics that influence the group's development and its productivity. One important influence is the context or purpose for which the group was formed. For example, if a group is formed to help members deal with a chronic illness such as diabetes, the purpose guides many of the activities of the group. Group process also influences how the group functions. Conflicts, anxieties, validations, agreements, and hopefulness are all byproducts of meeting together. Group dynamics, or how members of the group behave with each other, can be directed by helpers who understand the conditions that help a group run smoothly. Groups do develop unwritten rules and often resemble a family unit.

Alcoholics Anonymous (AA) is an example of a well-known group that illustrates these characteristics. Although many self-help groups formed during the late 1960s, AA is one of the more enduring ones, established in the late 1930s by founders who realized the effectiveness of individuals meeting together and interacting in such a way to support change (Gladding, 2003). Interaction among members is the foundation of AA meetings; for example, members share experiences and information. They also have a common goal, which is to gain and maintain control of their lives by remaining sober. To that end, members encourage, coordinate, evaluate, support, and lead, both in regular meetings and outside meetings. These techniques are similar to those used in other self-help groups such as Parents without Partners and Weight Watchers.

Groups are formed for reasons other than self-help. Today there are specialty areas in group work and a set of core competencies and standards that have been established for preparation for group work in these areas (Association for Specialists in Group Work, 2006). Identified specialty areas include task/work groups that are focused on accomplishing identified work goals, for example, task forces, planning groups, or community organizations. The teams described in Chapter 1 are examples of this type of group. Guidance/psychoeducational groups are another type of group whose focus is education, prevention, or both. In these groups, information may be shared about AIDS, bereavement, or divorce. The goal is to prevent the development of psychological disturbances. A third type of group is counseling/interpersonal problem solving, whose focus is the resolution of problems group members face. Examples may be test anxiety, relationship difficulties, or career decision making. Psychotherapy/personality reconstruction groups are most often found in mental health facilities such as clinics or hospitals and include individuals who have serious psychological problems of long-term duration. Both abusers and victims of abuse may benefit from involvement in such a group.

What is the role of the human service professional in a group? In natural groups, such as a family or a street gang, human service professionals enter as outsiders and must make a place for themselves (Brill & Levine, 2004). They are present because a member is in trouble or there are significant problems in the group or both. In formed groups, that is, those that are organized for a specific purpose or goal, the human service professional may have responsibility for getting people involved and getting the group underway. Organizational issues such as meeting times and places, purpose, and group structure must be addressed by members before the real work of the group begins. At this point the human service professional facilitates the work of the group toward its goal.

The foundation of all group functioning is communication skills. As stated earlier, interaction is key to the group's existence and involves the exchange of information and transmission of meaning (Johnson & Johnson, 2005). It is by means of effective communication that group members reach some understanding of one another, their goals, the division of labor, and other group tasks. Both verbal and nonverbal behaviors comprise effective communication and are every bit as complex in groups as they are in individuals. For example, silence may have many meanings: processing information, mulling over what was said, avoidance, or discomfort with the topic. Therefore, many of the points made earlier in the chapter about sending messages, listening, asking questions, and responding are critical for group work. In fact, the core skills identified by the Association for Specialists in Group Work (2006) include the communication skills to open and close group meetings, impart information, self-disclose, give feedback, and ask open-ended questions.

BOX 7.3	A CLIENT SPEAKS

Life was not very good for me about 15 years ago. I just hit rock bottom. I was a builder and an engineer by training and had established an excellent environmental consulting firm. In fact, during my consulting activities, I was fortunate enough to meet several individuals who helped me become a commercial land developer. Over a period of 5 years I amassed a fortune; I had increased my personal wealth to such a degree that I owned three homes—one in New York City; one in Lisbon, Portugal; and one in Miami, Florida. My kids attended private school; my family belonged to a prestigious country club; I was able to buy a home for my parents.

All of a sudden my financial situation began to deteriorate as the business began to crumble. Because of depressed economic conditions and a recession, the land value dropped and individuals and corporations were no longer interested in land investments. Because of stressful times and other complicating factors, my wife asked me for a divorce. She kept our family home and gained custody of our three children. The two dogs stayed with her as well. It seemed that I would have to file for bankruptcy and face the losses (financially, socially, and professionally) alone. My lawyer, who was handling the fight to avoid bankruptcy, recommended that I join a men's therapy group sponsored by Consumer Counseling Centers of America.

At the first meeting, I was scared to death. A million times during the day I changed my mind about going. I drove up to the meeting house at 6:45 P.M. and decided once again that I would have to skip the 7:00 P.M. meeting. My hands were sweaty, I had a

headache, my stomach hurt, and I had not had much sleep in months. I watched the participants enter one by one. My knees seemed to buckle as I stepped outside the car and headed for the door. The group met every week; this was an ongoing group that had been meeting for 10 years. I arrived awkwardly, sat in one of the chairs that formed a circle. I was asked to introduce myself and then I was welcomed by the other group members and the leader, a local psychologist.

The first night I talked was because I was challenged by one of the group members for coming, gaining from the group, and not really being willing to give. After I finally made my first contributions, I was able to participate in the meetings, although I never had a lot to say. One of the group rules was that we could not see each other socially. This was in part for confidentiality since we had to promise not to divulge the contents of the group discussion. We also could not acknowledge others who participated in the group. Another rule was that each person had to be honest when he spoke. There was no "B.S." allowed or tolerated.

My stay was 13 months. It was amazing what I learned in the group. I made some incredibly good friends, people that I would have never met in any other circumstance. A few I really did not like at all; we did not share many common values. The one thing that we did share was a tragic financial encounter. Some members were like me, caught in a very difficult financial situation due to the recession. Others, it seemed, had always been troubled by financial worries. I felt supported, and understood.

Groups are experiencing increased popularity at this time and focus on special populations. Examples are groups for individuals who are divorcing, adult offenders, overeaters, those with HIV/AIDS, adolescents, elderly living in institutions, unwed teenage fathers, and those who need support for any number of situations. This trend will continue.

SKILLS FOR CHALLENGING CLIENTS

Ideally, all clients of human services are motivated, cooperative, responsible, and like each of us; however, it is one of the challenges of this practice that not all clients fit that description. In your experience as a helper, you will likely meet clients who are different culturally or who are resistant, silent, overly demanding, or unmotivated. They may also be different from you in other ways, including background, religion, values, and life experiences.

You need to know something about these client groups because they often elicit in the helper feelings of uncertainty, hostility, and resentment. They are particularly difficult for many beginning helpers to work with, and it is important to realize that the client's behavior is not necessarily the helper's fault.

CULTURALLY DIFFERENT CLIENTS

Shifts in America's population will make the country far more ethnically diverse than ever before. By 2050, the Hispanic population will grow to 24% of the population and Asians to 9%. Non-Hispanic Whites will be reduced to 53%. This shift reflects a change in immigration patterns and differences in birth rates, combined with an overall slowdown in the growth of the country's population. Latinos and Asians will grow fastest in number, whereas African Americans will nearly double in number by 2050.

As these population shifts occur, it is increasingly likely that human service professionals will encounter clients whose cultural backgrounds differ from their own. The key to working with clients who are culturally different is awareness of and sensitivity to these differences. In Tucson, Arizona, for example, Suzy Bourque at the Family Counseling Agency emphasizes the need to hire workers who appreciate different cultures. Their client population is about 30% Latino and 10% African American. Native Americans are underrepresented because they tend to take care of their own. She is constantly looking for staff who are bilingual, bicultural, and/or African American (personal communication). For the case workers at Casita Maria Settlement House in the Bronx, sometimes getting people to accept help is difficult because accepting outside help is not part of their culture (personal communication). Instead of saying to a Latino client, "You need counseling," they find that a more acceptable phrase is "Maybe you need someone to talk with." Because many of their clients are Latino, they find that they can no longer refer to them as Hispanic or Latino. Now, it is important to recognize that Latino includes people from Puerto Rico, Nicaragua, Colombia, and Honduras—and they are all different.

Helpers must realize that culture shapes body language. Few gestures and body movements have universal meaning. For example, Arabs tend to cling or huddle together, whereas Americans like their space. Postures also vary by culture. The posture of the German male is stiffer than that of the American male, whereas the French male exhibits greater body limpness (Sielski, 1979). The direct eye contact that is so critical to standard American helping behavior may be offensive to people from Native American and Latino cultures. A helper with no knowledge of this may intend to communicate complete attention but be perceived by the culturally different client as disrespectful.

The beginning helper is cautioned against assigning too much meaning to a single gesture; instead, all means of expression—verbal, postural, facial, and cultural—should be considered. It is also wise not to generalize about cultural traits. Some Asian Americans may not like direct eye contact, yet some might.

Axelson (1999, p. 28) suggested that a multicultural approach to counseling should start with four steps to conceptualize the client who is culturally different.

1. Recognize that all human beings possess a similar capacity for thought, feeling, and behavior.
2. Be knowledgeable about several cultures; study both differences and similarities among people of different groups and their special needs and problems.
3. Gain an understanding of how the individual relates to important objects of motivation, what his or her personal constructs are, and how they are constructed to form his or her worldview.
4. Blend steps 1, 2, and 3 into an integrated picture of the distinctive person as experienced during the counseling process.

The following account, written by Michiko, a foreign student from Japan, may help you to begin thinking about culturally different clients in light of the preceding four steps.

MICHIKO

I am a foreign student from Japan who is studying at an American university. It has been more than a month since I arrived in the States, and still I am not making American friends. I usually hang around with my Japanese buddies, so that does not help either. I hardly have any time for socializing because of all of the assignments I have to do for class. I am tense and timid around people and feel uncomfortable most of the time because I do not know how to act in pleasing, acceptable ways. I miss my friends and family and often cry when I am alone.

I have two great needs. One is to feel accepted among Americans and to adjust to the American culture. The other need is for academic excellence, since I did not come all the way from Japan just to fool around. I would like to have American friends with whom I can talk and share experiences, who will like me the way I am. I find most of my classes large and impersonal and have hardly any hope of finding a friend there. I need someone who is interested enough to get past the language barrier to get to know me. As for the academics, my professors know that I am a foreign student and they will go out of their way to help me with any difficulties I might be facing. I appreciate the attention, but that is not enough. I need help with the report assignments because I am unfamiliar with formats in English writing. I also need to be advised on study skills, because even if I prepare well in advance for a test, the grades I get are Cs and Ds.

I have many fears. I am afraid being Japanese, a racial minority, makes me less desirable as a person worth knowing in the eyes of an American. I am in constant fear of saying wrong things at the wrong moments and acting weird in front of people. My language problem still persists. Conversational English is something I find difficult, and people must speak slowly and clearly for me. I am afraid this makes me boring to talk to and hard to discuss complex subjects with. The greatest fear of all is having to go back to Japan because I could not make it academically and socially at an American university.

The young woman in this case study is one among many culturally different clients. Axelson's four steps are useful in understanding Michiko as a unique, worthwhile individual. Michiko definitely has the capacity for thought, feeling, and behavior as she attempts to function successfully in a culture foreign to her. A helper would need to learn about the Japanese culture and the ways in which it differs from and resembles American culture. Michiko has established personal goals that focus on academic and social success and is frustrated by the barriers she is experiencing. To engage effectively in the helping process with Michiko, the helper would need to explore the relevant differences between American and Japanese cultures. For example, many Asian cultures are collectivist—the individual is less important than the group. Michiko may be fearful of not succeeding academically and socially because of the disgrace it would bring to her family.

The helper would also want to adjust his or her helping behaviors to the individual of a different culture and to assess appropriate strategies of intervention. In American culture, the individual is perceived as autonomous and separate from groups. Even though a person can be a member of many groups, no one group determines identity completely. In collectivist societies, however, the individual belongs to fewer groups, but the attachment is stronger; often the individual is defined by membership in a group. Taking this information into account, the helper would choose an intervention that would focus on Michiko in relation to her group rather than an intervention designed to promote independence.

THE RELUCTANT OR RESISTANT CLIENT

There are some distinctions between reluctant and resistant clients, but the principles for working with them are similar. The *reluctant* client is one who does not want to come in for help in the first place and is more or less forced to come. Such clients may be found in schools, correctional settings, court-related settings, and employment agencies (Egan, 2007). The *resistant* client may come more or less willingly but fail to carry through or participate actively in the helping process. Some of the causes of clients' **reluctance** and **resistance** are having negative attitudes about help, seeing no benefits in changing, feeling that getting help means admitting weakness or failure, and seeing no reason for going for help in the first place.

Reluctant clients may be embarrassed or angry that they are there for help. In many cases, they are there only because the court or some other authority has said they must be. These feelings are compounded by their unfamiliarity with the agency or the process. To attempt to lessen the reluctance, the helper can explain the process to the client. Discussing matters such as confidentiality, time limits, and expectations (for the client as well as the helper) can help demystify the process. Also, the manner in which the helper relates this can allow the client to see him or her in a role other than that of interrogator or advice giver. The following case provides an example.

JOSEPH

Joseph came into my office with his mother and father. He sat in the chair with his arms folded. His feet did not touch the floor. He was swinging one foot and then another. He looked at his knees. I talked with his mother and father first for a few minutes and then asked them to be excused so that I could talk with Joseph alone. I am used to working with young children who do not want to see a counselor. When I work with them the first time, many say nothing during a 35- to 45-minute period. Some just sit and stare at me. Some stare at the floor. Others pretend to be asleep or sing quietly to themselves. On rare occasions, they try to damage the room, me, or themselves in some way. Over the 20 years that I have worked with children, five of them have never talked with me, after weekly meetings for over six months to a year. Many of them will begin to relate to me after two or three weeks, mainly through games and drawing or watching short films or videos together. Some will finally talk with me and once they get started, they cannot stop. My foremost approach is to let them know that I care about them in whatever way I can. Even for those who never spoke, I was a consistent, caring presence in their lives for an extended period of time.

Resistance is slightly different from reluctance, because resistance can occur at any time in the helping process. Clients who come to the attention of human services agencies may initially feel threatened by the referral and application procedures. Resistance may also arise later in the helping process if the client feels threatened by the subject being discussed, by the helper, or even by the helping relationship.

What is resistant behavior? Missing appointments, rejecting the helper, and inattentiveness are examples of such behavior. Clients may try to protect themselves by denying the existence of a problem, claiming it is caused by other people or situations, or distancing themselves from it.

I feel that the counselor in my school has betrayed me. We have had a good relationship ever since I came to the high school. I have worked with her one-on-one to determine my school schedule. She has conducted groups in our high school. I have participated in ones on family life, balancing a checkbook, how to apply for a job, and how to maintain healthy friendships. Today I went to see her after basketball practice. I have not been feeling well. My coach is concerned and she asked me to go to see Ms. Sharpelli. You know what she asked me? "Do you think you might be pregnant?" I walked out without saying a word to her. Even though she might be right, I promise, I will never speak to her again.

The helper can use several strategies when working with a resistant client. First, recognizing and accepting the antagonism may defuse the situation. This type of action is very different from what the client might expect; a statement such as "You probably don't want to see anyone like me" may minimize the threat to the client. Second, asking for the client's perceptions of the problem will communicate support for the client's feelings. This does not mean that the helper must accept or believe everything the client says, but it does communicate support and respect. Asking what the client wants to happen in this situation is a third strategy. It engages the client in the helping process and also emphasizes the worker's support and respect for the individual. In addition, it can provide the client with some sense of control over his or her life. Finally, for resistance that occurs later in the relationship, changing the pace or the topic may temporarily lessen feelings of threat.

THE SILENT CLIENT

Particularly difficult for the beginning helper is the silent client. The uncomfortable silence may cause the helper to believe that nothing is taking place; in fact, silence can have many different meanings. It is the helper's responsibility to evaluate what a silence means so he or she can decide how to respond. Silence can mean that the client is waiting for direction from the helper. In this case, the client may feel that it is the helper's place to determine the topic of discussion or the direction in which the relationship should move. A second meaning of silence can be that the client is

TABLE 7.5 | SUMMARY POINTS: STRATEGIES FOR RESISTANCE

- Recognize and accept the antagonism.
- Ask for the client's perception of the problem.
- Ask the client for solutions.
- Change the pace or topic.

pondering what has been said. Resistance (discussed previously) may also manifest itself as silence; a change of pace or topic may be necessary until the client is ready to deal with what is happening.

MR. AND MRS. LOPEZ

Mr. Lopez and his wife were referred for counseling by their family physician. Mrs. Lopez is experiencing signs of dementia, and her deteriorating condition requires that Mr. Lopez be the caregiver. During the first session, Mrs. Lopez talked about her son, Enrique, and how he is learning to tie his shoes. Mr. Lopez volunteered the information that Enrique is 24 years old, lives in a neighboring state, and is a computer analyst. Other than this comment, he sat silently.

In this case Mr. Lopez may be silent for several reasons: despair over his wife's condition, confusion about her behavior, discouragement, or simply nothing to say. The helper will want to be sensitive to his behavior and to check out what he is feeling.

THE OVERLY DEMANDING CLIENT

Calling the helper at home, monopolizing time in the office, and scheduling frequent and unnecessary appointments are behaviors of an overly demanding client. Sometimes such clients become so dependent that they may want to be told what to do. When the client makes demands, the helper may become resentful of the time the client takes up and frustrated with the unsuccessful nature of the helping process. For these reasons, the helper must deal appropriately with the client's behavior.

I just called my case worker, Ms. Renfro, and she promised to come right over. I know that she usually goes to church on Sunday evenings, but I really need to see her. She is so good to me and tells me to call her whenever I need her. And she helps me all of the time. I have a regular scheduled appointment with her for 30 minutes every Tuesday morning, but I would not be able to get through a day without talking with her. Last Friday she called to tell me that she was going out of town next Tuesday and cancelled our regular Tuesday appointment. I have called her each day to urge her not to go.

Ms. Renfro will probably develop some resentment toward this client when her patience is exhausted. At some point, it will be in both their best interests for her to establish some boundaries for the relationship.

One strategy that may help with the overly demanding client is setting reasonable limits to decrease the client's dependence. Limiting client–helper contact to working hours only is one step toward decreasing dependence. A second strategy is to examine the helper's own need to be needed. Is the helper actually encouraging the demanding behavior of the client?

THE UNMOTIVATED CLIENT

Clients who are present because someone referred them or encouraged them to seek help may be unmotivated. They may not see the need for the service and may be showing up only because some authority such as their parents, the school, or the court is forcing them to attend. Unfortunately, the unmotivated client is often unwilling to change and only goes through the motions of the helping process. The helper may find that he or she is doing most of the work in the relationship and may come to feel resentful, frustrated, and even angry. Such clients may be classed as reluctant clients, and many of the same strategies previously suggested may be helpful in establishing rapport with them. A parolee is an example of a client who must have regular meetings with a parole officer.

> Many of my parolees come in to see me just because they have to. In fact, most of them come because it is one of the terms of their probation. They figure seeing me is not as bad as being returned to prison. Each day I try to see at least seven of them; and I also try to make two or three visits to see them at their work site. Most of the conversations are predictable: "How are you doing?" "Fine, I guess." "Looks like your job is going well." "Yep." "Tell me a little about your family." "They are fine." "I got some information about a new skills course ..." "Oh." "Is there anything that I can do for you ..." "... (offers no response and shrugs shoulders)." For these folks I am just a person that they must see or suffer the consequences.

INTERVENTION STRATEGIES

Now that you have learned about the helping process, it is important to look at two intervention strategies human service professionals are using. **Crisis intervention** is a helping process that is used to respond to stressful events and emergencies. **Resolution-focused brief therapy** is used when limited time or resources require a short-term intervention.

CRISIS INTERVENTION

Crisis intervention is a helping process that occurs at a much faster pace than other helping and incorporates many of the helping roles and skills that have been discussed in this chapter. You may find yourself engaged in crisis intervention when there is an emergency. For example, a crisis can be precipitated by suicide threats or attempts, the discovery of an unwanted pregnancy, abandonment, or natural disasters such as hurricanes or tornadoes. In this section, you will read a description of crisis intervention as a human service, including types of crises, the development of a crisis, the principles and skills of intervention, and the role of the human service professional in providing this service.

DEFINING CRISIS   Stressful events and emergencies are going to occur; individuals can probably handle some but may find themselves unable to cope with others. The inability to cope creates the potential for crisis. An individual's equilibrium is disrupted by pressures or upsets, and this imbalance results in stress so severe that the person is unable to find relief by using coping skills that have worked previously.

BOX 7.4	WEB SOURCES
	Find Out More about Crisis Intervention

http://www.wm.edu/TTAC/articles/

The Training and Technical Assistance Center (T/TAC) at the College of William and Mary is part of a statewide network funded by the Virginia Department of Education. T/TAC staff provide a variety of request-based support services and assistance to educational professionals serving school-age students with mild and moderate disabilities or transition needs in Eastern Virginia. The site describes how to develop a school-based plan for crisis intervention.

http://www.healingofnations.org/prevent.html

This site explores the ways that crisis intervention and suicide of Native Americans can be approached. The site provides information about statistics and incidence of suicide for this population, the psychology of suicide, how to cope, signs to look for, and risk factors.

http://www.apa.org/practice/

This web page of the American Psychological Association is a link to information about a

disaster response network. It includes a fact sheet and information on traumatic stress and managing traumatic stress.

http://main.edc.org

The Educational Development Center is an international, nonprofit organization that promotes health prevention. One area of focus is child violence and injury. Prevention issues are explored and services are provided.

http://www.crisishotline.org/

"Having a crisis? A crisis presents both a feeling of danger and an opportunity for growth by learning more effective coping skills. Explore strategies for working through this critical turning point." This paragraph introduces the website of Crisis Intervention of Houston, helping people in crisis through telephone crisis counseling, referrals, intervention, post intervention, and education.

When identifying crises, we need to distinguish between the event or situation and the person's response. The crisis is the individual's emotional response to the threatening or hazardous situation rather than the situation itself. Thus, the crisis lies in the individual's interpretation or perception of an event; the same event does not lead to crisis for all people. What one individual can handle may be a crisis for another person.

Crises can be divided into two types: developmental and situational. A *developmental crisis* is an individual's response to a situation that is reasonably predictable in the life cycle. Chapter 5 explained that as individuals grow and develop, they undergo periods of major transition such as childhood to puberty, puberty to adolescence, and adolescence to adulthood. Stresses can occur at each phase. For many people, the stresses are normal developmental problems with which they are able to cope. For those who cannot cope, the stresses of these stages can have destructive effects, such as suicide attempts, rejection of others, and depression. Such reactions constitute a developmental crisis in those circumstances.

Situational or *accidental crises* do not occur with any regularity. The sudden and unpredictable nature of this type of crisis makes any preparation or individual control impossible. Examples are fire or other natural disaster, fatal illness, relocation, unplanned pregnancy, and rape. Hazardous situations such as these may cause periods of psychological and behavioral upset. A crisis may result, depending on the individual's personal and social resources at the time of the event.

The skills and strategies that helpers use to provide immediate help for a person in crisis constitute *crisis intervention*. This is short-term therapy that focuses on solving the immediate problem and helping the individual to reestablish equilibrium. Common practice areas of crisis intervention are childhood and adolescence, mental health problems, marital and family conflicts, emergency hospitalization, suicide prevention, and substance abuse.

HOW A CRISIS DEVELOPS   Even a sudden or short-lived crisis has identifiable components that create a pattern of development. The case study that follows examines crisis in terms of its development. You may want to make note of the different roles the worker plays.

BEN AND JOAN MATTHEWS

Ben and Joan Matthews and their three children (ages 9 months, 2 years, and 5 years) left their trailer in rural Illinois to drive to Florida. Ben had lost his job because the factory where he worked for minimum wage closed down. He hoped to find a job in Florida working on some of the fruit farms. The hope for a job did not materialize in Florida, so they headed back to their trailer in Illinois and an uncertain future. Two of the children became ill, the car broke down twice, and Joan and Ben argued constantly about what they should do next. A couple of times, the arguments escalated into shouting matches that ended when Ben hit Joan.

By the time the Matthews were about halfway to Illinois, they had no money for food, lodging, or gas. They stopped at a fast-food place so that everyone could use the bathroom and have a drink of water. Joan gathered the children together and headed into the restaurant. When they returned, Ben and the car were gone.

According to Hoff (1995), crisis development has four identifiable phases. In the first, the person reacts to a traumatic event with increased anxiety. The individual then responds with problem-solving mechanisms to reduce or eliminate stress. Here is Joan's initial response:

Joan thinks that Ben has gone to get gas, so she returns to the restaurant. Selecting an out-of-the-way booth, she and the children sit watching and waiting for his return. After an hour, Joan begins to feel desperate. Joan fusses with the children and tries to look natural and unworried.

In the second phase, the individual's problem-solving ability fails. The stimulus that caused the initial rise in anxiety continues. In this case, the source of Joan's anxiety does not change: Ben is still missing. Her initial attempts to deal with the situation fail, and her anxiety continues to increase.

At this point the manager approaches and asks if he can be of any assistance. By now the children are crying. They are still hungry, are tired of sitting, and sense their mother's tension. Feeling frightened and alone, but not wanting to upset the children, Joan explains to the manager that her husband went to get some gas and that he will be back soon to pick them up. Joan leaves the restaurant with the children and begins to check the three nearby gas stations. No one has seen Ben. Joan decides to return to the restaurant.

TABLE 7.6 | SUMMARY POINTS: CRISIS DEVELOPMENT

- Reaction to a traumatic event with increased anxiety
- Problem-solving ability fails
- Additional attempts at resolution fail and anxiety increases
- Problem remains unresolved and tension and anxiety increase to an unbearable degree

Joan's anxiety level is increasing, and all attempts at resolution have failed. In the third phase, she uses every resource available to solve the problem and to lessen her anxiety. Joan tries several alternatives.

> During the next hour, Joan becomes more and more frightened that Ben is not coming back to the restaurant. The children are very hungry and tired. She is aware that people are staring at them, and she is afraid the manager will ask them to leave the restaurant. She decides to take the children and walk to the nearest gas station, again hoping to find Ben. There is no sign of Ben at the gas station. By this time, Joan is obviously very upset. She calls her mother collect in Illinois but gets a recorded message that the number is temporarily out of order.

At this point in phase three, the crisis may be prevented by redefining goals. Joan's original goal was to locate Ben or at least to wait for him to return to the restaurant. When she realizes that he is not returning, she attempts to resolve the situation by securing help from other known sources such as her mother.

> She asks the attendant if he knows of a shelter or a church that might take them in for the night. He suggests that she call the "welfare people." She is reluctant to call them. The children are getting hungrier and more irritable. Joan knows no one else to call. She does not want to call the local welfare office, but she feels that she really has no other choice.

This is phase four. A state of crisis results when the problem remains unresolved and the tension and anxiety rise to an unbearable degree. Both social support and internal resources to deal with the situation are lacking. All attempts on the part of the individual have failed to lessen anxiety or change the situation (see Table 7.6).

THE HELPER'S ROLE IN CRISIS INTERVENTION   At this point in the case study, the human service professional becomes involved. To illustrate the steps, principles, skills, and possible outcomes of crisis intervention, the focus of the case study will shift to the perspective of the helper. Before that happens, however, let us review some of the principles and skills of crisis intervention so that you will understand what is happening in the case.

Crisis intervention is a time-limited service. It occurs with a minimum of delay and focuses on the individual's current life situation. The helper must quickly establish trust and rapport with the client and support the client's self-esteem and self-reliance. Usually, more than one helper is involved in providing services so the client will not become dependent on a single individual. Two strategies important to crisis intervention are referral for needed services and activation of a social network for support and assistance.

Returning to Joan's situation, it is now 8:00 P.M. and the office of the Department of Human Services is closed. Her call is automatically referred to the emergency child abuse line. The human service professional who is on duty frequently gets calls such as the one Joan is making, because few resources are available after 5:00 P.M. The first step in crisis intervention is to assess the nature of the precipitating event and the problem. A key question to ask in this assessment is, "What level of danger does the person pose to himself or herself or to others?"

> Shirley, the helper on duty, answers the call in a pleasant but businesslike voice and introduces herself, attempting to establish a climate for positive communication. She listens as Joan describes her situation. Then Joan asks if the helper can do anything for her family and she explains that a number of options are available to her. Before she proceeds, however, Shirley asks Joan if she is in a safe place. Shirley tells Joan there is an opening at the women's shelter, and Joan and the children can take a cab there at the shelter's expense.
>
> When Joan arrives at the shelter, assessment continues as the case worker and the nurse on duty talk with her after dinner. The nurse completes a very basic physical assessment of Joan and each of the children, postponing a more extensive physical assessment until the next day. Joan and the children are taken to their room.

Once the initial assessment is completed, the second step, planning the intervention, begins. The purpose of this step is to restore the person to a precrisis state. Factors considered during this phase are the amount of disruption the crisis has caused in the person's life, the amount of time that has passed since the event, the individual's strengths and coping skills, and the presence or absence of supports in the person's life.

> In the morning, the family eats breakfast, and the children are allowed to go to the playroom with the other children at the shelter. Joan meets with the nurse and the case worker; they are concerned about a bruise on Joan's face, which has developed where Ben hit her the day before. Joan assures them that Ben's action was an isolated incident, caused by frustration, and that he has never hit her before. The caseworker encourages Joan to express her fears and frustrations and is supportive of the huge task Joan has before her.
>
> As they begin to talk about Joan's situation, the case worker is able to ascertain exactly what happened, when it happened, and how Joan has coped to this point. The case worker and Joan finally decide that the primary problem is transportation home to Illinois. Together she and Joan begin to explore some options. Joan wants to try to reach her mother's neighbor in hopes of getting a message to her mother.

The third step in crisis intervention is implementing the intervention. In this case, it may involve only the phone call to the neighbor, who may be able to reach Joan's mother. In other cases, the intervention may be more complicated, relying on the skills, creativity, and flexibility of the worker. During this phase, the helper must focus on reality and identify the clients' positive coping mechanisms and support systems. This may help clients deal with feelings that may have been suppressed (such as anger) or feelings that have been denied (such as grief).

The final step is the resolution of the crisis, in which the worker and the client plan for the future, reinforcing the new ways of coping. The worker also helps the client in planning for the future and preparing for any new crises that may arise. Here is how Joan's situation is resolved.

> Joan is able to reach her mother, who wires money for bus fare for Joan and the children. While they are waiting for the money to arrive, Joan talks with the helper, expressing her feelings about what happened and verbalizing her need for continued support. In response to Joan's need for support, the case worker gets the necessary information to refer her to a free counseling service at a mental health center near her home in Illinois.

As you reflect on the case study, what principles of intervention are illustrated? What roles did the helper play? What skills did the helper use in this situation? How would you describe the outcome? Finally, how is the helping process followed in this example?

At the conclusion of the crisis intervention, the client may need to continue with professional services. If the client shows little progress after the crisis intervention, the crisis helpers may recommend more traditional types of problem solving. If the help needs to be time-limited in scope, resolution-focused brief therapy might be recommended. The next section will explain how Joan benefited from receiving resolution-focused brief therapy from the counselor in Illinois.

RESOLUTION-FOCUSED BRIEF THERAPY

In response to the demands, guidelines, and funding constraints of managed care, brief therapy has emerged as a strategy to provide help that is limited in time and scope. This brief counseling intervention focuses on reaching specific outcomes in a relatively short time by making an immediate difference in the client's life, targeting behaviors that need to be changed and facilitating that change, and helping clients make new choices about thinking and behaving. Action is central to resolution-focused helping but takes place rather quickly. It now appears in treatment for chemical dependency, in children and youth services, and in mental health services.

Resolution-focused brief therapy is based upon client strengths with a focus on the present and the future. This orientation also advocates that small changes make a difference in the lives of clients. For success with each small change, clients begin to believe that they can effect change and continue to grow and develop on their own. The goals of the helping process are stated in positive, measurable terms, so that helpers and clients can measure the success of client progress.

There are several stages included in resolution-focused brief therapy (Ivey & Ivey, 2006). These stages are applied in the two resolution-focused brief therapy sessions Joan attends once she reaches Illinois.

1. Relationship building is still at the heart of this brief counseling process. The helper establishes rapport and uses listening skills to focus on a precise description of the problem. The helper also assesses client strengths and examples of past successful problem solving.

> At the beginning of the first session Mark introduces himself to Joan and asks her to sit down. From a short intake interview he is able to ascertain information about the crisis Joan and her children experienced. He explains to Joan that his role is to

provide a two-session helping experience that will focus on a specific problem she wants to address. Because they only have two sessions, he lets her know that he will ask questions and keep her focused on the present, the future, her strengths and her positive attributes. Joan explains that she is devastated by all of the responsibility that she is assuming without Ben. She is able to identify her strengths as an ability to problem solve, a commitment to caring for her children, and knowledge of other resources in the area such as her family.

2. The helper continues to identify client strengths by asking the client to talk about a time when she experienced positive outcomes. During this phase the client does not have to describe the problem in detail; in fact, the focus is really on what successes the client has had so far in dealing with the problem. The helper wants clients to be able to relate their own problems to normal "problems in living." During this time the helper and the client continue to look for resources such as client characteristics and skills, support of family and friends, and support of community organizations and institutions.

   Mark discovers that Joan has previous experience working as a secretary, has computer skills, is close to her family, makes friends easily, and believes that she is a good mother. Joan explains that she has survived the last few days because she has refused to blame herself, she has focused on loving her children, and she knows that she can support herself.

3. The helper and client establish specific goals that the client wants to achieve and that the helper can help the client achieve. Here the helper wants to know what the client expects. It is time to write down these goals in concrete and measurable terms.

   Joan wants to talk about how badly she felt when she discovered that Ben had really left. Mark is empathetic but draws her back to the task at hand, setting one goal for herself. He states that he wants her to leave the helping session with a positive, action-oriented goal. Joan decides that she wants to begin searching for a job.

4. The helper and the client begin to talk about how to reach the goal and the helper continues to talk about client success. The helper also provides the client with "homework" or a specific intervention that the client can work on after the session. Role playing and other strategies help the client practice new behaviors and try to link these behaviors to past successes that have already been discussed.

   Because Joan knows that she and her children can live with her family for a time, she is assured that their basic needs will be met. Mark and Joan work through a short action plan to conduct a job search. They practice each part of the plan that includes collecting newspapers, looking in the yellow pages, enlisting the help of her parents and some of their friends, and posting a letter asking for help in her parent's newspapers. Joan leaves with her homework.

   She returns for her next session. She reports on her progress. Mark asks her about her strengths and what helped her in her tasks. She identifies additional strengths such as being able to ask for help and listening well to what others have to say. She decides that she wants to practice interviewing since she has three interviews in the next week. By the time Joan leaves Mark's session, she has identified the strengths she brings to interviewing well, they have practiced an interview, and Joan has identified two individuals she will ask to conduct mock interviews with her. The session concludes as Joan articulates a list of strengths that she brings to her new situation.

The helping process is fundamental to the work of helping others. Understanding the nature of the process, the difficult clients one might encounter, how to help clients in a crisis, and how to apply group work and resolution-focused brief therapy guides your work as a human service professional.

KEY TERMS

attending behavior

crisis intervention

effective communication group

helping relationship

nonverbal messages

paraphrase

questioning

reluctance

resistance

resolution-focused brief therapy

responsive/active listening

termination

verbal messages

THINGS TO REMEMBER

1. Helping is always guided by two questions: (1) What is helpful? (2) How can the needs of the client be met?

2. The effectiveness of the helping process depends on the helper's ability to communicate an understanding of the client's feelings, clarify what the problem is, and provide appropriate assistance to resolve the problem.

3. Formal helping takes place in human service organizations and agencies.

4. Before the client arrives, the helper should attend to matters such as establishing the physical setting, deciding how to handle the paperwork, and determining how to gather information about the client.

5. During the helping process, the human service professional and the client set goals and determine how those goals will be reached to resolve the problem.

6. The way a helper listens and responds to the client is crucial in building a helping relationship with that person, "hearing" the client's verbal and nonverbal messages.

7. Attending behavior is a way to let the client know that the helper is listening.

8. There are four dimensions of attending behavior: eye contact, attentive body language, vocal qualities, and verbal tracking.

9. Beginning helpers should be wary of excessive questioning, which may hinder the helping process and make clients dependent.

10. The key to working with culturally different clients is awareness of and sensitivity to cultural differences.

11. Among the challenging aspects of human service practice is the reality that not all clients are cooperative and willing; helpers are likely to meet the resistant client, the silent client, the overly demanding client, and the unmotivated client.

12. Crisis intervention occurs at a very fast pace and incorporates many of the helping roles and skills.

13. Resolution-focused brief therapy is an intervention that provides focused, short-term, and concrete help to the client.

Additional Readings: Focus on Helping

Flannery, D.J. (2005). *Violence and mental health in everyday life: Prevention and intervention strategies for children and adolescents.* Lanham, MD: Alta Mira Press.
Case studies, readings, and websites are included in this resource about the impact of violence and victimization for parents, public health practitioners, and professionals in juvenile justice and law enforcement.

France, K. (2002). *Crisis intervention: A handbook of immediate person-to-person help.* Springfield, IL: Thomas.
The definition and philosophy of crisis intervention introduces the complex topic of working with clients in crisis. Interventions for suicide, crime victims, and groups are described in detail using in-depth case studies and words from clients and helpers.

Gibson, G. (1999). *Gone boy: A walkabout.* New York: Kodansha International.
This first-time author, an antiquarian bookseller and a father, has written a poignant and insightful chronicle of his attempts to make sense of his son's murder at the door of the college library.

Glicken, M.D. (2004). *Improving the effectiveness of the helping professions.* Thousand Oaks, CA: Sage.
This book covers the use of research and critical thinking to assist helping professionals make effective choices in treating clients. Topics include the use of evidence-based practice with PTSD, terrorism, abuse, mental illness, and bereavement.

James, R. K., & Gilliland, B. E. (2004). *Crisis intervention strategies.* Belmont, CA: Wadsworth.
The authors present the latest theories and techniques in crisis intervention. Case material from real situations illustrate theories and techniques.

Jamison, K. R. (1999). *Night falls fast: Understanding suicide.* New York: Alfred A. Knopf.
Suicide, a vast public health crisis, is the focus of this author, an internationally known authority on depressive illnesses and their treatment, who examines statistics, cases, survivors, and the media.

Meier, S. T., & Davis, S. R. (2005). *The elements of counseling.* Pacific Grove, CA: Brooks/Cole.
This book responds to the questions beginning helpers may have about the counseling process. It covers such fundamentals of counseling as explaining counseling to the client, noticing resistance, avoiding advice, listening for metaphors, and arranging the physical setting appropriately.

Mitchell, E. (Ed.). (2005). *Beyond tears: Living after losing a child.* NY: St. Martin's Griffin.
Nine mothers share what they have learned with parents experiencing a similar tragedy. Advice, reassurance, and the impact on their lives are some of the topics.

References

Association for Specialists in Group Work. (2006). *Home.* Retrieved November 4, 2006 from http://www.asgw.org/.

Axelson, J. A. (1999). *Counseling and development in a multicultural society* (3rd ed.). Pacific Grove, CA: Brooks/Cole/Thomson.

Brill, N., & Levine, J. (2004). *Working with people: The helping process* (6th ed.). New York: Longman.

Egan, G. E. (2007). *The skilled helper: A problem management approach to helping* (7th ed.). Pacific Grove, CA: Brooks/Cole.

Gladding, S. (2003). *Group work: A counseling specialty* (4th ed.). Boston: Prentice Hall.

Hoff, L. A. (1995). *People in crisis: Understanding and helping.* San Francisco: Jossey-Bass.

Ivey, A. E., & Ivey, M. B. (2006). *Intentional interviewing & counseling: Facilitating client development in a society* (5th ed.). Pacific Grove, CA: Brooks/Cole.

Johnson, D. W., & Johnson, F. P. (2005). *Joining together: Group theory and group skills* (9th ed.). Boston: Allyn & Bacon.

Negri, G., & Kramer, A. (1995). Mother Teresa brings message of love. *Boston Globe.* Retrieved January 28, 2006, from http://www.boston.com/globe/search/stories/nobel/1995/1995q.html/.

Okun, B. F. (2002). *Effective helping: Interviewing and counseling techniques* (6th ed.). Pacific Grove, CA: Brooks/Cole.

Perlman, H. H. (1983). *Relationship: The heart of helping people.* Chicago: University of Chicago Press.

Rogers, C. (1958). The characteristics of a helping relationship. *Personnel and Guidance Journal,* 37(1), 6–16.

Sielski, L. M. (1979). Understanding body language. *Personnel and Guidance Journal,* 57, 238–242.

Taylor, C. (1985). Carl Rogers and client-centered therapy. Unpublished manuscript. Knoxville, TN.

Weiten, W., & Lloyd, M. (2003). *Psychology applied to modern life: Adjustment in the 21st century* (7th ed.). Belmont, CA: Wadsworth.

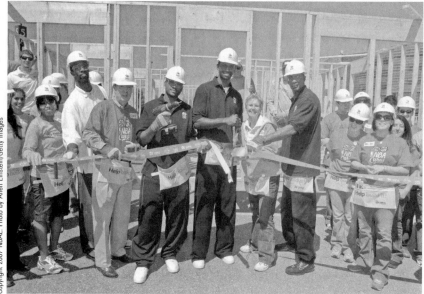

Copyright 2007 NBAE. Photo by Allen. Einstein/Getty Images

After reading this chapter, you will be able to:

- Describe the agency environment.
- Use the referral process.
- Build an information network.
- Identify the challenges in day-to-day human services.
- Define encapsulation and burnout in human services.
- Describe methods of promoting change.

Self-assessment

- Identify ways the professional can learn more about an agency.
- Explain the steps you would use to decide when to refer.
- What is a "good" referral?
- Describe the challenges the human service professional faces.
- How can professional development counter these challenges?
- How can human service professionals promote change?
- What are the pitfalls a professional may encounter while developing services in response to community needs?
- Why is the client empowerment model for change an effective one?

Many human services are provided within the context of an agency or organization in a community or a geographic area. This context or environment for human service delivery is important to those who work within its structure and boundaries. It would be difficult to assist clients, to deliver effective services, and to develop needed policies and services without an understanding of this context. This chapter will introduce the concept of the human service environment and its integral role in the work of human service professionals.

Agencies and organizations set the parameters or boundaries of the work of their employees. Concepts such as mission, structure, funding, and resources influence the world of human service agencies and organizations. Because agencies and organizations do not function in a vacuum, this chapter then introduces the larger environment of the community to help us understand the context in which the agency operates. Knowledge of the available resources in a community is part of the larger context. Some of the daily challenges encountered by human service professionals are also explored. Agencies and communities are dynamic, constantly shifting in response to social, political, and economic change. The chapter concludes with a look at ways in which the human service professional can facilitate change.

THE AGENCY ENVIRONMENT

The world of the human service agency is a complex one. In fact, when we talk about an agency's purpose or structure, it may almost seem like we are using another language. The purpose of this next section is to introduce the concepts that help define an agency. Understanding these concepts will increase your knowledge of human service delivery and the environment in which it occurs.

MISSION AND GOALS

One of the first questions you may have upon learning about an agency is "What does this agency do?" Several agency documents provide answers to this question. The first document is the agency's written **mission.** This is a statement that communicates the purpose of the agency by summarizing its guiding principles. Generally, it is relatively brief and appears in a prominent place at the agency, such as the entrance or reception area. It is usually included in all agency publications. A mission statement may identify the population served, the broad goals of the agency, sources of funding, the values that influence decision making, the agency structure, and agency priorities (Lewis, Lewis, Packard, & Souflee, 2006). It is also an important source of information about an agency's function and direction. An example of a mission statement is that of Aging with Dignity: "Our mission is to help you and your family plan and receive the care you deserve" (Aging with Dignity, 2006).

Other documents shed light on the work of an agency by clarifying rules and regulations, the work of the staff, and the standards of practice. These documents include goal statements, job descriptions, and policies and procedures. An example of a goal statement might read like this one from the Social Support Center in Abu Dhabi, United Arab Emirates: "Our goal: A Community without Crimes, A Stable Family, and A Safe Individual" (Social Support Center, 2006). To achieve this goal, Social Support Center Staff are guided by the following principles:

- Respect for human right and dignity of families and individuals
- Preservation and prevalence of law
- Keeping work as well as the parties related to the cases confidential
- Showing initiative and promptness in response, and fruitful work without limits
- Cooperation and coordination with various related parties and institutions, in order to ensure that all concerned categories are being supported
- To be wise and patient, and to discuss and consider carefully before making decisions (Social Support Center, 2006).

Another way to learn about an agency is by reading information about its job openings. When you apply for a position in a human service agency, the first exposure you will have to that position is the advertisement. Generally, it will include a brief job description, the qualifications, and sometimes a salary range or a statement that "salary is commensurate with experience." As you read the following position announcements, think about the questions you would ask if you were applying for one of these jobs.

Respite Counselor—Bachelor's degree in child development, human services, or related field. Minimum of one year experience working with children, youth, and families, and referral sources; good interpersonal skills working with seriously emotionally disturbed youth; flexible hours with occasional weekend work; some travel within a three-county region. Driver's license and safe driving record required.

Case Manager—Provide counseling, prevention services, mentoring, and case management services to adolescents in the community; facilitate parent and adolescent support groups; maintain accurate case records and reports; link youth and families to appropriate community resources; other duties as assigned. Qualifications: High school diploma or GED and five years experience working with youth and families; Associate's degree preferred and previous experience working with abuse, neglect, and special needs.

Children and Youth Crisis Treatment Team Member—Bachelor's degree in social sciences and one year professional experience working with children and youth preferred. Provide intensive case management services to mentally ill children, adolescents, and their families; work as part of a multidisciplinary team; position requires some flexibility with schedule.

If you want to learn more about a job, one request you might make is to read the official **job description** of the position. This is a written document that defines the duties and responsibilities and is much more extensive than a brief job announcement. For example, it lists the expectations for the person in the position, the job qualifications, and a salary range. Unfortunately, job descriptions are often general in nature, rarely capturing the realities of the day-to-day work. A job description may also change as a result of reorganization, changing client needs, and economic pressures. Still, it remains an important document that offers guidelines about agency expectations. The job description in Box 8.1 is for the case management position advertised. This position is with a nonprofit agency that serves children and families. As you read this job description, what additional information do you now have about the position? What else would you like to know?

Another source of important information is the policies and procedures that guide the work of the agency. An agency policy might detail how its governing board is selected or who the agency accepts for services. The school you are attending has policies about the number of hours you can take each term. An agency procedure reflects accepted standards of practice. For example, the steps necessary to spend agency funds for a client service or the rules regarding the release of client information provide a guide for the human service professional to do his or her job. Procedures at your school tell you how to register for courses or how to withdraw from school. It is important to be familiar with all policies and procedures.

Policies and procedures also influence the **organizational climate** of an agency. This term refers to the conditions of the work environment that affect how people experience their work. The range of responsibility and decision making and the intensity and frequency of supervision are examples of factors that contribute to the organizational climate. For example, is the human service professional free to determine his or her work schedule, make final recommendations for client treatment, or authorize expenditures for client services?

STRUCTURE

Another way to understand a human service agency is to learn about the way it is organized. This is the structure of the agency, and it refers to the relationships among the people who work there and the departments to which they are assigned. There are two helpful concepts that illustrate the structure of an agency. One is the **chain of command.** This refers to the layers of authority in an agency. For example, those at the

BOX 8.1	HELP WANTED: A CASE MANAGER

CHILD AND FAMILY SERVICES
Job Description

POSITION TITLE: Case Manager

Program: PARTNERS Teen Pregnancy and Responsible Parents

Effective Date: April 1

POSITION OBJECTIVE:

To provide case management services to adolescents, their families, and noncustodial parents. Case managers are advocates for customers and focus on goals that will move participants toward self-sufficiency.

ESSENTIAL FUNCTIONS:

- Provide counseling, mentoring, and case management services to adolescents
- Emphasize the importance of self-sufficiency to youth and responsibility to all parents
- Provide prevention services to youth in the community
- Facilitate parent and adolescent support groups
- Establish and maintain accurate case records and reports
- Link youth and families to appropriate community resources
- Assist with community presentations
- Assist noncustodial parents, youth, and their families with any barrier that they feel is preventing progress
- Monitor attendance and measure progress

- Maintain regular and predictable job attendance
- Work cooperatively with coworkers and residents
- Other duties as assigned

This list of essential functions is not intended to be exhaustive. Child & Family Services reserves the right to revise this job description as needed to comply with actual job requirements.

QUALIFICATIONS:

Required:

- High school diploma or GED
- Five years experience working with youth and families

Preferred:

- Associate's degree in social services—related field
- Previous experience working with abuse, neglect, and/or special needs children and their families

---

top of the chain control resources and actions. Lines of authority emanate from the top in most agencies. For some agencies, the chain of command is hierarchical with defined responsibilities and accountability from top to bottom. Each person is accountable for those under his or her supervision. Other agencies have a flatter chain of command. This means that there are fewer layers of authority from top to bottom so that decision making is more of a shared responsibility.

A second concept that is helpful in understanding the structure of an agency is a diagram known as an **organizational chart.** See Figure 8.1. At a glance, it is easy to see the boxes that represent offices, departments, and sometimes individuals. The organizational chart also illustrates the chain of command. The solid lines that connect the boxes clearly show lines of authority, information flow, and accountability. Often, lines connect vertically to represent departments or individuals that work closely together. The boxes identify different services and represent staff dedicated to providing those services.

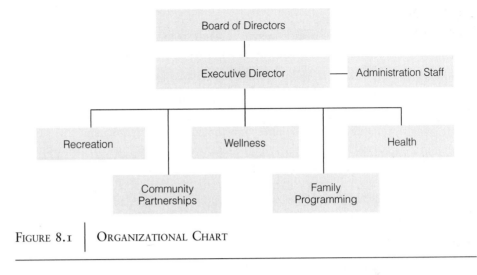

FIGURE 8.1 | ORGANIZATIONAL CHART

RESOURCES

Another source of information about an agency is its funding sources. These determine if an agency is public or governmental, not-for-profit (voluntary), or for-profit. The distinction between public and not-for-profit agencies is not always clear because not-for-profit agencies are increasingly providing services for public agencies on a contractual basis. The number of for-profit agencies is also increasing due to limited resources for voluntary agencies, reduced governmental spending, and changing political and economic times.

The term *revenue* refers to the money an agency receives from four primary sources of funding: federal, state, and local governments; grants and contracts; fees; and donations. It is not unusual for an agency to receive money from multiple sources. Public or governmental agencies receive funding from the federal, state, regional, county, and municipal governments. State government agencies such as a department of human services or a department of family and children are examples. Not-for-profit agencies such as the Red Cross and the Children's Defense Fund are funded by individual contributions, fund-raisers, foundation grants, and corporate donations. For-profit agencies are supported by contracts and fees. In some states, the prison system is run by an agency or organization for profit. This arrangement is often referred to as **privatization.**

These concepts are important in order to understand the context in which human services are delivered. They help human service professionals better understand their job responsibilities and how those responsibilities relate to the agency's mission and goals. They also allow human service professionals who operate within agency policies and procedures to provide effectively and efficiently the services their clients need. Finally, much of the planning and service delivery within an agency relates to funding. Staffing, the number of clients served, and the programs and services provided relate directly to funding.

Agencies have a number of other **resources** to use to develop services and provide them to clients. These resources include the obvious ones, such as available funds, buildings, land, staff, and short-term goods like equipment and supplies. An agency can also use resources that are not so apparent at first glance. One example is the skills and talents of the employees of the organization. These include artistic ability, physical strength, creativity, fund-raising ability, and a talent for advocacy. The skills and talents of patrons of the organization or individuals who volunteer also count as resources. Finding new resources to support agency work helps expand what the agency can do or balances deficits in funding. Homan (2004) suggests that new community resources may be identified by focusing on several aspects of those resources such as identifying major institutions, relevant community information, and personal connection to resources. Resources have a broader meaning than just staff, budget, and buildings. They include institutions, personal talents, relationships, and influences.

THE COMMUNITY CONTEXT

Just as human service professionals operate within the context of an agency or organization, human service agencies exist within the context of a larger framework—the community. For some agencies this may be a housing project or a neighborhood or a county; for other agencies, like state departments of human services or children's services, the community may be an entire state. Whatever the context, studying this larger framework is another way to understand the complexities of human service delivery.

The environments within which agencies exist influence the way they operate, the services provided, the clients served, and the professionals employed. The shared values of the community also influence the agency. The community environment may include other agencies, institutions, the specific missions and philosophies that guide their service delivery, and the specific needs that they address. Other influences include how individuals within these organizations communicate formally and informally with each other.

Community mapping is a strategy that human service professionals and the agencies they represent use to learn about other professionals and agencies. This strategy helps them connect their agencies to the life of the community and its citizens. The people employed by an agency may not be like the clients with whom they work—economically, racially, or ethnically. Yet their clients and the communities in which they live form a critical part of the helper's knowledge base.

How do agencies and their staffs connect with a community? The effective human service agency and its employees will become part of the communities where they are located. This means offering services within the context of client-identified needs; anticipating reactions to differences in race, ethnicity, attitudes, and roles represented by human service professionals; and planning for interactions among clients and helpers. Agencies accomplish this connection in several ways. Some choose to have clients represented on their governing boards or they appoint an advisory committee of clients. Locating the agency within the community is another strategy.

Youth-In-Need, the community organization you read about in Chapter 3, provides support for other agencies with whom it works and has become part of the larger community. Staff work with clients within the community, especially with teens who are homeless. Many staff spend their workdays meeting children and youth

TABLE 8.1	SUMMARY POINTS: AGENCY TERMS

- The brief mission statement of an agency communicates its purpose by summarizing its guiding principles.
- A job description is a written document that defines the duties and responsibilities of a particular position.
- The chain of command in an agency refers to the layers of authority.
- An organizational chart is a diagram that illustrates agency structure.
- Funding sources determine if an agency is public or governmental, not-for-profit, or for-profit.
- Human service agencies exist within the context of a community that influences operations, services, clients, and professionals.

on street corners, alleyways, and other street locations. Other agencies also meet clients where they are: home visits to residences in housing projects; intake interviews under bridges, at shelters, or wherever the homeless are found; meetings at residential centers or institutions for substance abuse, education, or mental illness; or even appointments at local fast-food restaurants.

Interacting in the community with residents, clients, and other professionals is another way that agencies connect with the community. This interaction serves two purposes. The first is to make connections; effective human service professionals who know the community know its resources. These include other human service agencies, religious organizations, service clubs, and businesses. And knowing these resources is the first step toward tapping them. The second purpose is to document the strengths of the community. What are the assets of the community? How can the agency support those assets in order to strengthen the community? How can these strengths be used to attack the problems?

Becoming a part of the community they serve should be the goal of human service agencies. However, the work is not over once this is accomplished. Remaining a part of the community requires continuity and interaction. The process is ongoing.

USING AVAILABLE SERVICES

An important part of the human service professional's responsibility is to work within the larger context of the human service delivery system and the client's environment. Knowledge of both agency and community resources is critical to fulfilling this responsibility. To facilitate this work, the professional will benefit from an understanding of the referral process and related issues.

Referral relates directly to the interaction between the human service professional and the environment by making use of the human service **network** during the referral process. In seeking services for a client, the helper often relies on other professionals both within and outside the agency to locate the needed services, negotiate introductions and meeting times, and establish the groundwork for the client to visit another agency. A successful referral results in the delivery of the services needed. The referral process is described in this section. The nature of and relationships among agencies and human service professionals contribute to the success of the referral.

REFERRAL

One of the most important roles of a human service professional is **brokering,** or referring a client to another agency or service. The actual referral involves a two-step process: (1) assessing the client's problems and needs, and (2) providing the link between the client and the needed service. To understand the process of referral, the worker must know when to refer, how to refer, where to refer, and how to develop the referral. Successful brokering requires considerable time and skill. Effective referral occurs when the referring professional knows what the clients may expect from another agency; it also helps the referral process if the professional has developed a cooperative relationship with other agency personnel. The human service professional and the client need to understand the services that are provided by the agency or the worker who is receiving the referral; it is important that their expectations match. Cooperation is another key ingredient in an effective referral. All the helpers involved must keep the client's needs as the primary focus. If difficulties arise, they need to remember that the goal is to serve the client well.

To make a successful referral, the helper must have information about a service or agency. This includes its history, possible legislation that affects it, its purpose or intent, and the specific client services it provides. Once the helper has this information, then an assessment begins to determine if the agency meets client needs. Several considerations about the agency need to be considered by the helper. The following questions may assist the helper determine if the agency under consideration is the correct one for the client.

- Will this agency be able to provide the service that the client needs?
- Does this agency accept referrals from us? Do we have a memorandum of agreement or an informal linkage?
- Is the client going to be able to travel to the agency's location?
- Is the intake process simple or streamlined?
- Are the eligibility standards difficult to meet?

In other words, if the services exist but are not readily available to your clients, the agency is not a good referral source.

WHEN TO REFER   A human service professional may send a client to another professional for several reasons. The referral may be client initiated—that is, the client may request a referral. The client may realize that other services would be helpful and thus suggests a specific referral. The client may request that the referral come from the worker in order to give the client more credibility with the new service, speed up the response, or both. In another case, the client may have come to the helper specifically to ask for help in working with other agencies.

Referral may also be appropriate because the helper is not able to provide the assistance necessary to solve the client's problems. The client may present requests or have problems that the worker cannot solve, or the worker may discover that the client has a major problem that must be addressed before the others can be solved and that requires more specialized assistance than the worker can provide. Another reason for referral is that the client may be in serious psychological distress—suicidal or violent—and require intensive therapy or crisis intervention that the worker cannot provide in the human services setting. The helper may also decide to refer the client because of lack of success with that particular client; a different professional would perhaps be more effective.

There are also reasons to consider what might make a referral difficult for the client. The client must want to be referred and be willing to accept services from another source. Second, the client must able to negotiate another agency setting and provide and receive information. If the client is ambivalent about the referral, then the helper must assess if the client can follow-up of his or her own.

How to Refer   Once the helper has decided that the client needs to be referred, the complex process of referral begins. A key word in the referral process is *communication*. The following four-step process provides guidelines for linking the client with another service.

1. *Explain.* The client needs to understand why the referral is taking place. Even if the client initiates the referral, the client must understand that he or she is not just being passed on to the next human service professional. Referral is a thoughtful activity, initiated for the good of the client.
2. *Describe the services.* The client needs to be informed about the referral agency and its services. The more information the worker can give about the intake process, the services available, the fee structure, and the professionals in the agency, the more comfortable the client will be in making the initial contact.
3. *Know the contact.* Talk to the agency and get the name of the contact person, the telephone number, the address, and directions to the agency. Help the client make the appointment for the initial visit to the agency.
4. *Transmit information.* Send appropriate information about the client to the new service, always considering what that agency needs to know about the client. This will allow the agency to plan. Sometimes information can be sent electronically, which speeds up the flow of information.

Where to Refer   To determine where to refer the client, the human service professional must first identify the client's problems. Then the worker must find services to meet those needs. The worker may use services that are familiar or may investigate other possibilities. Both formal and informal networks (described later in this chapter) are useful in determining what services are available and appropriate to meet the client's needs.

Home health services, a popular alternative today to hospitalization, depend on referral resources. The goals of these services are increasing client independence and minimizing the limitations of illness or disability. In many cases, this means knowing where needed services and products can be located. Home Health Source is an example of this community-based service (see Box 8.2).

BOX 8.2	HOME HEALTH SERVICES

According to the Bureau of Labor Statistics (2006), home health care services include skilled nursing care or medical services, primarily to the elderly, in the home of the patient. This service was created for dual purposes, to provide care to those who can not travel to care centers and to save financial resources. This was once a small component of the health care system, but its use and availability is increasing rapidly (Bureau of Labor Statistics).

Home health care services today include in-home nursing care, rehabilitation and therapy following hospitalization. They also includes assistance in daily living for those who can not provide care to themselves. Specific services include orthopedic-related treatment, fall-related assessment and treatment, cardiopulmonary disease management, rehabilitation services for traumatic brain injury and spinal chord injury, respiratory therapy, hospice, and consultation.

EVALUATING THE REFERRAL   The referral process does not end once the referral has been made; it continues with systematic follow-up. The helper can call the agency to learn whether the client has kept the appointment and can call the client to get the client's evaluation of the service. The worker needs to know if the service was effective and if the help received matched the worker's assessment of the problem. Such follow-up can be very time-consuming for the helper but will be valuable not only for this client but also for others in the future. It is especially good feedback for the professional and increases the client's faith in the system. The follow-up also reinforces the professional's care for and commitment to the client.

Making referrals is difficult for several reasons. Agencies are constantly changing, and maintaining an accurate picture of an agency, its current staff, and the services it provides is difficult. Sometimes services are not designed to meet the exact needs of the client, and the referring worker cannot guarantee treatment to the client. Each agency must independently assess the client's needs and the agency's ability to meet those needs. The service may not be provided because the client does not meet the eligibility criteria, because the services needed do not exist, or because there is a waiting list for assistance. The agency may not cooperate fully with the referring agency in the referral process or the follow-up. Many agencies also are so understaffed that they simply do not have the staff to provide follow-up.

BUILDING AN INFORMATION NETWORK

To make successful referrals, the human service professional must make effective use of all the resources in a community. First, the helper must know what services are available. The beginning professional is at a particular disadvantage because of a lack of experience in the system, a lack of personal contacts with other professionals in the system, and a lack of knowledge about the many problems that clients may have. Therefore, the helper must develop a systematic way of building a file of information about the human service network for referral purposes. The worker must first decide how to categorize the information to be gathered. Whether services are being organized by the physical, social, and emotional needs of the clients, the specific populations served, or one of the other organizational frameworks mentioned, the

TABLE 8.2	SUMMARY POINTS: REFERRALS

- The agency to which the client is referred must be able and willing to provide the service, be accessible geographically, and have reasonable eligibility criteria.

- A referral may be appropriate when the professional cannot provide the needed service or when the professional believes another helper might be more effective.

- When referring, the helper explains the purpose of the referral, describes the services, talks with the agency to identify a contact person, and sends appropriate client information to the agency receiving the referral.

- It is necessary to identify the client's problem prior to deciding where to refer.

- Follow-up to evaluate the success of the referral completes the referral process.

categories will help the worker think about how services are delivered in the community.

The helper can then begin to collect information and record it using computer software, a Blackberry or other hand held device, a card file, a file box, a loose-leaf notebook, or any other storage device that allows for easy additions and revisions. In reality the helper is building a database. The summary information needed includes a description of the agency or service, the types of clients it serves, the payment required for the service, the phone number and address, the e-mail address, the URLs for websites, and a contact person. The human service professional may collect information about community services from colleagues, clients, handbooks of agencies, newspapers, professional meetings, the phone book, the Web, and any community service directories produced by other agencies. The Internet has increased the access to information about other agencies, and e-mail and shared databases have facilitated communication between agencies.

Knowing more detailed information about each agency is helpful, including the purpose of the agency, eligibility requirements for services, its location and hours of operation, organizational patterns of staffing, and the nature of the agency funding. Prior to using an agency for referral, a human service professional should know what services it provides, to whom they are provided (individuals or families), whether it uses case management services, and whether it has a good record as a client advocate. Other helpful information includes the qualifications of the staff, their caseload, and their experience with specific populations. The human service professional will have a better knowledge of the agency after visiting the facility to determine its accessibility and its psychological and physical environment. Also critical is knowing how the agency receives referrals, if there is a waiting list, how long a client must wait for services, and what follow-up procedure is used to inform the referring agency of the disposition of the referred client's case. All this requires a detailed understanding of the organization and represents quite a bit of information to gather, but once you have this information, updates can be made with relative ease.

Understanding that creating the file is only one part of building a network, the worker should also begin to make personal contacts with other human service professionals. The worker should then try to establish communication as a cooperative effort—sharing information with other agencies, following up on referrals, and providing feedback to other agencies that have made referrals. These efforts will begin to build the new helper's credibility as a serious professional interested in building and maintaining networks among agencies.

Network building takes time, but it makes the referral process more effective. The better the worker knows the services available, the more appropriate the referrals will be. A network is difficult to maintain: It is a never-ending project, no matter how long the human service professional has been serving the community, because agencies are constantly in flux.

KNOWING THE FORMAL AND INFORMAL NETWORKS

A network represents informal and formal connections among individuals and agencies within the social service arena. In human service settings, the fabric of the system is formed by the elaborate channels of communication among the agencies and the workers. The securing takes place when both parties confirm that they wish to communicate, engage in two-way communication, and establish channels of communication. Human service delivery is a complex system containing two networks of communication: the formal and the informal. Both must be mastered if professionals are to participate fully in the system.

The formal network consists of organizations such as public and private human service agencies, self-help groups, schools, churches, businesses, and federal, state, and local government agencies. To understand this network, the worker must discover the answers to certain questions: What are the politics of these organizations? Who bears the major responsibilities within each? What are the formal ways to "hook up" the client to the services and resources available?

Beyond the formal network is a valuable informal network that is more difficult to recognize. It is not described in agency policy, formal reporting, or organizational diagrams. It is determined by an established history of agencies working together, personal friendships among workers, and political pressures, and it is maintained by mutual satisfaction and support. The informal network may also include informal helpers such as family and friends who provide needed support. Understanding this informal network is difficult, and accessing it takes time and effort.

There are three types of formal and informal networks: personal, professional, and organizational networks. Personal networks consist of individuals, families, and groups of people who are part of the helper's family or part of his or her social support. Individuals in this context often know the helper very well and can also reach out to a variety of others who can help in the referral process, including people in church, social clubs, and exercise and other activity-based environments. Professional and organizational networks consist of individuals with whom you work and include colleagues, teachers, and supervisors. Networking with these individuals can help reduce duplication and fragmentation of services and eliminate service gaps.

One example of formal and informal networks that human service professionals find in the client population is the formal human service system working to serve African American communities and the formal and informal religious and spirituality communities that support the development of identity, help balance emotions, provide a support system, and maintain overall wellness (Addison-Bradley, Johnson, Sanders,

Duncan, & Holcomb-McCoy, 2005; Constantine & Greer, 2003). The focus of spirituality emanates from family tradition and communal connectedness.

A human service worker who wants to help African Americans would need knowledge of the two networks. A special knowledge of the informal system allows the worker to build on the services that are already present rather than duplicate or attempt to replace them with formal services. The worker may learn about the special relationships between helpers in the informal and the formal networks by asking the following questions: What formal services are available? How do the informal and formal systems communicate? Who are the key individuals in both networks who provide services effectively or who assist the elderly in accessing the services?

CHALLENGES IN DAY-TO-DAY HUMAN SERVICE WORK

Human service professionals face many challenges throughout a typical day. They make decisions that affect their work, their clients, and their agencies. How to meet a client's need? What to tell an individual who is ineligible for services? How to stretch resources to cover the needs of three clients rather than one? Whether or not to recommend revocation of parole? At the time, some decisions are serious while others do not seem so serious; they appear to be merely choices about how professionals organize their work and spend their days. Yet, meeting these daily challenges represents survival in the human service world.

Let us examine some of the issues and their potential effects on helping professionals. You will read about the nature of issues such as allocation of resources, paperwork, and turf issues and their impact on human service professionals through the eyes and experiences of Barb LaRosa. She is the human service professional who worked with Almeada and Baby Anne in Chapter 1. She shares her perspective of these challenges and how they impact her work within the human service delivery system. Too many challenges may result in worker encapsulation or burnout. Ms. LaRosa shares her experiences of times when challenges become overwhelming. Professional development is suggested as a strategy that helps professionals meet the challenges they encounter.

ALLOCATION OF RESOURCES

Traditionally, administrators and boards of directors are responsible for allocating resources, such as staff, space, and money. It follows then that direct service professionals are solely involved in providing services once administrators have determined which services are to be provided, and where and to whom they are to be provided. In reality, however, human service professionals are also involved in resource allocation. Often they determine how they will spend their time, how much time they will spend with each client, and which services the client needs or is eligible to receive. Since resources are limited and the demands for resources often exceed their availability in many agencies and organizations, some of the decisions made by human service professionals determine the type of services that each client receives.

When you met Ms. LaRosa in Chapter 1, you were able to see her work with Almeada and appreciate her ability to support Almeada—providing her with information, services, and support during her prenatal care and after the birth of little Anne.

In that chapter the view of Ms. LaRosa was that of Almeada's helper. In the following paragraphs she talks about her own work during the days when Almeada was her client.

> Sometimes I think about my job during the time that I met Almeada. I was serving adolescents in the schools and also working with teenage dropouts. In addition, I was providing support for at-home young mothers. I had over 65 girls on my caseload at one time. I tried to keep track of all of them, but it was an impossible task.
>
> I started each day by making a list of everything I had to do. I saw the at-home young mothers weekly for one month, then monthly for six months. Then I would re-evaluate them to see if they could be referred to another service. During that time, the school wanted me to complete an in-depth intake interview with any girl who was pregnant. Then I would develop a plan and make appropriate referrals.
>
> The school referred about four girls to me each week. I tried to see all four the same week they were referred. Finally, I worked with teenage dropouts in a special program that identified irregular attendees who showed potential. I received about 10 referrals a week for this program, both boys and girls. Sometimes I would discover that these girls were pregnant or that the boys were fathers-to-be.
>
> I had two offices, one at the school and one at the welfare agency. I made it a point to begin each day at the school. That way I could check in with the office to see if I could gather any additional information about my clients. Unfortunately, when I began my work at the school, I did not get to hear the early-morning cries for help that I would occasionally receive from my young mothers. I also missed out on the "talk" with my colleagues at the welfare agency. For them, morning was an important time to check in with each other to discuss professional as well as personal business. So what I gained in helping my students at the school, I lost in helping my clients at the welfare office.
>
> The day I received the referral about Almeada, I also received seven other referrals. Almeada was the first student on the list. Taking the first person on the list is a technique of mine that I use to structure my day. I would also review the list of referrals and the list of students left from the day before for crisis situations. I would check with the assistant principal to see if he had any information about the students or if there were any problems that I needed to attend to immediately. I was so alarmed when I first talked with Almeada's parents that I became determined to find her. They told me she was pregnant, and they resented this inconvenience. I knew she needed my help; it was obvious that she had no support from her parents. That afternoon, I found Almeada at the grocery store. I canceled an appointment that evening so that I could meet her after work.

As Ms. LaRosa describes her work, it becomes obvious that she is involved in a daily allocation of her own resources. One resource is time. Like many other helping professionals, she is not able to spend as much time as she would like with each client. She constantly makes decisions about how she allocates her time. In general, she has decided that the pregnant teens and dropouts are a priority, so she spends the mornings of each day seeking them out and helping them plan for the future. When she began to gather information about Almeada, she discovered a very difficult situation. She determined that Almeada needed her immediate attention. She canceled an appointment with another client, so she could begin her work with Almeada. This meant that another client did not receive Ms. LaRosa's services that evening. Ms. LaRosa also describes some of the resources that Almeada received at the expense of some of her other clients.

TABLE 8.3 | SUMMARY POINTS: ALLOCATION OF RESOURCES

- Resources include staff, buildings, and money.
- Human service professionals are involved in resource allocation.
- When human service professionals determine how they will spend their time, they are involved in resource allocation.
- Decisions about implementation of a client plan also involve resource allocation.
- Special favors, extra attention, or concessions to clients also indicate involvement in resource allocation.

If you asked me about the most difficult part of my job, I would tell you it's not being able to give my clients all of the services that they need. So many times I discover programs that can serve my students or dropouts, especially the girls. Often though, the girls are not eligible for the services or there are not enough services for all of the girls who need them. I tried to find several options for Almeada to continue her education. I had a friend who ran an evening program, and she made an exception for me to accept Almeada because she did not really have enough credits to qualify for the night classes. In the end Almeada did not participate in the class, but the favor was granted and now I owe my friend the next favor.

I took Almeada to a family-planning clinic. Before the appointment we stopped at a fast-food restaurant to have a soda and talk about the appointment and what she could expect. The school believes that we should not buy our clients food—it is not a rule but a suggestion. The school personnel think that sharing food constitutes "friendly" relationships with students and is a use of time that cannot be documented. Honestly, Almeada was so worried about the appointment that I thought if we could just sit and talk in a place where she felt comfortable, then she might feel better about going. It worked, but it was not time that I could account for in my records.

It is obvious that Almeada received quite a bit of special treatment from Ms. LaRosa and other professionals. Almeada brought an intensity and interest to the helping process, and many professionals worked hard and "bent their rules" to help her. Again, decisions were made to provide Almeada with resources—resources that could have been provided to someone else. Ms. LaRosa "broke" the school suggestion not to take students "out" for lunch or a snack. She is aware that she is violating this protocol but feels that it was absolutely necessary to help Almeada prepare for her appointment at the family-planning clinic.

PAPERWORK BLUES

One demand on a human service professional's time is paperwork. It serves many functions, including providing a permanent record for the services received by the client. This is helpful to any agency employee who works with the client. It documents client history in the human service delivery system and is read by professionals who serve the clients at the same time or in the future. A thorough written record includes an intake interview, a social history, and medical, educational, and mental health records. As this information is obtained and carefully read by the helper, it also becomes a vehicle for organizing what is known about the client and what services are needed. In some cases, this organization may lead to possible solutions.

Paperwork involves a record of referrals and case notes of any client–helper contacts. It also documents the time that has been spent by an agency or professional, which is used for billing and accountability audits. Paperwork is becoming increasingly important in this time of strict professional accountability and scarce resources. Work with insurance and managed care companies has not only intensified and complicated the need for paperwork but has also created additional work for each professional who struggles with managing it all. If an agency is receiving state funds or support from a granting foundation, records are used in the evaluation process. Records provide documentation of the benefits of the work to clients and the community.

Clearly, the task of doing the paperwork signifies less time for client contact. Ms. LaRosa struggles with this problem.

> I have always liked to do my paperwork. Most of my co-workers do not like it and procrastinate. When I do my paperwork, it gives me a time to think about my clients, their problems, and how I can help them. I will admit that some of the paperwork drives me crazy, especially when I have to fill out multiple forms with the same information. Computers make the paperwork easier, although someone still has to enter the information. When I worked with Almeada, the paperwork actually became a nightmare for me because her case was complicated. Since I was working in three programs, I had to keep three sets of records, and all three were different. Sometimes I would try to complete one form for the right person in the wrong program. I would catch myself before I wasted too much time. Because I had two offices, it was also difficult to always have the information and records that I needed at the right office.

Each professional learns the importance of paperwork. Knowing how to handle it is a skill and a responsibility. Some helpers are very well organized, and they manage their paperwork successfully and still see a large number of clients. For most, the nature of the job, with its crises and unexpected client requests, works against any set time for paperwork. The best plans are often left unfulfilled. There is no doubt that the paperwork takes valuable time that could be used with the client. To solve that problem, human service professionals often take their paperwork home, working long after hours so that they can spend more time with their clients. They then shortchange themselves on time to focus on self, family, and others. Some helpers shorten the time they spend on paperwork, not being as thorough as they might. Incomplete or spotty records do not help the agency or the client in the long run. Still others take the time to keep excellent records and accept this as part of the job, but then they have less client contact.

TURF ISSUES

Within the context of the human service delivery system, there is a tension between competition and coalition building among agencies. For the most part, within communities, human service professionals find cooperation and goodwill among agencies as all strive together to meet common goals. This is a positive environment for human service professionals to work together for the good of the client. At times, however, either underlying tension or open conflict exists among organizations.

TABLE 8.4 | SUMMARY POINTS: THE IMPORTANCE OF PAPERWORK

- Paperwork has a variety of functions that include establishing a permanent client record, documenting client history, writing important assessments and reports, documenting referrals and billing units, and providing a record for accountability purposes.

- Professionals determine how much time and effort will go into their paperwork and report writing.

- Intensive time spent with paperwork means less time with clients.

This tension, commonly referred to as a dispute over **"turf,"** occurs for several reasons. Sometimes an agency operates in a competitive mode and sees other agencies as competing for the same resources and clients. This competition often occurs when more than one for-profit agency competes for clients; each believes there is room for only one or a few human service agencies to prosper. There are also times when an agency sees no real benefit from cooperating with another agency; it may believe there will be a loss of benefits for the organization. Because flexibility with each agency is essential for cooperation, an agency may not be able to cooperate because its mission and goals cannot change fast enough to work collaboratively. Finally, an agency may simply mistrust the intentions of those with whom they are working (Children's Alliance, 2006).

Working together becomes even more difficult when turf issues become turf battles. Strife in the human service sector can erupt over issues of inequality. For example, sometimes collaboration appears to benefit one agency more than another or one organization has access to more resources. Sometimes agencies feel they are dedicated to serving a particular area or a targeted population, and they are unwilling to share that responsibility. Agencies may also believe that the collaborative effort leads them away from their own mission and goals. Other times agencies do not agree on the methods to solve particular social problems. Finally, personality issues among individuals representing different agencies may interfere with the collaborative effort (Peck & Hague, 2006).

Ms. LaRosa has been involved in collaborative work throughout her career. Here she shares some of her experiences.

> For the most part, my experience with other agencies has been positive, since I usually work at the local level. What I mean by that is I contact other workers for help, and I help them in turn. I consider these people my colleagues. Sometimes we talk with each other every day, and other times we don't have contact for over a year. But usually we are always ready to help one another. Let me give you several examples that we have already talked about. My friend who runs the night classes and I maintain weekly contact. Sometimes I am able to help her with clients, and other times she is able to help me.
>
> I try to avoid the politics at the higher levels of agency work. The family planning clinic is a good example. I know that the superintendent of schools and his assistant tried working with five clinics in town to establish a coalition for teen pregnancy. The effort failed. My friend was able to tell the story from her perspective.
>
> She said that her boss opposed the mission of two of the clinics that were going to be in the collaborative. The first priority for those clinics is to promote adoption. They will not provide information about abortion, even when asked. They have a

TABLE 8.5 | SUMMARY POINTS: TURF ISSUES

- Collaboration among agencies benefits clients and the community.
- Turf issues arise among agencies over resources, power, and political issues.
- Turf issues can become turf battles and diminish opportunities for collaboration.
- Collaborative efforts are complex and need attention and continuous communication.

waiting list of clients who want babies, and they provide adoption services in concert with family planning. Evidently when the five clinics sat around the table, the issues of mission and goals were raised immediately. One director left the meeting early; the remainder continued to meet with the superintendent. At the end of the meeting, those present decided that no collaborative could be formed; each family planning clinic formalized individualized partnerships with the school system.

Of course I have some really positive examples to share. When I called Mr. Alvarez at the Department of Human Services (DHS), he was able to help Almeada right away because of the partnerships his organization had formed with several employers. In fact, they had formed the partnerships under the umbrella of the Chamber of Commerce and the City Development Council. That meant they did not have to form multiple partnerships; the Chamber and the Development Council, representing over 60 businesses, guaranteed cooperation among its members. Mr. Alvarez says that he has been able to provide vocational services much more effectively than ever before.

Ms. LaRosa provides two examples for us, one in which a collaborative effort was undermined by turf issues and one where a partnership was formed for the benefit of clients within the city. Agencies and organizations, human service professionals, clients, and the community all benefit when coalitions exist. Because the relationships are complex, continuous communication about goals, methods, and attention to turf issues helps resolve turf issues before they become turf battles.

Often, working within the human service delivery context can be very challenging. Professionals confront difficult issues every day; at times the organizational setting supports the human service work; at other times the bureaucracy contributes to the stress. Let us look at what happens to helpers when they face too many challenges.

ENCAPSULATION AND BURNOUT

Working as a human service professional is challenging and rewarding. Unfortunately, the enthusiasm can fade as workers become disenchanted, experience disequilibrium, and behave in ways that are less than professional. One reaction to the stresses and strains experienced by workers in helping professions is **encapsulaton**—retreating from the engagement of helping and becoming rigid, insensitive, uncaring professionals. Another result of the pressures of the job may be burnout, a syndrome that can result in poor work performance or a decision to leave the profession.

Helpers who become encapsulated may become static in their work as they face the difficulties of working within the human service delivery system. They may feel so threatened and frightened by the difficult tasks they are asked to perform that they quit learning, growing, and trying—thus becoming encapsulated. Such workers relate to clients in characteristic ways. First, they become rigid and inflexible, believing that there are enduring truths that must be upheld. Such truths can take many forms, such as "The system's rules are always right and just" or "Individuals who are unemployed do not deserve to be helped." If human service professionals are dynamic, their personal and professional experiences continually modify their ideas about clients and the entire delivery system. They grow, learning about the system and how it operates as well as learning about self. Clinging to the "truths" workers have at the beginning of their professional careers limits what they can learn from their experiences.

Ms. LaRosa talks about a time when she was encapsulated as a worker. She learned a lot during this time and believes that she is now a more committed professional as a result of the experience.

> Earlier I talked about my incredible schedule and workload. What I did not talk about was how much I enjoy my work. Working with adolescents is a great job. The preceding year, though, was a time of professional crisis for me. At this point I am able to see how much I have grown as a professional. Because I was once fairly rigid, today it is almost impossible to believe that I could have been an effective helper.
>
> I had been working with teenagers in a girl and boys club setting. I was so excited about my work when I began. I would get up and head to work at 7 A.M. just to be the first person in the building. By the time the young children arrived at 7:30 A.M., I was ready for them. I became involved in the lives of many of the families of my clients and worried about each and every one of them. I was also absolutely sure about what was best for them. I came from a wonderful family and was raised by loving parents. I was appalled by what I thought was inadequate and sometimes frightening care. Many of the parents were not at home for their children; babies were left with older siblings while parents worked. Single mothers were raising as many as five or six children. Some parents had extreme ways of disciplining their children. I tried to change the behaviors of these parents and became so frustrated when they refused to change.
>
> When I look back now, I think the only thing that saved my relationship with these parents was my absolute dedication to helping them. They knew they could depend upon me, even if I was constantly trying to show them a better way to raise their children. But, by the end of the school year, I really did not like the parents. I was not sure they deserved my attention since they were not changing their ways.

Encapsulated workers depend only on their own personal experiences and frames of references, which limits their understanding of their clients. Ms. LaRosa illustrates this limited understanding. There are many different types of clients and client situations, and it is difficult to be familiar with all of them. As a result, helping professionals should constantly read, discuss, and observe clients, so they can broaden the base from which they understand clients' experiences. Professionals who do not expand their knowledge remain limited in the ways in which they can serve their clients.

As mentioned, another result of the stress and strain new professionals experience is burnout. This condition results from negative changes in attitudes and behavior that are precipitated by job strain (Weiten & Lloyd, 2003). Like encapsulation, burnout effects the day-to-day work of the professional and results in behavior that has negative effects on the work environment as well as the helping process. There are identifiable pressures that lead to burnout. Loss of idealism and disappointment in

TABLE 8.6 | SUMMARY POINTS: ENCAPSULATION AND BURNOUT

Encapsulation occurs when:

- Professionals become static in their work;
- Professionals become rigid and inflexible and uphold their own beliefs or truths;
- Professionals support the beliefs of the traditional culture; and
- Clients are asked to accept norms of the traditional culture.

Burnout occurs when:

- There are multiple pressures at work over a long period of time;
- Professionals have unrealistic expectations about their job outcomes;
- Professionals begin to miss work, arrive late, denigrate their clients; and
- The bureaucracy does not support the professional or the client.

client motivations may result in a loss of commitment to both job and clients. Professionals who experience burnout may also be reacting to a less-than-perfect work setting—one that is too demanding, too frustrating, or too boring.

Some symptoms of burnout are a change in attitude about work, lower expectations of performance, severe emotional detachment from work, reduced psychological involvement with clients, and an intense concern with self. With burnout, helpers are likely to perceive work more negatively, resulting in sick days, tardiness, and clock watching. The syndrome also affects how workers perceive clients. They may call them names behind their backs, become angry with them, or feel that they are irresponsible and ungrateful for the help that is given them. These behaviors all impact negatively on the helper's ability to assist the client. They violate many of the basic values of helping, such as tolerance and acceptance of the client. In addition, individuals who are themselves involuntary clients are less likely to respond positively or see helpers in a positive light.

There are also some physical symptoms of burnout, such as chronic fatigue, frequent colds, serious illness, stomach trouble, lower back pain, and perhaps even substance abuse. Burnout may also affect the person's relationships with others outside of work, and the helper may be unable to take up new hobbies or concentrate on anything for long periods of time.

Ms. LaRosa has only experienced periodic burnout, but she has worked with a number of professionals who have severe cases of the syndrome. During the time she was working with Almeada, she had many of the symptoms. It was because she had such a large caseload and worked such long hours. Although she was never late or tardy, she began to resent her work. She would complain about her job to her friends and family, but she never took it out on her clients, or so she thought. Ms. LaRosa had begun to notice little things that denoted signs of burnout. As a result, she tried to adjust her pattern of unrealistic expectations for each workday. It is easy to lose your sense of professionalism when work demands exceed energy and resources.

Burnout is not temporary strain but rather a pattern of being and thinking that cannot easily be interrupted unless specific efforts are made to alleviate it. It is not just "poor adjustment" that can be corrected easily. Recovery from burnout is a long process that necessitates many changes in the life and work of the professionals who are affected.

PROFESSIONAL DEVELOPMENT

One approach that counters the devastating effects of encapsulation and burnout is professional development. In fact, this is a positive approach to address the challenges that affect the day-to-day work of helpers. A commitment to professional development is a means of keeping positively engaged and well-supported while delivering services.

Critical to improving one's professional standing is a commitment to developing new knowledge and skills. The ultimate goal is to be a more effective helper and to be able to respond to each helping opportunity in a way that positively supports the client. If the helper is involved in learning new knowledge about clients, developing and improving skills, and reflecting on current practice, then the services he or she is delivering are more effective. Within the field of human services, new information is always available about the problems of clients' experiences. New methodologies are constantly being developed to help professionals address client needs. As the field of human service delivery constantly changes, professionals need to assess what these changes mean for their work with clients. Professional development means helpers do not serve clients in the same way, year after year, but recognize that their clients' problems change, the world in which they live shifts, and new ways of helping continually emerge.

Both formal and informal approaches to continuing education are important to professional growth. Returning to school for an advanced degree—whether it be an associate, baccalaureate, master's, doctorate, or specialist degree—is a legitimate way to continue professional education in the human services. Such formal education will also open alterative career paths and allow helpers to increase their qualifications and competence. Workshops and conferences are also available within an organization or within the working radius of the professional to broaden his or her understanding of client needs and the changing times. Other educational opportunities may focus on developing one or two specific skills in greater depth. Ms. LaRosa shares with us her own experiences with professional development.

> I am indebted to a summer educational experience I had when I worked with the boys and girls club. My fellow students allowed me to see the "client experience" from another perspective. As they talked about their work with helpers and their frustrations with the helping process, I felt shame for the way in which I had treated the parents with whom I had worked. But we learned in class how to avoid treating clients in such a disrespectful way, so I was able to replace one set of thoughts and behaviors with another. Since that summer, I have continued to believe that professional development is a critical part of becoming a professional.
>
> Sometimes it is easy to be involved in professional development. Other times it seems impossible to take the time to attend a workshop, lecture, or class. I know the times that I think I am too busy to go are the very times that I should quit what I am

doing and sign up for that seminar or workshop. I am always so glad once I am there. There is an excitement I feel when I am involved in learning. It is also a good way to share ideas with other professionals and to expand my professional network. The last workshop that I attended was three months ago. The focus was substance abuse, which is a common problem among my clients. I learned how the very latest brain research impacts the ways in which we now deliver treatment to this population. Three professionals I met at the workshop volunteered to establish a "group counseling" experience for my pregnant girls.

Commitment to the profession is also a part of professional development. When human service professionals become active in an organization or become active members of the community, they expand their professional associations and their professional awareness. Anytime they study political issues or become deeply involved in solving individual or community problems that are difficult to comprehend, they are expanding their professional understanding. Even the continuous updating of their knowledge of the community, its professionals, and its resources is an informal professional development process.

PROMOTING CHANGE IN A DYNAMIC WORLD

One continuous theme throughout this text is that the world is changing rapidly. We are experiencing the globalization of the economy, increased immigration, the development of new technologies, and the emergence of new methodologies for approaching the problems in this third millennium. For a human service professional to be effective with and responsive to clients, and knowledgeable about and sensitive to community needs, it is increasingly important to function as a change agent. Becoming involved in change is often difficult for the beginning professional.

This section will present three contexts in which professionals can promote change. The first is within the arena of the local community, becoming involved in developing specific services in response to community needs. The second is also within the context of the community, initiating and participating in **community organizing.** The focus on this type of change occurs with the development of a new vision or a new focus for the community. Community organizing occurs when the development of a coalition of individuals and communities is powerful enough to continue to create and promote change. The third approach centers around the **empowerment** of a specific population with little previous status or power. The empowerment occurs once the population is identified and a team of professionals and other interested individuals work with that population to build the skills that allow them to advocate for themselves and facilitate their own change. A description and examples of each of these three approaches follow.

DEVELOPING SERVICES IN RESPONSE TO HUMAN NEEDS

In developing, maintaining, and reevaluating human service delivery, a primary consideration is the response to community needs. The community has a dual role in the causation and resolution of client problems. On one hand, the community is a source of client problems. On the other hand, it provides many of the resources needed for resolving problems. The World Bank announced a project beginning in 2007 to

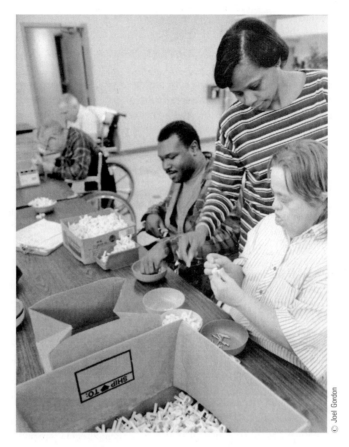

© Joel Gordon

empower women in developing countries as a way of addressing community needs (World Bank, 2006). The project links women's economic power with education, reduction of infant mortality, improved health, and the reduction of HIV/AIDS. Two issues, advocacy for nonexistent services and planning based on community needs, are integral components of fostering change.

Advocating the establishment of services that are nonexistent is one of the most difficult responsibilities of the human service professional. The **advocate** is one who speaks up for the rights of others and defends those who cannot defend themselves. When helpers discover that their clients have needs that cannot be met through the human service delivery system, they have a responsibility to work with others to develop alternative ways of meeting those needs. To do so requires skills that incorporate working with the individual, agencies, and legal and legislative bodies. Regardless of the type of advocacy, the process is much the same:

- Identify the needs of the individual or the population.
- Determine how to meet the needs.
- Work with a network of individuals or agencies to provide the services.
- Identify the barriers that must be overcome.

BOX 8.3	INTERNATIONAL FOCUS

World Bank: Gender Equity as Smart Economics

The World Bank is working to address the economic needs of women in developing countries. The focus is on working with countries, donors, and other development agencies to further the economic empowerment of women by encouraging women's participation in government and business infrastructures, finance, and agriculture. The project also supports research about the factors that restrict gender equity and those that encourage women's participation in the economic sector. One story that illustrates the power of economic involvement comes from the island of Char Montaz, Bangladesh.

Women in this small and isolated island, with funding and support from the World Bank and the United Nations, began a small company whose goal was to create battery-powered lamps. The women, defying the long-held custom of women remaining in the home, built these lamps to use in the home, replacing kerosene lanterns and reducing pollution. This effort resulted in the usage of over 1,000 lamps, businesses remaining open longer, more children staying in school, and incomes increasing over 30%.

The World Bank believes that the programs will reflect the needs of each country. For example, in many countries women are more educated that ever before, but they are still having difficulty finding jobs

so they can support themselves. Because there is a strong link between women's economic status and poverty, level of education, health, and infant mortality, the World Bank's directors believe that this project, by creating opportunities for women, will help eradicate poverty in developing countries. Some specific objectives the World Bank has targeted for this project include:

- Providing the women access to financial services and business education
- Providing women with school-to-work transition training
- Providing women with legal training to understand both women's issues and economic issues
- Teaching women technical skills needed for their businesses, whether small industry or agriculturally related
- Supporting the revision of discriminatory laws that restrict women's economic activity

Source: Adapted from the *World Bank: Empowering women, boosting economies*. (2006, October 4). Retrieved November 11, 2006, from http://web.worldbank.org/WBSITE/EXTERNAL/NEWS/0,contentMDK:21079590~menuPK:34457~pagePK:34370~piPK:34424~theSitePK:4607,00.html

- Teach clients about the advocacy process and give them a role.
- Negotiate to meet goals and objectives.
- Develop a framework that continues the success of the advocacy process.

Many professionals are successful in acting as advocates for their individual clients and can use their networking skills to find food where no food services exist, glasses and other special medical needs where resources are unavailable, and housing for those who temporarily need shelter. More difficult is the advocacy as an individual that involves developing a political voice for the larger issues that require community, state, or national attention. Colin Powell's championing of America's Promise and the lobbying efforts of Nancy Reagan and Michael J. Fox for funding for stem cell research are examples of advocacy in the community, state, and national arenas for issues of concern.

A critical component in developing services is knowing both the needs and the characteristics of the populations in need. The following case study illustrates the importance of being able to identify the problems and develop programs that address those specific problems when planning for services. A change project in Redwood City, California, did just that.

Community organizers in this mid-size city near San Francisco were interested in improving the lives of youth who lived in their community. They had always worked from a community collaboration model, but when it came to identifying the needs of the youth in their community, they realized that they were not clear what those needs were. Not only would they ask these youth what they needed, they also involved the youth in the data gathering process.

To begin the project, they asked eighth graders to help them collect information about the youth in their city using the research methods that they were learning in their social science classes. The youth would then help design programs and evaluate them. In other words, their involvement would span the entire life of the program. These middle school students would work with adults from community organizations and schools to develop services and programs to meet the needs identified.

The interviews that the middle school students collected surprised the adult participants of the project. Instead of just raising youth-related issues, these young interviewers uncovered a concern for broader community issues among their interviewees. For example, the youth talked about the lack of fun in their communities and wished they had some place to just hang out and be with each other. But they also talked about the high cost of food and housing, little access to transportation, and violence.

The youthful participants were able to contribute to the dialogue about the planning and programming to address the issues identified. And they advocated for services that would help other populations, not just themselves. Specific recommendations included concrete suggestions for improving the community, such as an archway ramp across a busy street so that all members of the neighborhood could cross without harm. They also asked for broader participation in the political process. (Fernandez, 2002, pp. 1–8).

Suppose you are a human service professional planning services to reduce youth-related violence in your city or rural area. What needs must be considered? How would you discover what those needs are? What problems might you anticipate in implementing new programs in the community? What actions might you take to ensure successful planning and implementation?

In answering these questions, you may realize how difficult planning is. Your responses should consider a variety of viewpoints and take into consideration how the services fit within the context of the current environment.

ORGANIZING TO PROMOTE COMMUNITY CHANGE

Promoting community change relies on the development and use of a network or larger confederation to advance the cause, mobilize individuals and agencies in the community, and create a financial resource base and a willing workforce of professionals and volunteers. Although promoting community change is a broader activity than just creating services, the change that you want to create must be defined, and numerous issues could benefit from the effort and focus. Read any national or local newspaper, listen to conversations between friends, tape dialogues in a teacher's lounge, or monitor the exchanges in a human service agency and organization lounge. In all of these settings you will hear numerous issues being raised. Unfortunately, most of these communications end with frustration, hopelessness, some humor, but no hope for action. The difficulties seem too challenging to overcome. (See Table 8.7).

BOX 8.4   WEB SOURCES

Find Out More about Community Organizing

http://uac.utoledo.edu/Links/comdev.htm

This comprehensive community organizing on-line site is housed at the University of Toledo. The mission of this organization is to help connect people who care about the craft of community organizing. This organization is also committed to finding and providing information that organizers and scholars can use to learn, teach, and do community organizing.

http://www.uwm.edu:80/Library/arch/findaids/mss011.htm

This website provides a fascinating history of a community organizing effort in Milwaukee, Wisconsin, that of the Eastside Housing Action Committee. The records of activities were kept from 1972 to 1978.

http://www.gamaliel.org/

This is the website of The Gamaliel Foundation, originally established in 1968 to support the Contract Buyers League, an organization in the African-American community on Chicago's West Side. The league was fighting to protect homeowners who had bought their homes on contract because financial institutions had red-lined the area. In 1986, the foundation was revamped as an organizing institute, with a mission to support grassroots leaders in their efforts to build and maintain empowerment organizations in low-income communities. The purpose of this website is to link those in need with existing community organizing resources.

http://www.grassrootsworks.net/

GrassRoots Organizing Works is an organization that supports the development of volunteer organizing for low income individuals and people of color. This organization supports target organizations and works with them on a two-year cycle to foster community development skills and projects.

http://www.cfls1.org

Community Family Life Services in Washington, D.C., is active in making changes within the environments of those in need. The CFLS Community Organizing Program develops and implements strategies for neighborhood participation and revitalization in low-income sections of Washington, D.C. Working closely with the residents and housing developers in the Galveston Place and Brandywine Street neighborhoods in Ward 8, CFLS has helped residents take pride in and take charge of their communities.

TABLE 8.7   PRINCIPLES OF COMMUNITY ORGANIZING

- Individuals and organizations identify a common goal.
- Like-minded individuals and organizations consolidate themselves to have a more effective voice in the community.
- All individual members of the community are welcome to participate in the effort, including politicians, business leaders, citizens, and others.
- Organizations and agencies are welcome to form a network of the concerned. This network includes schools, financial institutions, social service organizations, political organizations, nonprofit organizations, and others.
- The combined effort of many voices has the power to facilitate change.
- Basic to the work is organizing as a team and gathering information to understand the community and its needs.
- Basic to the work is developing an action plan.

The process of community action begins with a community action plan (CAP). The Presidents' Summit for America's Future prepared material that outlines the steps in developing a community action plan (America's Promise, 2006). It is during the development of this plan that the concerned coalition answers the question "How will this initiative be carried out?" To answer that question fully, the following questions adapted from the America's Promise plans for promoting change (America's Promise):

- What will be the community effort focus?
- Where can we find the resources we need?
- What knowledge and skills do we need to support our effort?
- What offices, technology, and equipment do we need?
- How will we gather support?
- What are the benefits of being in this coalition?
- How do we promote ourselves?

The CAP will address these questions, develop a plan of action, make assignments, and create a timeline to ensure that the plan will be implemented.

The development of the CAP focuses on meeting the goals and objectives. It begins to bring people together to talk about issues. For the first time, individuals from every corner of the community are talking together. The action plan becomes the forum for the conversation; a strong community network is being built. Not all conversation has to occur when individuals are meeting together. There are new models of community organizing that use technology to bring people together to discuss major issues and develop CAPs. These programs are developed to teach organizers how to effectively use technology to allow individuals in remote areas to participate in the community action process.

In summary, work within the community to promote change is an important part of the human service professional's responsibility. It can be a rewarding way to improve client environments and services and can expand the helper's network to include many individuals and organizations outside the human service.

USING A MODEL OF CLIENT EMPOWERMENT

Throughout this text we have discussed the importance of both advocacy for the client and empowerment of the client. Using a model of client empowerment is another approach to facilitating change, a model that is commonly used in many developing countries. The primary goal of this model is to ultimately place the advocacy and empowerment in the hands and voices of the clients or those in need. The basic thrust of this model is to educate and train those in need to organize, establish their agenda, and work for their own cause by organizing campaigns, networking with government and business leaders, proposing legislation, and participating in the political, economic, and social processes of the community. How does an effort like this begin?

One such example is the Women's Bean Project (WBP), a not-for-profit effort begun 16 years ago in Denver, Colorado. It is an on-site packaged food business (Haynes, Ryan, & MacDonald, 2006).

TABLE 8.8	SUMMARY POINTS: PROMOTING CHANGE

- Promoting change is an important role for the human service professional.

- One way of supporting change is to develop services in response to community needs, including establishing services that are nonexistent.

- The process to promote change involves identifying needs, deciding how needs can best be met, working with a network of individuals or agencies to provide services, identifying barriers that must be overcome, and teaching clients the advocacy process.

- Negotiating the meeting of goals and objectives and developing plans for future services are also part of the process.

- Community involvement to promote change uses a confederation of individuals and organizations committed to the same cause.

- One model of client empowerment focuses almost entirely on supporting clients to develop their own agenda, support structure, plan for change and evaluation, and the recruitment of new members.

This project prepares women for the world of work by teaching them basic job skills and basic life skills. Each woman commits to enrollment in the project for at least six months and for as long as a year. Women with backgrounds of chronic poverty and unemployment are eligible to enroll. Success stories include Mary, who kicked a 2-year old heroin addiction, left prison, and is now a productive worker and an involved grandparent for the children she wasn't able to care for. Or Barbara who came to the Bean Project when she was living in a homeless shelter and had no job skills to help her obtain employment and has now been employed at the same place for seven years. She owns a home and a car (Haynes et al., 2006).

The WBP uses the Results Oriented Management and Accountability (ROMA) method that helps link project goals to outcomes, indicates measures of success, and demands a data collection and data analysis process. In line with the commitment to empowerment and advocacy, the agency itself has changed with its use of ROMA. Successes include participants who focus on improving their lives, an increased graduation rate in the program and an increased in the rate of employment. The program offers women an opportunity to develop skills, stabilize their lives, and in turn begin to help others. (Haynes et al., 2006)

There are many ways the human service worker can become involved in change. You do not have to spearhead a movement or fight single handedly for your clients. Just look around your neighborhood, city, or organization to find efforts you wish to support to ultimately improve the lives and environments of your clients.

KEY TERMS

advocate	empowerment	network	referral
brokering	encapsulation	organizational chart	resources
chain of command	job description	organizational climate	turf
community organizing	mission	privatization	

BOX 8.5	INTERNATIONAL FOCUS
	Disha Kendra

Disha Kendra was established in 1978 by Jagrut Bhaubandhi Sangatana to help village tribal people in India fight their socioeconomic and political oppression. Tribals are indigenous people who live in remote rural areas in India. Each tribe has a different culture, speaks a unique dialect, and lives according to long-standing traditions.

The first phase of the organization's work (1978–1983) focused on economic and human rights development. One example of this work was the two-year process of breaking the economic hold of the moneylender on the 35-household village of Chadhawadi and substituting a six-year bank-loan program to support local farming efforts. During this initial phase, education was also enhanced with the formation of preschool and adult education programs. From 1983 to 1991—the second and third phases of the organization's history—the effort determined long- and short-term needs of the village and assessed the outcomes of past efforts. In addition, the organization promoted the tribal people's ability to lead their own political organizations as they struggled to increase the availability of water, electricity, and employment opportunities.

The fourth phase of the agency's work is underway and includes strengthening political organization and leadership training, improving community organization, and improving the lives of tribal women. The emphasis is on helping tribals help themselves.

During the authors' visit to the village, the agency's political action director, Bunsi, conducted a meeting of the village committee, a group of six men from surrounding villages. Their task was to prepare for a meeting the following week with the police superintendent inspector who would rule on a land-access dispute. A wealthy Mumbai businessman had bought a large track of land near the village and was denying access to their farmland, water supply, and firewood. Bunsi asked those in attendance to decide who would speak for the committee, and he explained the hearing process. They then role-played what the spokesman would say at the hearing.

The agency workers visit the villages weekly or live in the villages themselves. They are available to help with whatever issues arise that affect the rights of tribals as a protected class of people in India.

THINGS TO REMEMBER

1. The work of the human service professional occurs within an agency or organization.

2. An agency's written mission statement communicates an agency's purpose by summarizing its guiding principles.

3. Goal statements, job descriptions, and policies and procedures are other agency documents that clarify the work of an agency and its employers.

4. The relationships among the individuals who work in an agency and the departments to which they are assigned describe an agency's structure.

5. Chain of command, often illustrated by an organizational chart, refers to the layers of authority in an agency.

6. Funding sources determine if an agency is public or governmental, not for-profit (voluntary), or for-profit.

7. Human service agencies exist within the context of a community that influences agency operations, services, clients, and professionals.

8. One of the most important roles of a human service professional is brokering, or referring a client to another agency or service.

9. The referral process involves the worker, the client, and the other agency to which the client is referred.

10. In referral, the beginning human service professional is at a disadvantage because of a lack of experience in the system, a lack of personal contacts with workers in the system, and a lack of knowledge about the many problems that clients may have.

11. The beginning professional must develop a systematic way of building a file of information about the human services network for referral purposes.

12. Challenges such as allocation of resources, paperwork, and turf issues influence the work of the human service professional.

13. Responses such as encapsulation and burnout leave workers unable to be effective helpers.

14. Professional development strategies such as attending workshops and participating in professional organizations help professionals respond to changes in human services.

15. An important responsibility of the human service professional is to be an advocate for change.

16. In developing, maintaining, and reevaluating the delivery of human services, it is important to consider human services as a response to community needs.

17. Empowering clients to advocate for their own change is one model of responding to client needs.

Additional Readings: Focus on Organizations

Bolman, L. G., & Deal, T. E. (2003). *Reframing organizations: Artistry, choice, and leadership.* San Francisco: Jossey-Bass.
A consistent bestseller, this book offers practical ways of thinking about today's challenges.

Homan, M. S. (2004). *Rules of the game: Lessons from the field of community change.* Pacific Grove, CA: Brooks/Cole.
The author offers practical wisdom and 135 guidelines for community change as readers explore what they need to know about themselves, others, and the change process.

Hull, G. H., & Kirst-Ashman, K. K. (2004). *Generalist practice with organizations and communities.* Belmont, CA: Wadsworth.
This text applies the generalist practice model to work with larger systems, including organizations, neighborhoods, and communities.

Sen, R. (2003). *Stir it up: Lessons in community organizing and advocacy.* Hoboken, NJ: Jossey-Bass.
This text provides the steps of building a constituency and organizing for social justice. There are multiple case studies to illustrate the concepts presented.

Smith, M. B., Graham, Y., & Guttmacher, S. (2005). *Community-based health organizations: Advocating for improved health.* New Brunswick, NJ: Jossey-Bass.
This text presents basic principles to create community-based health organizations. Included is a history of community-based care and a structured outline of developing services in communities.

References

Addison-Bradley, C., Johnson, D., Sanders, J. L., Duncan, L., & Holcomb-McCoy, C. (2005) January). Forging a collaborative relationship between the black church and the counseling profession. *Counseling and Values, 49,* 147–154. Retrieved November 11, 2006, from Academic Search Premier.

Aging with Dignity. (2006). *Home.* Retrieved October 11, 2006, from http://www.agingwithdignity.org/.

America's Promise. (2006). *Home.* Retrieved November 11, 2006, from http://www.americaspromise.org/.

Bureau of Labor Statistics. (2006). *Health.* Retrieved November 11, 2006, from http://www.bls.gov/oco/cg/cgs035.htmhttp://www.bls.gov/oco/cg/cgs035.htm.

Children's Alliance. (2006). *Voice of Washington's children, youth and families.* Retrieved November 11, 2006, from http://www.childrensalliance.org/.

Constantine, M. G., & Greer, T. M. (2003). Personal, academic, and career counseling of African American women in college settings. In M. Howard-Hamilton (Ed.), *Meeting the needs of African American women: New directions for student services* (pp. 41–51). San Francisco: Jossey-Bass.

Fernandez, M. A. (2002). *Creating community change: Challenges and tensions in community youth research.* Palo Alto, CA: John W. Gardner Center for Youth and Their Communities.

Haynes, S., Ryan, T., & MacDonald, B. (2006). *The Women's Bean Project: Defining the mission and measuring outcomes to better serve the needs of women.* Unpublished manuscript, Denver, Colorado.

Homan, M. (2004). *Promoting community change* (3rd ed.). Pacific Grove, CA: Brooks/Cole.

Lewis, J. A., Lewis, M. D., Packard, T., & Souflee, F. (2006). *Management of human service programs* (3rd ed.). Pacific Grove, CA: Brooks/Cole.

Peck, G. P., & Hague, C. E. (2006). *Turf issues* (CDFS 12). Retrieved November 11, 2006 from http://ohioline.osu.edu/bc-fact/0012.html.

Social Support Center. (2006). *Community policing department.* Abu Dhabi, United Arab Emirates Ministry of Interior, Abu Dhabi Police G. H. Q.

Weiten, W., & Lloyd, M. (2003). *Psychology applied to modern life: Adjustment in the 21st century* (7th ed.). Belmont, CA: Wadsworth.

World Bank. (2006). *Gender equality as smart economics: A World Bank Group Gender Action Plan.* Retrieved November 11, 2006, from http://siteresources.worldbank.org/INTGENDER/Resources/GAPQ&AOct5.pdf.

| # PROFESSIONAL CONCERNS

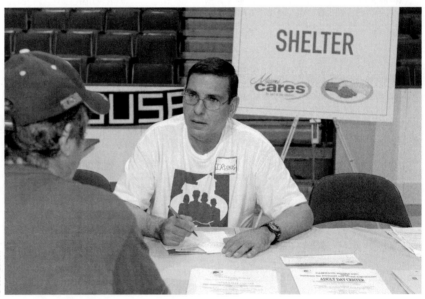

© Joel Gordon

After reading this chapter, you will be able to:

- State the purpose and limitations of codes of ethics.
- Summarize the influence of law, diversity, and technology on codes of ethics.
- Write vignettes to illustrate the concerns of competence, responsibility, confidentiality, and client's rights.
- List the steps in the ethical decision-making model.
- Apply the ethical decision-making model to an ethical dilemma.

Self-assessment

- Identify the purposes and limitations of codes of ethics.
- Why are competence and responsibility ethical issues? How will each influence a human service professional's relationship with a client?
- Describe the components of the Ethical Standards of Human Service Professionals.
- What is difficult about the practice of confidentiality? Why is it important?
- What rights do clients have?
- How do professionals make ethical decisions?
- How might a human service professional use the model for ethical decision making?

This final chapter focuses on the ethics of human service practice. The helper is continually faced with ethical decisions. Sometimes these issues arise between the professional and the client and other times there are multiple individuals and even agencies with a stake in the decisions made. The helper's responsibilities are not simply to recognize an ethical situation and make the "right" decision. In fact, ethical practice and decision making require that the helping professional consider the situation from all points of view, develop a list of issues that represent multiple viewpoints, generate possible decisions, and weigh carefully the consequences of each decision. This type of ethical practice demands that the helper have knowledge of the professional code of ethics, critical thinking skills, an understanding of human behavior, good communication skills, the ability to establish rapport, and decision-making skills.

In this chapter you will use your knowledge of the history of human services, the work of the professional, and the nature of clients and settings to imagine yourself in the role of the helper. The chapter includes an introduction to codes of ethics, definitions of competence and responsibility, a discussion of confidentiality, a description of the client's rights, ethical standards of human service professionals, and a model for ethical decision making.

ETHICAL CONSIDERATIONS

As you deliver human services, situations will arise in which you may be unsure about the appropriate action to take. A third party requests information about a client; you observe a colleague joking about a client in the break room at work; a client requests information about obtaining an abortion, but your agency opposes providing this type of information. These situations represent **ethical dilemmas** for the human service professional. Even though education and training in human services emphasize the values of confidentiality, acceptance, individualism, self-determination, and tolerance, situations will inevitably occur in which simply possessing these values will not be enough to determine the right course of action.

The foundation of ethical behavior is based upon principles that are shared by members of the profession. Professions such as medicine, nursing, psychology, counseling, health, and human services adhere to similar principles that undergird practice. These principles focus on the way in which professional helpers work with clients. They include autonomy, nonmaleficence, beneficence, justice, fidelity, and veracity.

Autonomy represents the commitment to respect a client's right to define his or her own problems, help choose interventions, and help evaluate successes and satisfactions. Helpers who provide the client with autonomy foster self-determination and support client independence.

Nonmaleficence essentially means that the professional will not harm the client. This means that human service workers will not take risks that might, in the short or long run, hurt the client.

Beneficence defines an act that is in someone's best interest. Helpers guided by this principle provide services or serve as advocates with what the client needs in mind. At times, family considerations or agency rules and regulations clash with perceived client needs.

Justice as a principle means that the human service professional works tirelessly to promote equality of access for clients, is fair in all interactions, and is obligated to adhering to the principles of nondiscrimination.

Fidelity is respecting the trust that clients place in their helpers and guarding against an erosion of that trust. Helpers are careful to fulfill their responsibilities, keep promises, and be honest in their interactions with clients.

Veracity means being honest with clients. Human service workers commit to providing clients with all of the information that they need and to providing fair and honest feedback.

In the past decade, increased public awareness of professional behavior, coupled with the passage of federal and state legislation controlling the helping professions, has underscored the importance of ethical concerns in service delivery. The Family Educational Rights and Privacy Act of 1974, state legislation requiring the reporting of child abuse, and *Tarasoff v. Regents of the University of California* (1976), which imposed a duty to warn potential victims, are examples of government action that directly affects the ethics of service provision. A more recent example is the Health Insurance Portability and Accountability Act (HIPPA) that went into effect in 2003 and has greatly impacted informed consent practices. The human service professional must obey the law and also be cognizant of the implications of the law.

An exploration of codes of ethics or statements of standards of behavior as guides for professional behavior begins the next section. Some major areas of ethical concern for the human service professional follow. Then we describe an ethical decision-making model that can be applied to dilemmas for which there is no relevant guideline. Vignettes are used to illustrate the range of dilemmas that may arise.

Codes of Ethics

Professionals have responded to the dilemmas of service provision by developing **codes of ethics,** or statements of ethical standards of behavior for the members of their profession. Codes of ethics or ethical standards reflect professional concerns and define the guiding principles of professional activities. As an aid to ethical decision making in dilemmas arising in service delivery, such standards or codes help clarify the professional's responsibilities to clients, to the agency, and to society. Typically, a code of ethics includes items that state the goals or aims of the profession, that protect the client, that provide guidance to professional behavior, and that contribute to a professional identity for the helper. A complete understanding of a code of ethics or ethical standards requires knowledge of the code's strengths and purposes as well as its limitations.

PURPOSES AND LIMITATIONS The primary functions of a code of ethics or ethical standards are to establish guidelines for professional behavior and to assist members of the profession in establishing a professional identity (Corey, Corey, & Callanan, 2007; Welfel, 2006). Other purposes include providing criteria for evaluating the ethics of a professional's practice and serving as a benchmark in the enforcement of ethical standards.

Ethical codes do have limitations; they cannot cover every situation. They do, however, present a framework for ethical behavior, although their exact interpretation will depend on the situation to which they are being applied. As a result of this vagueness, codes may have a limited range, and some codes of ethics will likely conflict with others regarding some standard of behavior. Such conflicts pose problems for professionals who are members of more than one professional organization.

Other entities that set standards may also issue ethical standards that conflict. For example, a code may not include a statement relating to the duty to warn, but the California Supreme Court has ruled in *Tarasoff* (1976) that there is a duty to warn potential victims of danger. Members who are bound by a code of ethics must be alert to the possibility that other forums may reach conclusions that differ from their code. Of course, this is especially critical when the other forum is a court of law or a legislative body.

Some other limitations of codes of ethics are beyond the scope of this text; however, human service professionals must be aware that such limitations exist. The professional must develop ethical reasoning skills to help resolve ethical dilemmas that may arise. A first step in this process is differentiating ethical dilemmas from situations in which the guidelines are clear. For resolving problem situations for which there are no specific guidelines, an ethical decision-making model is presented later in this chapter.

ETHICS AND THE PROFESSION A code of ethics is binding only on the members of the group or organization that adopts it. Several organizations in human services have issued codes of behavior expected of their membership—organizations such as the American Counseling Association, the National Council for Social Work Education, and others in the fields of corrections, mental health, gerontology, and education. Most codes of ethics stipulate that the helper's first responsibility is to enhance and protect the client's welfare. Codes also give guidance about the helper's responsibilities to employers, to colleagues in the profession and other fields, and to society in general.

BOX 9.1	WEB SOURCES

Find Out More about Codes of Ethics

http://www.counseling.org/Publications

This site provides the Code of Ethics of the American Counseling Association as well as cross-cultural counseling competencies and objectives.

http://www.apa.org/ethics/code2002.pdf

This site provides ethical considerations articulated by the American Psychological Association.

http://www.nbcc.org/etras/pdfs/ethics/nbcc-codeofethics.pdf

This site presents ethical consideration of counseling presented by the National Board of Certified Counselors.

http://www.nationalhumanservices.org

The site of the National Organization for Human Services includes the Ethical Standards of Human Service Professionals adopted in 1996.

Ethical codes adopted by a professional association are usually based on the premise that a profession polices itself. Members of helping professions are assumed to be responsible, sensitive persons who are accountable for their behavior and the behavior of their colleagues. Self-regulation involves two types of discipline: informal and formal. Informal discipline is seen in the subtle and not-so-subtle pressure that colleagues exert on one another in the form of consultations, client referrals, and informal and formal discussions. Formal discipline occurs when professional associations publicly criticize or censure their members—in extreme cases, barring them from membership.

CODES OF ETHICS AND THE LAW   The law is generally supportive of, or at least neutral toward, ethical codes and standards. It is supportive in that it enforces minimum standards for practitioners through licensing requirements and generally protects the confidentiality of statements and records provided by clients during service provision. It is neutral in that it allows each profession to police itself and govern the helper's relations with clients and fellow professionals. The law intervenes and overrides professional codes of ethics only when necessary to protect the public's health, safety, and welfare. One instance of legal intervention occurs when the profession's standards of confidentiality (deemed necessary to ensure effective treatment) call for the suppression of information that government authorities require to be disclosed to prevent harm to others.

The California Supreme Court's ruling in the case of *Tarasoff* (1976) legally supported a "duty to warn" possible victims of clients once counselors have this information. The court stated that

> when a therapist determines, or pursuant to the standards of his profession should determine, that his patient presents a serious danger of violence to another, he incurs an obligation to use reasonable care to protect the intended victim against such danger. The discharge of this duty may require the therapist to take one or more steps, depending on the nature of the case. Thus, it may call for him or her to warn the intended victim or others likely to apprise the victim of the danger, to notify the police, or to take whatever other steps are reasonably necessary under the circumstances. (p. 340)

ETHICS AND DIVERSITY   Ethical concerns in providing human services in a diverse society occur on two levels. One is at the individual level. The unintentional bias of a human service professional may encompass hidden beliefs and attitudes that can be a harmful influence on the helping relationship. Sometimes human service professionals may even consciously endorse prejudiced beliefs and attitudes. Behaving in such a way is unethical.

On a more general level, the basic tenets or underlying principles of some codes of ethics may not always apply to all cultures. For example, the United States is recognized as an individualist culture where the focus is on the individual or the self. Think of the words in English that begin with self: self-actualization, self-disclosure, self-concept, self-acceptance, self-esteem, self-control, and so forth. Other cultures are collectivist in nature, emphasizing the importance of the family, the extended family, or even a larger group. These associations take precedence over the individual. In practical terms, one illustration of this difference is the health and well-being of the individual versus the health and well-being of the group. In the past, failure to take culture into account and to acknowledge individual differences within cultures has contributed to the ineffectiveness of human services with diverse groups.

Today, codes of ethics emphasize cultural competence that encompasses three broad dimensions: awareness, understanding, and skill (Sue & Sue, 2003). Later in this chapter you will read the Ethical Standards of Human Service Professionals. The preamble recognizes "an appreciation of human beings in all their diversity." Specific standards address the "respect, acceptance and dignity" due each client (#2), the need to be advocates (for the rights of all members of society, particularly those who are members of minorities and groups at which discriminatory practices have historically been directed) (#16), and the provision of services "without discrimination or preference based on age, ethnicity, culture, race, disability, gender, religion, sexual orientation, or socioeconomic status" (#17). Human service professionals are also "knowledgeable about the cultures and communities within which they practice" (#18), and they are "aware of their own cultural backgrounds, beliefs, and values" (#19). Other professional helping associations and organizations have indicated that helpers who work with other cultures without culture-specific awareness about those cultures are behaving in an unethical manner (Pedersen, 2000).

But ethics in a multicultural society are more complex. For example, self-disclosure, encouraged in European-American culture and often considered necessary for understanding by the helper, is taboo in other cultures. Asian Americans, American Indians, and Hispanic Americans do not value self-disclosure as many of us do,

TABLE 9.1	SUMMARY POINTS: CODES OF ETHICS

- Reflect professional concerns
- Define guiding principles of professional activities
- Clarify responsibilities to clients, the agency, and society
- Do not address every situation
- Are binding only on members of the group that adopts it

believing that it reflects negatively not only on the individual but also the family. Also prized in western culture is eye contact and directness. Other cultures perceive these as signs of rudeness that should be avoided. A final example is the express prohibition of dual relationships in the ethical standards of many helping organizations, for example, Statements 6 and 7 in the Ethical Standards of Human Service Professionals found later in this chapter. In some cultures like India, for instance, it is likely that dual relationships may be more normal and acceptable (Nagpal, 2001). For example, meetings with clients at their homes rather than an office may be expected. Clients may also be people who are known to the helper through relatives or friends, and it is these very associations that make it acceptable for the client to seek help from the helping professional.

So how do human service professionals provide human services ethically in a diverse culture? Here are several guidelines (Corey, Corey, & Callanan, 2007; Sue & Sue, 2003; Welfel, 2006):

- Develop an attitude of openness, respect, and appreciation toward other cultural views; expand your comfort zone with cultural differences.
- Acquire knowledge of specific cultures other than your own.
- Learn to modify interventions so that they are appropriate and effective with other cultures.
- Develop a tolerance for ambiguity and divergent philosophies, worldviews, and problem-solving behaviors that may be different from your own.

ETHICS AND TECHNOLOGY   The rapidly changing world of technology and its impact on human service delivery have created a number of concerns for both professionals and constituents. These concerns include access to personal information, online instruction, the electronic transmission of records, Internet use, web counseling, and teleconferencing. Faxes, answering machines, voice mail, and e-mail also raise issues regarding privacy, confidentiality, and security. These concerns have prompted professional associations to respond through revisions of ethical codes, statements, or guidelines, such as:

- American Counseling Association: Standards for the Internet
- ACES Guidelines for Online Instruction in Counselor Education
- National Board for Certified Counselors Standards for the Ethical Practice of Web Counseling
- APA Statement on Services by Telephone, Teleconferencing, and Internet
- NCDA Guidelines for the Use of the Internet for Provision of Career Information and Planning Services

As indicated by these professional organizational responses previously listed, using technology in the human service arena means focusing on several concerns such as a lack of confidentiality, limited training, and at times, unequal access to technology and its accompanying resources. As mentioned earlier in Chapter 3, privacy is not guaranteed when individuals and organizations use listservs, e-mail, and the World Wide Web. This means that client information, related treatment documents, agency records, and correspondence may become more public than warranted in service delivery. At best, the professional must make every effort to secure information and communication between professionals and those being helped. Clients should be warned of the potential for violation of privacy. They should also be informed of the steps that they can take to increase the likelihood of privacy from their end of the electronic communication.

Professional human service workers are encouraged to help within their own scope of expertise. If helpers are to use technology to implement treatment strategies, gather data, record data, or make assessments, then they will need training to use technology in service delivery. Technology continues to change so rapidly that training needs to be ongoing. As helpers integrate computers into their work, they need to be encouraged to try new approaches and new ideas.

Because helpers are ethically obligated to provide quality services or use best practice, they need to study the effectiveness of the use of these new technologies. Also, helpers need to be sensitive to their clients' comfort with technology and client access to the Internet. For some clients, access is not possible, or at best, difficult. Maintaining this sensitivity will help human service workers use technology to actually support clients and not to create additional barriers for them.

COMPETENCE AND RESPONSIBILITY

Before any involvement with clients, helpers must concern themselves with two areas: their competence as professionals and their responsibility to the individuals, groups, or organizations with whom they are affiliated or with whom they serve as clients. Ethical concerns of competence and responsibility pervade all areas of professional practice.

Competence is a difficult concept to define from an ethical standpoint. One way to define it is by identifying the standards for practice within the profession. Most codes of ethics in helping professions include statements about academic training, practical training, or supervised experience and areas of specialization in which the helper is most knowledgeable or competent. During their training, human service professionals must acquire knowledge about the helping process, professional ethics, the limits of professional practice, and the pertinent legislation that governs practice.

In addition to the competence acquired through preparation to be a professional, the human service professional in practice also has an obligation to ensure that available services meet acceptable standards. Helpers have a further obligation to improve services and skills through activities such as involvement in ongoing research and study, participation in peer consultation, and review of the current professional literature. All these activities contribute to the competence of the helper.

TABLE 9.2 | SUMMARY POINTS: COMPETENCE

Standards for professional practice include:

- Academic training
- Supervised experience
- Areas of specialization
- Obligation to improve services and skills

The second concept that pervades all phases of service delivery is **responsibility.** This means that the helping professional is committed to helping clients develop to the best of their abilities and to protect them from harm. Helpers also have obligations to support the profession. Furthermore, human service professionals value their work within a social services environment that promotes social justice for society as a whole. The idea that helpers have obligations to others in addition to the client may present dilemmas for the helper in cases of conflict. It is important for the helper to understand the nature of the conflict and be able to explain to the client how this may limit the client–helper relationship.

To fulfill their commitment to being responsible, helpers must know the ethical and legal procedures that are pertinent to their service delivery functions. These include the profession's code of ethics, its standards of behavior, and the consequences of failure to conform to codes and standards.

In many instances, ethical standards of competence and responsibility are compatible. For example, human service professionals are obligated to provide high-quality service to their clients. Discharging this obligation relies to a certain extent on the competence of the worker, as the worker is expected to provide only those services he or she is trained and qualified to deliver. If the client has needs beyond the competence of the worker, then the worker has a duty, according to codes and standards of professional behavior, to locate alternative services from a coworker or another agency. In this situation, the competence of the human service professional is reflected in an awareness of available services and knowledge of how those services relate to the client's problems.

The responsibility of the helper extends beyond client contact. The helper is also concerned with having sufficient time to work with a client and the resources necessary for effective practice. Should these not be present, the helper is responsible for locating or developing resources such as grants for additional funding or increased staff for specialized caseloads. The overriding concern, of course, is the obligation and commitment to provide good quality services to whomever needs those services.

The vignettes that follow illustrate some of the dilemmas that a helper might face while working with human service clients. The primary issues in these vignettes are competence and responsibility.

CASE 1

Sue is a night counselor for a cerebral palsy group home. She works five nights a week, arriving at 4 P.M. and staying until 7 A.M. the next day. Right now the group home is in the process of hiring three new staff members: a van driver, an evening visiting nurse, and a day teacher/counselor. Until these professionals are hired,

TABLE 9.3	SUMMARY POINTS: RESPONSIBILITY

Helpers must know the ethical and legal procedures, including:

- Profession's code of ethics
- Standards of behavior
- Consequences of failure to uphold codes of ethics and ethical standards

BOX 9.2	ETHICAL STANDARDS FOR PSYCHOLOGISTS

American Psychological Association

2. Competence

2.01 *Boundaries of Competence*

a. Psychologists provide services, teach, and conduct research with populations and in areas only within the boundaries of their competence, based on their education, training, supervised experience, consultation, study, or professional experience.

b. Where scientific or professional knowledge in the discipline of psychology establishes that an understanding of factors associated with age, gender, gender identity, race, ethnicity, culture, national origin, religion, sexual orientation, disability, language, or socioeconomic status is essential for effective implementation of their services or research, psychologists have or obtain the training, experience, consultation, or supervision necessary to ensure the competence of their services, or they make appropriate referrals, except as provided in Standard 2.02, Providing Services in Emergencies.

c. Psychologists planning to provide services, teach, or conduct research involving populations, areas, techniques, or technologies new to them undertake relevant education, training, supervised experience, consultation, or study.

d. When psychologists are asked to provide services to individuals for whom appropriate mental health services are not available and for which psychologists have not obtained the competence necessary, psychologists with closely related prior training or experience may provide such services in order to ensure that services are not denied if they make a reasonable effort to obtain the competence required by using relevant research, training, consultation, or study.

e. In those emerging areas in which generally recognized standards for preparatory training do not yet exist, psychologists nevertheless take reasonable steps to ensure the competence of their work and to protect clients/patients, students, supervisees, research participants, organizational clients, and others from harm.

f. When assuming forensic roles, psychologists are or become reasonably familiar with the judicial or administrative rules governing their roles.

Source: Material from "Ethical Principles of Psychologists and Code of Conduct." Copyright © 2002 by the American Psychological Association, Inc.

much of the responsibility falls to Sue. She does not mind doing all that she can for the group home and the clients, but she feels that she is not qualified to do some of the things asked of her.

CASE 2

George has a job as a case worker for a mental health outpatient service. He provides individual and group counseling for adult clients. One of his clients, Kim, is having trouble relating to her husband, her son, and her father. George suggests to Kim that she practice various forms of sexual intimacy with him as a part of her therapy to improve her relationships with men.

| BOX 9.3 | ETHICAL STANDARDS FOR SOCIAL WORKERS |

Code of Ethics of the National Association of Social Workers

5. Social Worker's Ethical Responsibilities to the Social Work Profession

 5.01 Integrity of the Profession

  a. Social workers should work toward the maintenance and promotion of high standards of practice.

  b. Social workers should uphold and advance the values, ethics, knowledge, and mission of the profession. Social workers should protect, enhance, and improve the integrity of the profession through appropriate study and research, active discussion, and responsible criticism of the profession.

  c. Social workers should contribute time and professional expertise to activities that promote respect for the value, integrity, and competence of the social work profession. These activities may include teaching, research, consultation, service, legislative testimony, presentations in the community, and participation in their professional organizations.

  d. Social workers should contribute to the knowledge base of social work and share with colleagues their knowledge related to practice, research, and ethics. Social workers should seek to contribute to the profession's literature and to share their knowledge at professional meetings and conferences.

  e. Social workers should act to prevent the unauthorized and unqualified practice of social work.

Source: Material from "Code of Ethics of the National Association of Social Workers." Copyright 2006 NASW.

CASE 3

Dim Su is a social service worker in a health care facility for the elderly. He is in a dilemma because several of his clients are requesting that he provide them with cigarettes even though smoking has been discouraged by the doctor. Dim Su's colleague, Betty, laughs when he tells her of his dilemma. She tells him that there is no dilemma. She has provided cigarettes for patients for the past three years.

CASE 4

Jim, the sports program director for the Millerville Home for Boys, walks by a group of new workers who are discussing their recent orientation session. They mention the newest rule that prohibits workers from transporting a client in a private car. Jim had heard about the new rule, but so far he has ignored it, hoping to plead ignorance if someone were to challenge his behavior. Many of the relationships he forms with the children are established during one-on-one private outings to the mall, movies, and out to dinner. He hates to give them up.

CASE 5

Bradley's job as coordinator of the hospice program in a local hospital is very demanding. His hours are 8 A.M. to 5 P.M., Monday through Friday, but the needs of the clients do not follow these regular hours. He is operating the program with little help: one half-time secretary to answer the phone and one hospice nurse. He often works 15 to 18 hours a day. He feels committed to his work but is often so tired that he is afraid he cannot be effective.

CASE 6

Susan Deerpath is a traveling health department worker in a rural area. She is the only worker serving clients in 12 counties. Once every two weeks, she meets with other health department officials from the district, but for the most part she has limited contact with other professionals. She read her last professional magazine two years ago, and she has attended only one in-service meeting in the past five years.

CASE 7

Luis works for an outpatient AIDS clinic whose major goals include prevention and therapeutic counseling. Luis feels that meeting the demands of his clients is the most important service he provides, and he has difficulty ignoring the clients. Consequently, he is booked solid each day, seeing individual AIDS victims and their families. The director thinks he should spend more time on preventive efforts to promote the agency's other main goal.

CASE 8

Enrique has a new client with a psychiatric diagnosis that is new to him. Even though the agency has a *Physician's Desk Reference,* Enrique searches the Internet for information and finds a site on herbal remedies that he believes will be helpful to both him and the client.

In each of these situations, the helper faces a dilemma regarding worker competence and responsibility for which there is no easy solution. Competence is a personal issue that demands professional self-assessment and then commitment to professional development. Responsibility involves the interpersonal relationships the helper has with individual clients or groups and human service agencies. The common ground between responsibility and competence is the helper's primary commitment to serving the client.

CONFIDENTIALITY

Confidentiality is the helper's assurance that information the client divulges will remain between the two of them. If information is to be shared, it will be shared only with those designated by the client. These two statements regarding the concept of confidentiality provide only general guidelines for the helper. In some situations, laws require confidentiality to be breached: Parents have the legal right to information about their offspring in most circumstances. Courts may require the disclosure of information that would otherwise be confidential; and helpers have a duty to alert authorities if they suspect child abuse (Remley & Herlihy, 2005). The concept is a complex one. This section provides an introduction to confidentiality and gives examples of the complex situations workers may encounter in human service practice.

Confidentiality is a complex concept. For example, a term often associated with confidentiality is **privileged communication.** Both terms address the commitment to keep a client's identity and communications secret. There is a basic difference. *Confidentiality* is a moral obligation grounded in values and ethics (Welfel, 2006); *privileged communication* is a legal term that allows practitioners to legally refuse to release certain information in response to a subpoena. The term *legally* is used because privileged communication is a right granted to a group of professionals by state lawmaking bodies. Examples of situations in which helpers are ethically or legally obligated to breach confidentiality include but are not limited to the following:

1. When the client is dangerous to self or others
2. When there is suspicion of abuse or neglect
3. When the client brings charges against the counselor
4. When the client has already introduced privileged material into litigation

A second example of the complexity of confidentiality is a type often called **relative confidentiality**. This term refers to the informal sharing of information that occurs in an agency or organizational setting among coworkers or treatment team members and supervisors. The client's permission is not required for this type of exchange to take place. Typically, agency policy will also guide this sharing by determining who has access to confidential information. The Federal Privacy Act of 1974, which governs confidentiality in federally funded and administered programs such as the Department of Veterans Affairs and the Social Security Administration, states that clients have access to their records and establishes procedures for this to occur. It also supports the concept of relative confidentiality by providing for the sharing of information among those workers within the agency who need the information in the performance of their duties.

An issue that has recently emerged is maintaining confidentiality within the technological environment. One concern is the safety of records that exist in large management information systems. Organizations and agencies that maintain their records in networks adopt policies and software to ensure limited access. In other words, no one has access to the client files without a security clearance, a password, and the need to know. Personal communication with clients via e-mail must also be regarded as confidential exchanges. Helpers take care to ensure the security of their e-mail systems. Several professional organizations have adopted guidelines for technology-related helping.

In summary, privileged communication and relative confidentiality illustrate the complexity of confidentiality. Privileged communication rarely exists for the beginning human service professional, but relative confidentiality is a concept that deserves the worker's attention. Agency guidelines, the profession's code of ethics, and the laws of the state in which one practices are important considerations in the delivery of services. A professional should be familiar with all three as guides to circumstances that may arise. Communication via the Internet brings an additional set of issues regarding confidentiality. The following vignettes provide examples of confidentiality dilemmas that you may face as a beginning human service professional.

CASE 1

Sue Lee works for the Department of Human Services in Child Protective Services and visits families once a week to review the status of the home environment. Yesterday she received a subpoena and will be required to testify in court that the father in one of the families in her caseload was not at home the last two times she visited. He is charged with armed robbery and states in his defense that he was at home during the time of the crime. That time coincides with her visit.

CASE 2

Joe Cullinane works in a small agency that provides educational services to children with developmental disabilities. He promises clients that his records are confidential and is very careful not to divulge the names of the clients or the nature of their problems. The mother of one of his young clients reports to him that "someone at her church" had heard that her child was receiving his services. If it was not Joe who breached confidentiality, it might be the secretary who answers the phones or the typist who keeps the records.

CASE 3

Faye Goldstein is a counselor/recreation specialist working in an after-school recreation facility. One of her favorite teenagers has just told her "in confidence" that she is pregnant. Should she keep this confidential?

CASE 4

Betsy needs to reschedule an appointment she has with a new client tomorrow. When she called the client, she got voice mail. Knowing that anyone can access message, she decides not to leave one; instead she e-mails her at her workplace.

CASE 5

David Root is a recovering alcoholic and has not had a drink in the last two years. He understands and practices confidentiality in his human service work, but he cannot help but wonder how well he would do in this regard if he were to go on a drinking binge.

CASE 6

Cynthia Loomis works in a high-stress hospice program. Working with the dying patient and family and friends is emotionally draining, and she often "takes her work home." Many of her clients communicate with her via e-mail, since clients and caregivers are homebound. How does she ensure confidentiality?

CASE 7

Jefferson Smith works with adults on probation and has just heard one of his clients tell how she abuses her 6-month-old child. Does he report this information? To whom does he report it?

CASE 8

Raphael Sanchez is a vocational rehabilitation counselor working with a Vietnam veteran. His client has been very depressed during the last month, and during his last individual conference with Raphael, he talked of "ending all the agony." Raphael wonders what he should do and whom he should tell.

These are just a few examples of the many conflicts that can arise over the issue of confidentiality. Many of the troublesome dilemmas result from the constant tension between worker responsibilities, agency policies, and client needs. Privileged communication and relative confidentiality are difficult principles to follow. The preceding cases illustrate the problems helpers may encounter as they translate their values into action in the workplace. An equally complex issue that human services professionals encounter concerns clients' rights.

CLIENTS' RIGHTS

Clients are first and foremost citizens of a democratic society; as such, they have certain rights and privileges. In a helping situation, the client's trust in the helper is important for the development of the helping relationship. In exchange for the trust of the client, the helper is ethically obligated to protect the rights of the client. Two examples of clients' rights are the right to privacy and informed consent.

Clients have the right to share whatever information they wish with a helper. They also have the right to withhold information they do not want to share. The helper is ethically bound to respect clients' **right to privacy** by not pressuring them to reveal things they do not wish to reveal.

Informed consent is another example of the rights of clients involved in the helping process. It is the client's right to know about the qualifications of the helper, treatment procedures, costs of services, confidentiality, and access to records. The concept of informed consent extends beyond simply telling the client about such matters. The client must comprehend this information and consent voluntarily. In some cases, the helper must educate the client about his or her rights with regard to consent.

Informed consent is a particularly critical aspect of client rights with respect to decision making. In the helping process, the client is an active participant who has a voice in what is happening. In the absence of informed consent, the client's right to self-determination is compromised. The helper has an ethical obligation to ensure that clients receive and understand the appropriate information.

One way the client can become informed about the helper is for the helper to write and to share with the client a **professional disclosure statement.** This form should include information about the worker and the worker's credentials, which will allow the client to make an informed assessment of the worker's competence. In addition to name, business address, and telephone number, other information may include education and training competency areas, and the name, address, and telephone number of the state government agency that regulates human service delivery.

Developing a personal professional disclosure statement has several benefits. As the helper shares the statement with the client, it promotes the development of a helping relationship. Not only does it signal to the client that this relationship is different from informal helping relationships, but it also acquaints the client with the person in whom the client will soon place his or her trust. While working out the statement, the helper has an opportunity to think about and put into words exactly who he or she is as a human service professional. It also allows the worker to define himself or herself as a professional and links the individual to the common knowledge, skills, and values of the profession.

TABLE 9.4 | SUMMARY POINTS: PROFESSIONAL DISCLOSURE STATEMENTS

- Introduces the helper to the client
- Provides opportunity for the helper to clarify his/her professional identity
- Promotes the development of a helping relationship

The following sample professional disclosure statement was written by Carmen Rodriguez, the vocational evaluator introduced in Chapter 6.

CARMEN RODRIGUEZ

My name is Carmen Rodriguez, and I am involved in vocational rehabilitation of the handicapped. My purpose is to help my clients understand who they are and what they can do to make their lives more satisfying. Specifically, I evaluate clients to determine what knowledge, skills, and abilities they possess and explain to them what potential work opportunities are available for them.

Once a client meets the eligibility requirements established by the agency, there is no charge for my services. I have worked for this agency for four years as a vocational evaluator. I received training in college for this work and frequently attend workshops to update my knowledge.

Evaluations can take from two weeks to six weeks. This may depend on the client, the disability, and what we want to know. I often refer my client to other team members in my agency and to other professionals in the community. The clients I see usually have such complex problems that I cannot address them all by myself, so I work with a team. Because my agency uses this team approach, I may share information about clients with coworkers within the agency but not with outsiders or other clients. The agency has strict guidelines about how information is shared and prohibits communicating any client information via voice mail, answering machines, cellular phones, faxes, and e-mail.

Now that you have read Carmen's statement, can you write one of your own? It may be easier to write such a statement if you imagine that you work in a specific agency with a well-defined population.

Protection is another of the helper's obligations to clients. Clients have the right to expect the helper to protect them from harm. It is the helper's responsibility to be sensitive to situations in which the client risks economic or physical harm, and, if possible, to prevent harm from occurring. If there is a clear and imminent danger to a third party, the helper has a duty to take action to protect the individual at risk. Determining when a situation warrants action may be difficult for the human service professional; when questionable occasions arise, consultation with colleagues or supervisors will be helpful in deciding on a course of action.

The following cases provide examples of dilemmas that a human service professional may encounter in relation to clients' rights. Several of the cases present ethical situations in which the human service professional is confronted with a difficult decision about what action to take. In other cases, the dilemma is one over which the worker has little or no control.

CASE 1

Susan Yew and her client, Mr. Rodriguez, have agreed on what referral information should be sent to a local educational reading clinic. The clinic, however, wants more information. Specifically, they want to know whether Mr. Rodriguez is a veteran, but he feels they will treat him "special" if they know that he fought in Vietnam. Susan has agreed that the file to be sent should include a short note explaining why he does not want to answer that particular question.

BOX 9.4 | CODE OF PROFESSIONAL ETHICS FOR REHABILITATION COUNSELORS
Confidentiality

SECTION B: CONFIDENTIALITY
B.1. RIGHT TO PRIVACY

a. **Respect for Privacy.** Rehabilitation counselors will respect client's rights to privacy and will avoid illegal and unwarranted disclosures of confidential information.

b. **Client Waiver.** Rehabilitation counselors will respect the right of the client or his/her legally recognized representative to waive the right to privacy.

c. **Exceptions.** When disclosure is required to prevent clear and imminent danger to the client or others, or when legal requirements demand that confidential information be revealed, the general requirement that rehabilitation counselors keep information confidential will not apply. Rehabilitation counselors will consult with other professionals when in doubt as to the validity of an exception.

d. **Contagious, Fatal Diseases.** Rehabilitation counselors will become aware of the legal requirements for disclosure of contagious and fatal diseases in their jurisdiction. In jurisdictions where allowable, a rehabilitation counselor who receives information will confirm that a client has a disease known to be communicable and/or fatal. If allowable by law, the rehabilitation counselor will disclose this information to a third party, who by his or her relationship with the client is at high risk of contracting the disease. Prior to disclosure, the rehabilitation counselor will ascertain that the client has not already informed the third party about his or her disease and that the client is not intending to inform the third party in the immediate future.

e. **Court-Ordered Disclosure.** When court ordered to release confidential information without a client's permission, rehabilitation counselors will request to the court that the disclosure not be required due to potential harm to the client or counseling relationship.

f. **Minimal Disclosure.** When circumstances require the disclosure of confidential information, rehabilitation counselors will endeavor to reveal only essential information. To the extent possible, clients will be informed before confidential information is disclosed.

g. **Explanation of Limitations.** When counseling is initiated and throughout the counseling process as necessary, rehabilitation counselors will inform clients of the limitations of confidentiality and will identify foreseeable situations in which confidentiality must be breached.

h. **Work Environment.** Rehabilitation counselors will make every effort to ensure that a confidential work environment exists and that subordinates including employees, clerical assistants, and volunteers maintain the privacy and confidentiality of clients.

i. **Treatment Teams.** If client treatment will involve the sharing of client information among treatment team members, the client will be advised of this fact and will be informed of the team's existence and composition.

j. **Client Assistants.** When a client is accompanied by an individual providing assistance to the client (e.g., interpreter, personal care assistant, etc.), rehabilitation counselors will ensure that the assistant is apprised of the need to maintain confidentiality.

Source: Material from "Code of Professional Ethics for Rehabilitation Counselors," adopted June 2001, effective January 1, 2002.

<table>
<tr><td>BOX 9.5</td><td>AMERICAN COUNSELING ASSOCIATION CODE OF ETHICS
AND STANDARDS OF PRACTICE
Client Rights</td></tr>
</table>

B. 1. Respecting Client Rights

B. 1. a. Multicultural/Diversity Considerations

Counselors maintain awareness and sensitivity regarding cultural meanings of confidentiality and privacy. Counselors respect differing views toward disclosure of information. Counselors hold ongoing discussions with clients as to how, when, and with whom information is to be shared.

B. 1. b. Respect for Privacy

Counselors respect client rights to privacy. Counselors solicit private information from clients only when it is beneficial to the counseling process.

B. 1. c. Respect for Confidentiality

Counselors do not share confidential information without client consent or without sound legal or ethical justification.

B. 1. d. Explanation of Limitations

At initiation and throughout the counseling process, counselors inform clients of the limitations of confidentiality and seek to identify foreseeable situations in which confidentiality must be breached. (*See A. 2. b.*)

Source: Material from "American Counseling Association Code of Ethics and Standards of Practice." Reprinted by permission of the American Counseling Association. Approved by the ACA Governing Council 2005.

CASE 2

Once a week, the staff members at the battered women's shelter discuss the cases in which they are involved. One client, age 56, told the worker "in confidence" that she had an abortion when she was 13. She asked the worker not to tell the other staff members.

CASE 3

The local mental health institution has a new professional staff member: the patient advocate, who has been hired by the mental health association to protect the rights of the clients in the institution. The patient advocate explains to each patient his or her rights when he or she enters the institution, but many patients forget or are unable to comprehend how they might use the services of the advocate. Sometimes Ron, a social worker on a treatment team serving the men's locked ward, sees clients' rights being abused, but to recommend that a client see the advocate might cause trouble for the treatment team to which Ron belongs.

CASE 4

Youvella is a patient in a health care facility. She wants to see her medical records before they are examined by the team of specialists who will decide what protocol to prescribe for the treatment of her cancer-ridden pancreas. Although Youvella is entitled to review these records, the nurse questions the wisdom of this decision because of Youvella's emotional instability. The nurse requests assistance from the hospital social service worker in this dilemma.

CASE 5

Emile is a human service student working with rehabilitation services. For the next two weeks, he will be administering vocational aptitude tests to new clients. He is unsure whether he should tell his clients that he is a student. He wants them to trust him and have confidence in him, as they would if he were a seasoned worker.

CASE 6

The adoption agency is reviewing the files of a young couple considering adoption. Unfortunately, the adoption counselor has received some damaging information from the couple's landlord of 10 years ago that will make it impossible for the agency to consider them suitable as parents. The counselor really respects this couple and believes that they would make wonderful parents, but she also knows that the information cannot be withheld. The adoption counselor must tell the couple of the agency's decision not to consider them "fit" to adopt and must tell them of the negative recommendation.

CASE 7

The Annas are involved in marital therapy; the stated purpose of the counseling is to "save the marriage." They receive individual counseling once a week, and once a month they participate in counseling sessions together. Ms. Anna has recently told the counselor of her desire to harm Mr. Anna. The counselor wonders how to handle this information, since it was given in confidence and also may jeopardize the goal of saving the marriage.

In clients' rights issues, the helper's judgment and the agency's judgment are often not the only considerations. Legal rulings must also be taken into account. Sometimes legal pronouncements, ethical standards, and personal commitments conflict, presenting a difficult dilemma for the worker. The professional then must decide what action is most ethical.

ETHICAL STANDARDS OF HUMAN SERVICE PROFESSIONALS

In 1995 the National Organization for Human Service Education (NOHSE) approved ethical standards for human service professionals (see Box 9.6). Previously, students and graduates were guided by the codes of ethics or ethical standards of various other professions, some of which have been excerpted in this chapter. These codes did not reflect the unique history or philosophy of the human service profession. As you read these ethical standards, you will note that they address the topics discussed at the beginning of this chapter. The preamble introduces the goals or aims of the profession. The ethical standards then divide professional responsibilities in six areas: to clients, to the community and society, to colleagues, to the profession, to employers, and to self.

These ethical standards and those in other helping professions provide guidelines only. They do not provide answers to all ethical dilemmas. The ethical decision making that follows the ethical standards is helpful when these situations arise.

ETHICAL DECISION MAKING

Clearly, no code of ethics or statement of standards can provide a course of action for every situation that might arise in the practice of human services. What does the human service professional do in situations for which there are no guidelines or guidelines that conflict? In such ethical dilemmas, the conflict is in determining the

BOX 9.6 | ETHICAL STANDARDS OF HUMAN SERVICE PROFESSIONALS

National Organization for Human Service Education
Council for Standards in Human Service Education

Preamble

Human services is a profession developing in response to and in anticipation of the direction of human needs and human problems in the late twentieth century. Characterized particularly by an appreciation of human beings in all of their diversity, human services offers assistance to its clients within the context of their community and environment. Human service professionals and those who educate them, regardless of whether they are students, faculty or practitioners, promote and encourage the unique values and characteristics of human services. In so doing human service professionals and educators uphold the integrity and ethics of the profession, partake in constructive criticism of the profession, promote client and community well-being, and enhance their own professional growth.

The ethical guidelines presented are a set of standards of conduct which the human service professionals and educators consider in ethical and professional decision making. It is hoped that these guidelines will be of assistance when human service professionals and educators are challenged by difficult ethical dilemmas.

Although ethical codes are not legal documents, they may be used to assist in the adjudication of issues related to ethical human service behavior.

Section I—Standards of Human Service Professionals

Human service professionals function in many ways and carry out many roles. They enter into professional–client relationships with individuals, families, groups and communities who are all referred to as "clients" in these standards. Among their roles are caregiver, case manager, broker, teacher/educator, behavior changer, consultant, outreach professional, mobilizer, advocate, community planner, community change organizer, evaluator and administrator (SREB, 1967). The following standards are written with these multifaceted roles in mind.

The Human Service Professional's Responsibility to Clients

STATEMENT 1 Human service professionals negotiate with clients the purpose, goals, and nature of the helping relationship prior to its onset as well as inform clients of the limitations of the proposed relationship.

STATEMENT 2 Human service professionals respect the integrity and welfare of the client at all times. Each client is treated with respect, acceptance and dignity.

STATEMENT 3 Human service professionals protect the client's right to privacy and confidentiality except when such confidentiality would cause harm to the client or others, when agency guidelines state otherwise, or under other stated conditions (e.g., local, state, or federal laws). Professionals inform clients of the limits of confidentiality prior to the onset of the helping relationship.

STATEMENT 4 If it is suspected that danger or harm may occur to the client or to others as a result of a client's behavior, the human service professional acts in an appropriate and professional manner to protect the safety of those individuals. This may involve seeking consultation, supervision, and/or breaking the confidentiality of the relationship.

STATEMENT 5 Human service professionals protect the integrity, safety, and security of client records. All written client information that is shared with other professionals, except in the course of professional supervision, must have the client's prior written consent.

STATEMENT 6 Human service professionals are aware that in their relationships with clients power and status are unequal. Therefore they recognize that dual or multiple relationships may increase the risk of harm to, or exploitation of, clients, and may impair their professional judgment. However, in some communities and situations it may not be feasible to avoid social or other nonprofessional contact with clients. Human service professionals support the trust implicit in the helping relationship by avoiding dual relationships that may impair professional judgment, increase the risk of harm to clients or lead to exploitation.

STATEMENT 7 Sexual relationships with current clients are not considered to be in the best interest of the client and are prohibited. Sexual relationships with previous clients are considered dual relationships and are addressed in Statement 6 (above).

continued

BOX 9.6 | ETHICAL STANDARDS OF HUMAN SERVICE PROFESSIONALS *continued*

STATEMENT 8 The client's right to self-determination is protected by human service professionals. They recognize the client's right to receive or refuse services.

STATEMENT 9 Human service professionals recognize and build on client strengths.

The Human Service Professional's Responsibility to the Community and Society

STATEMENT 10 Human service professionals are aware of local, state, and federal laws. They advocate for change in regulations and statutes when such legislation conflicts with ethical guidelines and/or client rights. Where laws are harmful to individuals, groups or communities, human service professionals consider the conflict between the values of obeying the law and the values of serving people and may decide to initiate social action.

STATEMENT 11 Human service professionals keep informed about current social issues as they affect the client and the community. They share that information with clients, groups and community as part of their work.

STATEMENT 12 Human service professionals understand the complex interaction between individuals, their families, the communities in which they live, and society.

STATEMENT 13 Human service professionals act as advocates in addressing unmet client and community needs. Human service professionals provide a mechanism for identifying unmet client needs, calling attention to these needs, and assisting in planning and mobilizing to advocate for those needs at the local community level.

STATEMENT 14 Human service professionals represent their qualifications to the public accurately.

STATEMENT 15 Human service professionals describe the effectiveness of programs, treatments, and/or techniques accurately.

STATEMENT 16 Human service professionals advocate for the rights of all members of society, particularly those who are members of minorities and groups at which discriminatory practices have historically been directed.

STATEMENT 17 Human service professionals provide services without discrimination or preference based on age, ethnicity, culture, race, disability, gender, religion, sexual orientation or socioeconomic status.

STATEMENT 18 Human service professionals are knowledgeable about the cultures and communities within which they practice. They are aware of multiculturalism in society and its impact on the community as well as individuals within the community. They respect individuals and groups, their cultures and beliefs.

STATEMENT 19 Human service professionals are aware of their own cultural backgrounds, beliefs, and values, recognizing the potential for impact on their relationships with others.

STATEMENT 20 Human service professionals are aware of sociopolitical issues that differentially affect clients from diverse backgrounds.

STATEMENT 21 Human service professionals seek the training, experience, education and supervision necessary to ensure their effectiveness in working with culturally diverse client populations.

The Human Service Professional's Responsibility to Colleagues

STATEMENT 22 Human service professionals avoid duplicating another professional's helping relationship with a client. They consult with other professionals who are assisting the client in a different type of relationship when it is in the best interest of the client to do so.

STATEMENT 23 When a human service professional has a conflict with a colleague, he or she first seeks out the colleague in an attempt to manage the problem. If necessary, the professional then seeks the assistance of supervisors, consultants or other professionals in efforts to manage the problem.

STATEMENT 24 Human service professionals respond appropriately to unethical behavior of colleagues. Usually this means initially talking directly with the colleague and, if no resolution is forthcoming, reporting the colleague's behavior to supervisory or administrative staff and/or to the professional organization(s) to which the colleague belongs.

STATEMENT 25 All consultations between human service professionals are kept confidential unless to do so would result in harm to clients or communities.

continued

The Human Service Professional's Responsibility to the Profession

STATEMENT 26 Human service professionals know the limit and scope of their professional knowledge and offer services only within their knowledge and skill base.

STATEMENT 27 Human service professionals seek appropriate consultation and supervision to assist in decision-making when there are legal, ethical or other dilemmas.

STATEMENT 28 Human service professionals act with integrity, honesty, genuineness, and objectivity.

STATEMENT 29 Human service professionals promote cooperation among related disciplines (e.g., psychology, counseling, social work, nursing, family and consumer sciences, medicine, education) to foster professional growth and interests within the various fields.

STATEMENT 30 Human service professionals promote the continuing development of their profession. They encourage membership in professional associations, support research endeavors, foster educational advancement, advocate for appropriate legislative actions, and participate in other related professional activities.

STATEMENT 31 Human service professionals continually seek out new and effective approaches to enhance their professional abilities.

The Human Service Professional's Responsibility to Employers

STATEMENT 32 Human service professionals adhere to commitments made to their employers.

STATEMENT 33 Human service professionals participate in efforts to establish and maintain employment conditions which are conducive to high-quality client services. They assist in evaluating the effectiveness of the agency through reliable and valid assessment measures.

STATEMENT 34 When a conflict arises between fulfilling the responsibility to the employer and the responsibility to the client, human service professionals advise both of the conflict and work conjointly with all involved to manage the conflict.

The Human Service Professional's Responsibility to Self

STATEMENT 35 Human service professionals strive to personify those characteristics typically associated with the profession (e.g., accountability, respect for others, genuineness, empathy, pragmatism).

STATEMENT 36 Human service professionals foster self-awareness and personal growth in themselves. They recognize that when professionals are aware of their own values, attitudes, cultural background, and personal needs, the process of helping others is less likely to be negatively impacted by those factors.

STATEMENT 37 Human service professionals recognize a commitment to lifelong learning and continually upgrade knowledge and skills to serve the populations better.

Section II—Standards for Human Service Educators

Human service educators are familiar with, informed by, and accountable to the standards of professional conduct put forth by their institutions of higher learning; their professional disciplines, for example, American Association of University Professors (AAUP), American Counseling Association (ACA), Academy of Criminal Justice (ACJS), American Psychological Association (APA), American Sociological Association (ASA), National Association of Social Workers (NASW), National Board of Certified Counselors (NBCC), National Education Association (NEA), and the National Organization for Human Services (NOHS).

STATEMENT 38 Human service educators uphold the principle of liberal education and embrace the essence of academic freedom, abstaining from inflicting their own personal views/morals on students, and allowing students the freedom to express their views without penalty, censure or ridicule, and to engage in critical thinking.

STATEMENT 39 Human service educators provide students with readily available and explicit program policies and criteria regarding program goals and objectives, recruitment, admission, course requirements, evaluations, retention and dismissal in accordance with due process procedures.

STATEMENT 40 Human service educators demonstrate high standards of scholarship in content areas and of pedagogy by staying current with developments in the field of human services and in teaching effectiveness, for example, learning styles and teaching styles.

STATEMENT 41 Human service educators monitor students' field experiences to ensure the quality of the placement site, supervisory experience, and

continued

| BOX 9.6 | ETHICAL STANDARDS OF HUMAN SERVICE PROFESSIONALS *continued* |

learning experience towards the goals of professional identity and skill development.

STATEMENT 42 Human service educators participate actively in the selection of required readings and use them with care, based strictly on the merits of the material's content, and present relevant information accurately, objectively, and fully.

STATEMENT 43 Human service educators, at the onset of courses, inform students if sensitive/controversial issues or experiential/affective content or process are part of the course design; ensure that students are offered opportunities to discuss in structured ways their reactions to sensitive or controversial class content; ensure that the presentation of such material is justified on pedagogical grounds directly related to the course; and differentiate between information based on scientific data, anecdotal data, and personal opinion.

STATEMENT 44 Human service educators develop and demonstrate culturally sensitive knowledge, awareness, and teaching methodology.

STATEMENT 45 Human service educators demonstrate full commitment to their appointed responsibilities, and are enthusiastic about and encouraging of students' learning.

STATEMENT 46 Human service educators model the personal attributes, values and skills of the human service professional, including but not limited to, the willingness to seek and respond to feedback from students.

STATEMENT 47 Human service educators establish and uphold appropriate guidelines concerning self-disclosure or student-disclosure of sensitive/personal information.

STATEMENT 48 Human service educators establish an appropriate and timely process for providing clear and objective feedback to students about their performance on relevant and established course/program academic and personal competence requirements and their suitability for the field.

STATEMENT 49 Human service educators are aware that in their relationships with students, power and status are unequal; therefore, human service educators are responsible to clearly define and maintain ethical and professional relationships with students, and avoid conduct that is demeaning, embarrassing or exploitative of students, and to treat students fairly, equally and without discrimination.

STATEMENT 50 Human service educators recognize and acknowledge the contributions of students to their work, for example, in case material, workshops, research, and publications.

STATEMENT 51 Human service educators demonstrate professional standards of conduct in managing personal or professional differences with colleagues, for example, not disclosing such differences and/or affirming a student's negative opinion of a faculty/program.

STATEMENT 52 Human service educators ensure that students are familiar with, informed by, and accountable to the ethical standards and policies put forth by their program/department, the course syllabus/instructor, their advisor(s), and the Ethical Standards of Human Service Professionals.

STATEMENT 53 Human service educators are aware of all relevant curriculum standards, including those of the Council for Standards in Human Service Education (CSHSE), the Community Support Skills Standards, and state/local standards; and take them into consideration in designing the curriculum.

STATEMENT 54 Human service educators create a learning context in which students can achieve the knowledge, skills, values, and attitudes of the academic program.

Source: Ethical Standards of Human Service Professionals. (2000). *Human Service Education, 20*(1), 61–68. Reprinted with permission of National Organization of Human Service Education.

right thing to do regarding obligations to two or more constituencies. They occur in situations when a choice exists between contradictory directives or standards or "when every alternative results in an undesirable outcome for one or more persons" (Loewenberg & Dolgoff, 1996, p. 8). The areas of confidentiality, role conflict, and counselor competence frequently present ethical dilemmas. Rather than attempt to provide possible solutions to every situation that comes to mind, this subsection will introduce steps for ethical decision making that can be applied to many dilemmas to determine a course of action.

Determining the best action under the circumstances and with the individuals involved is at the crux of ethical decision making. To accomplish this, the helper must assume an attitude of **moral responsibleness.** This should be distinguished from the kind of responsibility discussed earlier. That responsibility is imposed by some higher authority, such as the profession or the government; it may be interpreted as one's duty. Moral responsibleness, on the other hand, comes from within the individual, who assumes that there is a course of action that is morally right. A commitment to rational thinking and a knowledge of moral principles are necessary components of moral reasoning.

A number of ethical decision-making models exist. Although the process is not necessarily linear in that some steps may need to be repeated, there are steps that many models share:

1. *Identify the problem.* This may involve gathering additional information, considering the legal, ethical, moral, and professional perspectives, and determining the issues involved. It is also prudent to think about relevant cultural factors and, of course, to review ethical standards.
2. *Consult with colleagues or experts.* Legal counsel, co-workers, and supervisors are some of the resources that can be tapped to obtain different perspectives about the dilemma. In addition, consultation is also evidence that a worker has acted in good faith if there is a legal challenge to the decision.
3. *Identify and explore options.* Both brainstorming and consulting are techniques that increase the numbers and types of options worth consideration. An important part of this step is thinking about the desired outcomes and the advantages and disadvantages or risks and benefits of each option.
4. *Choose a course of action and act.* Then evaluate both the process and the choice.

We have discussed dilemmas that involve competency and responsibility, confidentiality, and clients' rights and have presented short cases to illustrate problems that might arise in actual practice. As you consider how you would respond to each case, review the steps in the previous paragraph and follow them as you deliberate. The following questions may be useful as you consider how you would respond to each case.

1. State the dilemma clearly. There may be more than one; if so, please think of all that you can.
2. What options are available?
3. What are the disadvantages and advantages of each option?
4. What action do you choose?
5. What factor most influenced your decision?

Another place to use the ethical decision-making model is with dilemmas that are unique to a specific setting, for it provides a purposeful way of thinking about them. Human services in a correctional setting provides examples of such ethical conflicts.

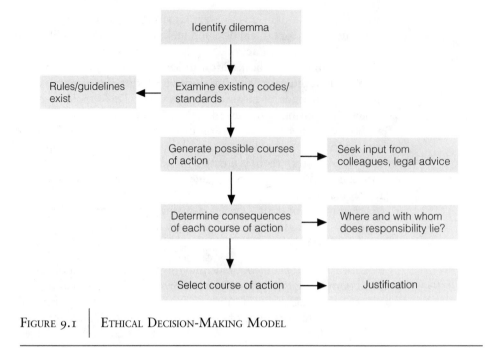

FIGURE 9.1 | ETHICAL DECISION-MAKING MODEL

The dilemmas that correctional workers face illustrate the conflict between human service professionals' responsibilities to the client, to the agency, and to society. As an officer of the court, the corrections worker has the primary role of ensuring that clients do not break the law or injure others. This role places the professional in the position of judge, evaluator, and reporter, making establishing and maintaining helping relationships difficult. The following two dilemmas arise from a conflict between this primary role of the corrections worker and the human service professional's overriding concern for the welfare of the client.

One dilemma may arise when the courts mandate counseling sessions for public offenders. The fact that counseling is imposed will probably impede the helping relationship. The second dilemma, which further complicates the relationship, occurs when the worker explains what confidentiality means in the corrections setting. If a client has violated an institution's rules or any state or federal law and tells the worker of the violations, the professional is expected to report this information to the appropriate authorities. Many clients never develop the trust needed for a good helping relationship, refusing to share problems with the worker. Other clients may be reluctant to disclose real problems they are experiencing, as the worker is often in a position to provide information and make recommendations about clients. Thus, clients may tell the helper only good news, in hopes of securing a positive recommendation.

In situations like these, the professional should begin by identifying exactly what the conflict is. After reviewing ethical guidelines, the helper then considers possible courses of action and the consequences of each. It may be helpful at this point to ask coworkers for input and clarification as the professional explores what each course of

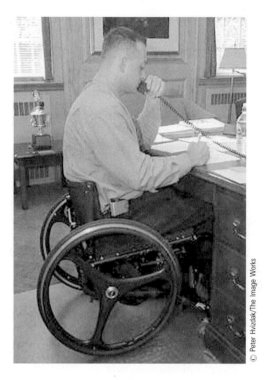

© Peter Hvizdak/The Image Works

action will mean to the client, to the agency, and to the helper. At some point, the helper will have to select a course of action. This ethical decision-making model provides only a structure for thinking about a dilemma; selecting a course of action may still be difficult.

The situations that follow are actual dilemmas that human service professionals encountered. During interviews with human service professionals in urban multicultural areas in the United States, ethical dilemmas were often mentioned as one of the most difficult challenges that they face day to day. As you read these situations, apply what you have learned about ethical decision making. What steps would you take to resolve each one?

SITUATION 1   Our agency was built on volunteers. Many of our clients come into care, love their experience with case management, and then they want to volunteer. In a volunteer role, they may participate in some of our groups, so they may get some privileged information about other clients. They all sign confidentiality statements but signing a statement for some people does not necessarily mean that they adhere to policies or standards. (Atlanta)

SITUATION 2   A problem we often encounter is illegal aliens. In our area, many are industrial workers or food service workers. We don't have migrants who work in agriculture. I guess we should pick up the phone and call the INS but we don't. It comes up when they want benefits and need a social security number. There is actually a black market in social security numbers. We don't advocate that; on the other hand, though, it hasn't been our policy to pursue it or encourage it. (Providence)

SITUATION 3   I live and work in a small rural community. Most people have lived here for generations, so everyone knows everyone else's business. This is particularly difficult for me as a human service worker, a member of the largest church in town, and president of the PTO. Sometimes it's hard to separate what I know as a person in this community from what I learn about clients as a professional. (Maynardville)

In this chapter we explored many of the ethical issues and dilemmas that human service professionals encounter. Professionals use codes of ethics, state statutes and regulations, judicial rulings, and agency policies and procedures as guides as they determine their responses to these issues. After exploring the issue and, at times, using the ethical decision-making model, the human service professional acts, ultimately guided by the principles of moral responsibleness.

KEY TERMS

code of ethics

competence

confidentiality

ethical dilemmas

informed consent

moral responsibleness

privileged communication

professional disclosure statement

protection

relative confidentiality

responsibility

right to privacy

THINGS TO REMEMBER

1. In the course of delivering human services, the professional may encounter numerous ethical dilemmas; for some of these, the worker may be unsure of the appropriate action to take.

2. Professionals have responded to the dilemmas of service provision by developing codes of ethics or statements of ethical standards of behavior for the members of their profession. Items are included that state the goals or aims of the profession, protect the client, provide guidance as to professional behavior, and contribute to a professional identity for the worker.

3. Most codes of ethics indicate that the helper's first responsibility is to enhance and protect the client's welfare.

4. The California *Tarasoff* case establishes the professional's responsibility to warn others if a client threatens harm to self or others.

5. The human service professional has an ethical obligation to respect, understand, and use knowledge of the culture of the client in defining problems and developing treatment plans.

6. Most codes of ethics emphasize that the helper must have adequate knowledge, values, and skills to address the client's needs.

7. Human service professionals have the responsibility to help clients develop their potential and to keep them from harm.

8. Belonging to professional organizations and participating in professional development are

ways the helping professional keeps abreast of current trends and develops new methods of helping.

9. Privileged communication is a legal concept that protects the confidentiality between client and helper.

10. Human service professionals write professional disclosure statements that include training, theoretical framework, and

experience. They share this information with their clients early in the helping process.

11. Human service professionals have a code of ethics that articulates guidelines for professional behavior.

12. An ethical decision-making model delineates steps that human services professionals can use to consider ethical issues.

ADDITIONAL READINGS: FOCUS ON PROFESSIONALISM

Ball, J. R. (2001). *Professionalism is for everyone: Five keys to being a true professional.* Reston, VA: Goals Institute.
This guide addresses five key areas to being a true professional.

Crowell, W. (2006, September 1). Ethics and technology in human services. *Policy and Practice,* 64(3), 30.
A digital document from *Policy and Practice,* a journal published by Thomson Gale, this article addresses the intensifying trend of using technology, its implications for security, privacy, and acceptable use, and the changes in doing business.

Pack-Brown, S. P., & Williams, C. B. (2003). *Ethics in a multicultural context.* Beverly Hills, CA: Sage.
This book identifies culturally troublesome issues, encourages culturally appropriate interpretations of existing ethical guidelines, and promotes ethical behavior in multicultural contexts. Extensive case studies explore ethical dilemmas, critical decision making, and cultural competency.

Sajoo, A. B. (2004). *Muslim ethics: Emerging vistas.* Montreal: Institute for Islamic Studies.
This is one of a series of papers that explores Muslim ethics and the challenges presented by recent political and social events and advances in science and technology.

Skovholt, T. M. (2001). *The resilient practitioner: Burnout prevention and self-care strategies for counselors, therapists, teachers, and health professionals.* Needham Heights, MA: Allyn & Bacon.
The author identifies and explains practitioner stress and provides remedies for self care.

REFERENCES

Corey, G., Corey, M. S., & Callanan, P. (2007). *Issues and ethics in the helping professions.* Belmont, CA: Thomson Brooks/Cole.

Loewenberg, F. M., & Dolgoff, R. (1996). *Ethical dimensions for social work practice* (5th ed.). Itasca, NY: Peacock.

Nagpal, S. (2001). Through the cultural looking glass. *Counseling Today, 42.*

Pedersen, P. (2000). *A handbook for developing multicultural awareness.* Alexandria, VA: American Counseling Association.

Remley, Jr., T. P., & Herlihy, B. (2005). *Ethical, legal, and professional issues in counseling.* Upper Saddle River, NJ: Pearson Merrill Prentice Hall.

Sue, D. W., & Sue, D. (2003). *Counseling the culturally diverse: Theory and practice.* Boston: John Wiley.

Tarasoff v. Regents of the University of California. (1976). *Pacific Reporter,* 2nd Series, 551, 340.

Welfel, E. R. (2006). *Ethics in counseling and psychotherapy* (3rd ed.). Pacific Grove, CA: Brooks/Cole/Thomson.

GLOSSARY

acceptance The ability of the worker to be receptive to the client regardless of factors such as dress or behavior.

administrator A human service professional whose primary responsibilities are planning and organizing services.

advocacy Speaking out on behalf of clients who cannot speak for themselves.

advocate A human service role that involves speaking on the client's behalf.

AFDC A federally funded public assistance program, titled Aid to Families with Dependent Children, that was replaced in 1996 as a result of welfare reform.

almshouses Workhouses for the mentally ill, the elderly, children, able-bodied poor, criminals, and other groups of people who needed care.

Americans with Disabilities Act Legislation passed in 1990 to enable people with disabilities to have equal access to goods, services, and employment.

antianxiety drugs Psychotropic medications prescribed to relieve anxiety, fear, or tension.

antidepressant drugs Psychotropic medications that relieve depression.

antipsychotic drugs Psychotropic medications that are effective in managing psychotic disorders.

assisted living Residential living that matches level of care to individual need.

asylums Institutions for the mentally ill.

attending behavior Verbal and nonverbal components that describe listening: eye contact, vocal qualities, verbal tracking, and body language.

barriers Factors or experiences that prevent clients from seeking help.

brokering Referring a client to another agency or service.

case management The activities of planning and coordinating treatment strategies.

Centers for Faith-based and Community Initiatives (CFBCI) Created by President George W. Bush to strengthen the partnership between faith-based social services initiatives and the federal government and to provide financial support for these activities.

chain of command Layers of authority in an agency.

client An individual, small group, or larger population that needs help.

code of ethics A statement of ethical standards of behavior.

community-based services Services available in the community that enable clients to interact with their environments in the least restrictive setting in which they can function.

community mental health centers Multiservice centers established to provide a variety of community-based services for the mentally ill, including inpatient and outpatient care, emergency services, assistance to the courts, and services for the mental health of children and the elderly.

community organizing Activity based on like-minded people joining together to promote change.

competence Knowledge and skills that meet established professional standards.

confidentiality The worker's assurance to clients that their cases will not be discussed with others.

conservatism A political trend that supports freedom, market solutions, and less government.

consumer A term that designates the recipient of human services.

continuum of care A managed care service delivery strategy that provides care as needed along a continuum of intensity of intervention.

counselors Individuals who help people deal with a variety of problems, including personal, social, educational, and career concerns.

crisis intervention The skills and strategies that helpers use to provide immediate help for a person in trouble.

deinstitutionalization The movement that promoted the transfer of patients

283

from institutions to the community for outpatient care.

developmental process The process of engaging in certain tasks or activities that occur at different life stages.

diversity Refers to many demographic variables, including age, color, disabilities, gender, national origin, race, religion, and sexual orientation.

effective communication The result when the receiver interprets a message the way the sender intended.

E-mail A convenient communication mode that allows for the transfer of messages via the Internet.

electroshock therapy The administration of electricity to the brain to diminish problem behaviors.

empathy Acceptance of the client that allows the worker to see the situation or understand feelings from the client's perspective.

employee assistance programs Programs that address the needs of workers and are available to the employees of companies and corporations.

empowerment Providing services based on client strengths and moving clients to self-sufficiency.

encapsulation When a human service worker retreats from the engagement of helping and becomes rigid, insensitive, and uncaring.

environment The client's surroundings, which include both the physical and the interpersonal (other people).

e-therapy Counseling and other support services provided online.

ethical dilemmas Situations with two or more values in conflict.

ethical standards Guidelines for the behavior of human service professionals.

ethnicity A common culture, heritage, and shared meaning.

external reviews Ways that managed care organizations influence human service delivery, including authorization for services and continuous review.

fee-for-service The standard charge for a specific service.

flexibility Multifaceted trait that allows human service professionals to shift their perspectives of helping, clients, problems, and interventions.

frontline helper A human service professional who focuses on direct services to the client.

full-service schools A partnership between human services and education designed to provide more comprehensive services to children, youth, and families.

gang Two or more individuals who form a group that engages in illegal activities.

gatekeeping A method used in managed care to control access to services.

generalist A human service professional with diverse skills and functions that are applicable in a number of settings with a variety of client groups.

generic focus General helping knowledge and skills to serve individuals with a variety of problems in different settings.

gentrification Urban renewal to revitalize the downtown area of cities.

group A number of individuals who interact with each other sharing values, a social structure, and cohesiveness.

helping relationship The medium through which help occurs.

hierarchy of needs A pyramid of the needs of individuals that identifies lower-order needs such as food, clothing, and safety, and higher-order needs such as social relationships and self-esteem.

homelessness An urban and rural problem that describes single men, women and children, and families who are without the basics of shelter, food, and clothing.

human service model A treatment approach that utilizes problem solving to work with clients and their problems within the context of the environment.

human service system The combination of several parts of the social welfare system, including resources, policies, programs, and knowledge.

individualism The belief that hard work by any individual is the way to success.

individuality The qualities or characteristics that make each person unique and distinctive from all other people.

informed consent The client's right to know about the helper and the helping process.

involuntary clients Individuals who do not freely choose the services they are receiving.

job description A written document that defines the duties and responsibilities of a particular position.

laissez-faire An economic concept that advocated a society or government with little responsibility to those in need.

managed care A set of tools or methods designed to manage resources and deliver human services, especially in the areas of health care and mental health.

Medicaid An amendment (Title 19) to the Social Security Act that provides grants to states to assist them in helping medically indigent citizens receive medical and hospital care.

medical model A system of treatment that suggests that mental disorders are diseases or illnesses that impair an individual's ability to function.

Medical Prescription Drug, Improvement, and Modernization Act of 2003 (MMA) Provides outpatient prescription drug benefits for individuals on Medicare.

Medicare An amendment (Title 18) to the Social Security Act that provides health insurance for those over age 65.

Mental Health Patient Bill of Rights A list of rights that clients should expect when they receive mental health services.

mission The purpose of an agency as summarized by its guiding principles.

mood stabilizers Psychotropic medications primarily used in the treatment of bipolar disorders.

moral responsibleness A commitment to rational thinking and an orientation to moral principles.

multiracial A term that refers to individuals with mixed ancestry.

National Institute of Mental Health (NIMH) A federal agency created in 1946 to help states develop programs for increased training, research, and practice.

network Channels of communication among human service agencies and professionals.

networking Establishing links among human service professionals and agencies to deliver quality services.

neurosis A disorder of the mind or emotions.

New Federalism An approach advocated by Richard Nixon to limit federal spending and human services.

nonprofessional helpers Individuals who engage in helping with little training and agency responsibility.

nonverbal messages Behaviors or body language.

organizational chart A diagram illustrating an agency's structure.

organizational climate Conditions of the work environment.

paraphrase A helper statement that is interchangeable with the client's statement.

paraprofessional helpers Individuals who perform some traditional counseling functions as well as advocacy and mobilization in their work with professionals.

partnerships When two or more human service organizations work together to better serve the client.

patient Recipient of services in the medical model.

Personal Responsibility and Work Opportunity Reconciliation Act (PRWORA) The primary welfare reform legislation that ended the welfare system created by the Social Security Act of 1935.

physicians Medical doctors who perform medical examinations, diagnose illnesses, treat injured or diseased people, and advise patients on maintaining good health.

poor relief Food and protection for the poor provided by the church.

prevention A component of the public health model to improve the present and future quality of life and to alleviate health problems.

privatization Arrangement in which an agency or organization provides a human service function for profit.

privileged communication The legal right of some professionals to refuse to release certain information.

probation Term of supervision given to individuals who break the law but are not incarcerated.

problem solving A five-step approach to solving problems that focuses on the present.

problems Situations, events, or conditions that are troublesome for the client.

problems in living The term used to describe problems that focus on the client, the environment, and the interaction between them.

profession An occupation that is important to society, is based on academic training, and is bound by ethical standards.

professional disclosure statement A form that includes information about the helper and the helper's credentials.

protection A helper's ethical obligation to prevent harm to clients.

psychiatrist Physician concerned with the diagnosis, treatment, and prevention of mental illness.

psychiatry A medical specialty that diagnoses and treats mental, emotional, and behavioral disorders.

psychoanalytic method A method of therapy for investigating unconscious mental processes and neuroses.

psychologists Helping professionals who have advanced degrees in the study of human behavior and who provide counseling, perform assessments, and conduct research in that field.

psychopharmacology The study of the effects of drugs upon mental health.

psychotherapy Process concerned with thinking, emotion, and behavior disorders.

psychotropic drugs Drugs that act on the brain.

public health model A service delivery model that extends health care beyond the medical model, applies a multicausal approach to studying the causes or origins of problems, and emphasizes a preventive approach.

questioning A common verbal technique used to elicit information.

referral Important role where professionals link clients to another service.

rehabilitation The process of returning an individual to a prior state of functioning.

relative confidentiality The informal sharing of information that occurs in an agency or organization among co-workers or treatment team members and supervisors.

reluctance Hesitancy to seek help.

resistance Behavior that can occur at any time in the helping process with a client who is unwilling to participate in the helping process.

resolution-focused brief therapy A counseling intervention that is focused on specific outcomes in a short time.

resources The funding, personnel, volunteers, buildings, and other assets at an agency's disposal.

responsibility The obligation to promote and safeguard the dignity, well-being, and growth of clients, colleagues, the profession, and society.

responsive/active listening The behaviors of helpers as they attend to the words and behaviors of their clients.

right to privacy An individual's right to withhold information he/she does not wish to share.

self-awareness The process of learning about one's self.

self-determination The act of deciding for one's self a course of action or resolution to a problem.

self-sufficiency The ability to care for one's self.

selling A relationship approach to helping that emphasizes a partnership.

settlement house A large house in a slum area that serves as a community center, sponsoring classes, vocational training, and child care.

situational problems Difficulties individuals experience that occur without any predictability and may result in both short-term and long-term problems.

social care Assistance to clients in meeting their social needs, especially those clients who either temporarily or long-term cannot care for themselves.

social change Individuals experience problems as a result of the breakdown of many traditional forms of society.

social control Assistance for those individuals who could provide for themselves but have failed to do so or have done so in a manner that deviates from society's norms for appropriate behavior.

Social Darwinism The belief that the fittest of society would survive through the process of natural selection.

social security Public assistance to those in need that was provided as part of the American welfare state created by Roosevelt's New Deal legislation, the Social Security Act of 1935.

social workers Professionals with training in social welfare, human behavior, and the social environment who work with individuals, families, and groups.

standards of good practice An approach to service delivery that emphasizes the provision of appropriate services for clients and the matching of services to specific outcomes.

TANF (Temporary Assistance to Needy Families) Federal funding that was available to states in block grants to replace the federal AFDC program.

teaming Working together in groups or units to provide efficient and effective client services.

teleconferencing A way in which human service professionals in different locations can communicate with each other.

termination The final stage of the helping process.

terrorism Unlawful use of force or violence against persons or property to intimidate or coerce a government, the civilian population, or both to further political or social objectives.

tolerance The worker's ability to be patient and fair with each client.

turf The clients, services, and resources that an agency or organization believes it controls or serves.

urbanization A long-term global trend that describes population movement from rural areas to cities.

values Statement of beliefs about what guides behavior and provides direction to people's lives.

verbal messages Words spoken by a person.

war on poverty Program initiated by President Lyndon Johnson in 1964 to eradicate poverty by providing means for the poor to improve their economic situation.

web logs Sites where individuals can post their diaries, journals, thoughts, and opinions.

welfare reform Legislation passed in 1996 to end the federal government's six-decade guarantee of aid to the poor.

whole person The many components of a person, such as psychological, social, physical, financial, and vocational, that comprise the total individual.

World Wide Web Online method of expanding communication and information about individuals and organizations through the use of web pages.

Index

Acceptance, 164
Accountability, 71
Active listening, 200–201
Addams, Jane, 39, 41
Administrative work, 176–177
Administrator, 181–182
Advocacy, 89, 245–246
Advocate, 175, 179
Agency structure, 224–226
Aging, 81–83
  web sources on, 84
Aid to Families with Dependent
  Children (AFDC), 43
AIDS, 142, 149
Alcoholics Anonymous, 205
Allocation of resources, 235–237
Almshouse, 33
American Counseling Association, 271
  code of ethics, 271
American Psychological Association, 262,
  275
American Red Cross, 65, 88
Americans with Disabilities Act, 65, 66, 91
Anthropology, 10–13
Antidepressant drugs, 101
Antipsychotic drugs, 101
Assessment, 175
Asylums, 29–30, 36, 38
Attending behavior, 220

Barriers to help, 150–152
  cultural factors as, 150
  friends as, 152
Beers, Clifford, 57
Behavior changer, 175–176, 181
Bethlehem Hospital, 30
Bipolar disorder, 101, 123
Body language, 198, 202, 208
Bombay, 77
Booth, William, 36

Brief counseling, 218
Broker, 175–178
Burnout, 240–243
Bush, George H. W., 50, 65
Bush, George W., 55–57, 65, 90
  ADA, 57, 65

Caregiver, 175–176, 181, 183
Carter, Jimmy, 48,117
Case management, 19–20, 69–70,
  224–226
  managed care, 67–75
Case manager, 18, 20, 74, 75, 160, 163–164,
  226
Catholic Church, 29–30
Chain of command, 225–226
Challenging clients, 190
Change
  advocacy for, 244–247
  client empowerment as, 249–250
  community organizing for, 247–248
Charity Organization Society, 38–39
Child abuse, 136–137, 148
Child welfare, 37
  for homeless, 140
Church as provider, 29–30, 33, 56, 90
Civilian Conservation Corps (CCC), 42
Client, 127–157
  challenging, 207–213
  definition of, 127
  empowerment of, 249–251
  expectations of, 152–153
  problems of, 130–144
  responsibility of, 88–89
  satisfaction of, 154–155
  strengths of, 143–144
Client problems, 130–131
  definition of, 130–131
  help for, 146–150

  perceptions of, 130–131
  perspectives on, 131–144
Clients' rights, 268–269
  ethical standards, 271
  managed care, 73
Clinical psychology, 41
Clinton, Bill, 50–51
Closed questions, 204
Codes of ethics, 256–272
  professional, 257–259
Cognitive messages, 199–200
Colonial America, 32–33
Commitment, 168–169
Communication, 66–68, 167–168, 169, 175,
  177, 181 197–204, 206
  computers in, 66–68
  group, 206
  nonverbal, 198–199, 201
  questions in, 203–204
  responding in, 200–203
  technology for, 66–70
  verbal, 199–200
Communicator, 176–177
Community
  change in, 247–248
  environment of, 228–229
  mapping of, 228
  needs of, 244–248
Community Action Plan (CAP), 248
Community-based services, 61–62
Community mental health centers,
  45, 117
Community Mental Health Centers
  Act of 1963, 45
Community organizing, 244, 248
  web sources on, 250
Community planner, 175–176,
  179–181
Community Support Skill Standards, 24, 175
Competence, 22, 261–265

Computer technology
  email, 66
  for communication, 66–70
  information management, 68
  LISTSERVs, 67
  teleconferencing, 67
  World Wide Web, 67–69
Confidentiality, 165, 265–272
  computers and, 70
  ethics of, 270–271
Conservatism, 90–91
Consultant, 175–176, 179–180
Consumer, 127
Continuing education, 23–25, 243
Continuous review, 73
Continuum of care, 72–74,
Corrections, 98
Council for Standards in Human Service Education (CSHSE), 47, 276
Counseling, 68–70
Counselors, 173–174,
Crisis, 213–218
  development of, 215–216
  helper's role in, 177, 216–218
  intervention in, 216–208
  phases of, 215–216
Crisis intervener, 177, 181
Crisis intervention, 213–218
  roles in, 216–218
  web sources on, 214
Cultural sensitivity, 208–210
Culturally different clients, 208

Data manager, 175–178, 180–181
Deinstitutionalization, 47, 102
Developmental crisis, 214
Developmental perspective,
  131–134
Developmental theory, 127, 131–134
Direct service, 176–177
Diversity, 83–88
  ethics of, 255–257
  ethnicity as, 85
  religious differences as, 85
  sexual orientation as, 86
  and world view, 84
Dix, Dorothea, 34, 36
Documentation, 175, 177–178,
  180–181
Duty to warn, 256, 257, 258

Early history, 28, 29
Education, 22–24
Educator, 14–15, 175–177
Effective communication, 198
Eight stages of man, 131–134
Elderly people, 81–83, 84, 149
Electroshock therapy, 98–99
Elizabethan Poor Law of 1601, 31–32
E-mail, 65–67
Empathy, 168–169
Employee assistance programs, 64, 66
Empowerment, 244, 246, 249
  Disha Kendra, 251
  evaluation of, 18
  model for, 249
Encapsulation, 240–243
Environment, 140–143
  agency, 223–232
  client, 142–143

  human service professional,
Erikson, Erik, 131–134
E-therapy, 70
Ethical considerations, 255–280
  clients' rights, 268–272
  codes of ethics, 256–261
  competence, 261–265
  confidentiality, 265–267
  responsibility, 261–265
  web sources on, 258
Ethical decision making, 272, 276–280
  steps in, 277–278
Ethical dilemmas, 255
  in corrections, 278
Ethical principles, 262
  Ethical standards, 25, 256–272.
    See also Codes of ethics
  diversity, 84–85
  for counselors, 281
  for human service professionals,
    273–276
  for psychologists, 262
  for rehabilitation counselors, 270
  for social workers, 264
Ethics, 255–280
  codes of, 256–261
  of human service professionals,
    272–276
Evaluator, 175–178, 180–181, 183
External reviews, 72, 76

Facilitator of services, 176, 177, 178
Family Educational Rights and Privacy Act of 1974, 256
Family Support Act, 49–50
Federal Privacy Act of 1974, 266
Follow-up studies of graduates, 21
Ford, Gerald, 48
Formal network, 234–235
Fox, Michael J., 246
Franklin, Benjamin, 33
Freud, Sigmund, 99
Friendly supervision, 36
Friendly visiting, 37–38
Frontline worker, 181–182, 184
Full service schools, 63
Future projections, 76–77

Galbraith, John K., 45
Gangs, 145–146
  case study of, 144–145
  web sources on, 146
Gatekeeping, 75
Generalist, 20–22
Getting help, 146–147, 149, 153
  barriers to, 152–153
  inadvertent services for, 149–150
  involuntary placement, 156
  referral, 147–149, 155–156
Government involvement, 31, 33–39, 39–46,
  47–56
  decline of, 56
  increase of, 42–43
  in welfare reform, 50–54
Great Society, 46
Groups, 204–207
  role of human service professional in, 206

Harrington, Michael, 45–46
Healthy people initiative, 110–111

Healthy People 2010, 111
Help
  barriers to, 140, 152, 153
  client evaluation of, 153–155
  client expectations of, 152–153
  client perspective on, 152–155
  inadvertent, 149
  involuntary, 148–149
Helper
  characteristics of, 168
  communication skills of, 169
  empathy of, 169
  philosophy of, 160
  responsibility and commitment
    of, 169
  self-awareness of, 168–169
Helping, 160
  case study of, 196–197
  in crisis intervention, 213–218
  Maslow's view of, 167
  process of, 191–197
  skills for, 197–213
  stages of, 193–197
Helping relationship, 4, 13,
  190–194
  characteristics of, 4
Helping skills, 192
  in communication, 197–198
  in crisis intervention, 213–220
  in groups, 205
  listening as, 200–203
  multicultural, 209
  questions as, 203–204
  responses as, 202–203
Hierarchy of needs, 136, 137
Hippocrates, 28–30
History, 28–59
  Colonial America, 32–33
  early, 28–32
  early 20th century, 39–43
  late 20th century, 47–54
  mid-20th century, 43–47
  Middle Ages, 28–30
  19th century, 33–39
  reform movements, 37–39
  social philosophies, 34–35
  welfare reform, 50–54
HIV/AIDS, 110, 139, 245
Home health source, 232
Homeless people, 138, 140
  children, 137–140
Homosexuality, 84, 86
Hull House, 34, 39
Human service agency, 223–225
  community, 223–225
  goals of, 224
Human service delivery, 235–244
  day-to-day, 235–244
  professional issues in, 237–244
  referral in, 230–232
Human service environment, 223
Human service model, 97, 114–121
  case study of, 119–121
  characteristics of, 117–118
  definition of, 114–116
  philosophy of, 117–118
  problem solving in, 116
Human service movement, 46–47
  and professional organizations, 47
Human service professional, 159–188

categories of, 170–171
characteristics of, 167–170
crisis intervention by, 216–218
ethical standards for, 273–276
in managed care, 74–75
motivations of, 161–162
networking by, 232–234
philosophy of, 166
roles of, 175–183
skills of, 88–90
values of, 162–167
Human service professional organizations
Council for Standards in Human
Service Education, 47
National Organization for Human Services, 47
Human service roles, 175–183
administrative, 177–179
case study of, 183–184
direct service, 176–177
generalist, 4, 167–170
Human Services Research
Institute, 24
Hypnotics, 101

Idiots, 29, 30
Immigrants, 37
Immigration, 78–79
Inadvertent services, 149
Individualism, 34–35, 37
Individuality, 163–164, 166
Industry, 64–65
Informal networks, 231, 234
Information management, 68
Information network, 232
Informed consent, 256, 268
Insane asylum, 30, 98
in 1902, 41
Institutional settings, 61
International focus
on children, 12, 103
Disha Kendra, 251
Peace Corps, 79, 80
International human services,
76, 77, 79
challenges of, 76, 83
models of service design, 98
Peace Corps, 79, 80
International migration, 76
Intervention strategies, 195, 213
crisis intervention, 215,
217–218
multicultural, 209
resolution-focused brief therapy, 218–220
Interviewing, 193
Involuntary placement, 147

Johnson, Lyndon B., 45–46
Joint Commission on Mental Illness
and Health, 44

Kennedy, John F., 57–58

Laissez-faire, 34–35, 37–38
Less eligibility, 34
Life expectancy, 110
Listening, 200–201
LISTSERV, 67

Managed care, 68–69, 71–76, 79
and human service professional, 74–75
Management principles, 4, 15–20
Manic depression, 101
Maslow, Abraham, 14, 136–138,
156, 167
McPheeters, Harold, 16
Medicaid, 46
Medical model, 96–99, 102, 104
case studies of, 104–107
definition of, 96–97
history of, 96, 100
managed care, 103
Medicare, 46
Mental health, 40–41, 43–47
legislation for, 43–47
Mental Health Association, 40
Mental health counselor, 174
Mental health movement, 39, 40
Mental Health Study Act of 1955, 44
Mental illness, 36, 38, 40–41, 98–103
case studies of, 104–107
international, 38
psychotropic drugs for, 101
Mental institutions, 32, 36, 40, 57
Middle Ages, 28, 30, 33
Military, 64–66
Mission, 223–224, 227, 229
Missionaries of Charity, 192–193
Mobilizer, 175–176, 179, 181
Models of service delivery, 96–123
human service, 96–97, 116–118, 120–122
medical, 96–104, 107–108
public health, 96–98, 107–111
Mood stabilizers, 101, 102
Moral responsibleness, 277
Mother Teresa, 191–193
Multicultural counseling, 83, 209
Multi-racial, 78
Mumbai (Bombay), 77

National Association of Social Workers, 264,
275
National Institute for Mental Health, 44
National Mental Health Act of
1946, 43
National Organization for Human Services
(NOHS), 47, 275
Networker, 179, 181
Networking, 15–17, 175
Networks, 234–235
New Deal, 42
New Federalism, 47
Nixon, Richard, 47–49, 57–58
Non compos mentis, 29–30
Nonprofessional helpers, 171
Nonverbal messages, 198

Occupational Outlook Handbook,
171–172
Older adults, 81–82, 84, 156
web sources on, 84
Online counseling services, 69–70
Open questions, 204
Organizational chart, 226–227, 229
Organizational climate, 225
Organized charity movement, 37, 38
Outreach worker, 175–176,
179–181
Overly demanding client, 212

Paperwork, 193, 196, 237–239
Paraphrase, 202
Paraprofessionals, 46, 170–171
Participant empowerer, 176, 177
Participant empowerment, 175
Partnership, 18–19
goals of, 18
with clients, 19
Pasteur, Dr. Louis, 109
Patient, 97
Peace Corps, 79, 80
Peer helpers, 170
Personal Responsibility and Work
Opportunity Reconciliation Act
(PRWORA), 50
Philosophy of helping, 160
Physicians, 172, 174
Planner, 176–178, 181
Poor Law Reform Bill of 1834, 34
Poor relief, 30, 32
Population, 78, 144–146
aging, 81–83
as clients, 144–146
shifts in, 208–209
Poverty, 37–39, 44–46
case study of, 142–143
organized charity movement and, 37–38
social philosophies of, 34–35
war on, 46
Powell, Colin, 246
President's Commission on Mental Health, 48
Prevention, 108–110
Primary influences, 141–142
Privatization, 227, 250
Privileged communication, 265,
266, 267
Probation, 34–35, 37, 39
Problem solving, 13, 114, 118,
121–122
Problems, 127–146
cultural, 136
defining, 4, 130–131
identification of, 130–131
modern, 7
understanding, 131–144
Problems in living, 5–7
Professional development, 70–71,
243–244
Professional disclosure statement,
268–269
Professional helpers, 160, 170–172, 174
Professional issues
burnout, 240–243
paperwork, 237–239
professional development, 243–244
resources, 234–237
turf, 239–240
Proposition 13, 49
Psychiatrists, 172–173
Psychiatry, 99–100
Psychoanalytic method, 99
Psychologists, 173–174, 262
Psychology, 10–11
Psychopharmacology, 121–123
Psychotropic drugs, 101–104
side effects of, 102, 106
Public health model, 96–97, 107–108
definition of, 107
history of, 109
Public Health Service, 108–110

Quality of care, 72–73
Questions, 201, 203, 206
  closed, 204
  open, 201, 204, 206

RAM, 113, 114
Reagan, Nancy, 241
Reagan, Ronald, 49–50
Red Cross, 79, 227
Referral, 147, 195–196, 229–233, 238
  evaluation of, 232
  how, 231
  when, 230
  where, 231
Reform movements, 37
Rehabilitation, 9–10
Rehabilitation counselor, 174
  code of ethics, 270
Relative confidentiality, 266–267
Religious differences, 85
Reluctant clients, 152, 240–241
Remote Area Medical Volunteer Corps
  (RAM) 113–114
Report writer, 176, 180
Resistance, 211–212
Resolution-focused helping, 218–220
Resource allocator, 177, 179
Resources,
  agency, 223–234
  allocation of, 235–236, 252
Responding, 197, 200
Responsibility, 169, 175–184, 261–265
  administration, 177–179, 181–183
  direct service, 19, 176–177
Responsive listening, 200–201, 220
Revenue, 227
Richmond, Mary, 29,
Rogers, Carl, 195
Roles, 88–90, 175–181
  advocate, 179
  behavior changer, 176
  broker, 178
  caregiver, 176
  communicator, 177
  community and service
    networker, 179
  community organizer, 180
  community planner, 180
  consultant, 180
  crisis intervener, 177
  data manager, 178
  educator, 177
  evaluator, 178
  facilitator of services, 178
  generalist, 20–24
  new, 88–90
  outreach worker, 180
  participant empowerer, 177
  planner, 178
  report writer, 178–179
  resource allocator, 179
  teacher/educator, 177
Roosevelt, Franklin, 42, 57

Rural services, 61
Rush, Benjamin, 32, 34, 36, 43

Salvation Army, 36, 58
Scheuer Subprofessional Career Act
  of 1966, 45
School-based services, 63
Schools, 63
Secondary influences, 141, 143
Self-awareness, 170
Self-determination, 165–166
Self-help groups, 205
Self-sufficiency, 7–9
Selling, 89–91
September 11, 2001, 86–87
Settings,
  community-based, 62, 66
  industry, 65
  military, 65, 66
  rural, 62–64
  school, 62–63
Settlement house, 37–39
Settlement house movement,
  37–39
Sexual orientation, 83–84, 86
Shattuck, Lemuel, 109, 111
Silent client, 212
Situational crisis, 214
Situational perspective, 134, 138
Skills,
  advocacy, 89, 91
  changing, 83–85
  selling, 89–91
Social care, 9–11
Social change, 138, 140
Social control, 9–11
Social Darwinism, 34–35
Social engineering, 38, 39
Social philosophies, 34–35
Social reform, 36, 39
  child welfare, 37
  Dix, Dorothea, 36
  movements inc, 36, 39
Social Security Act of 1935, 42
Social work, 39, 40
Social worker, 171–173
Sociological era, 39
Sociology, 10–11
SOLER, 201
Stages of helping, 193–197
Standards of best practice, 73–74
Strengths, 143–144, 191–192,
  218–219

Tarasoff v. Regents of the University
  of California, 281
Tardive dyskinesia, 102
Teacher/educator, 175–177
Team approach, 17–19
Teams, 17–19, 225
Technology, 66–71
  communication, 65–68

confidentiality, 265–268
  counseling, 63–71
  information management, 66, 71
  professional development, 66, 70–71
  service delivery, 66–69
Teen pregnancy, 8
Teleconferencing, 67, 69, 71
Telemedicine, 69, 71
Temporary Assistance to Needy
  Families (TANF), 51
Termination, 196
Terrorism, 86–88
Tolerance, 163–164
Trends,
  aging, 81–83
  diversity, 83–86
  international, 75–79
  managed care, 71–75
  settings, 61, 63, 66
  skills, 88–90
  technology, 66–71
  terrorism, 87–88
Turf issues, 238–240
Typology, 170–174
  human service professional,
    170–172
  other, 172, 175, 179–180,
    183–184

U.S. Department of Health and
  Human Services, 48
U.S. Sanitary Commission, 111
Unemployment, 138–139
Unmotivated client, 213
Urbanization, 77

Values, 160–164
Verbal messages, 190, 199–200
Violent crime, 134, 135
Vocational rehabilitation, 193
Volunteer, 170

War on Poverty, 43, 46
Web sources,
  client problems, 133
  codes of ethics, 258
  community organizing, 250
  crisis intervention, 214
  gangs, 146
  human services, 12
  older adults, 84
  psychotropic medication, 103
  technology, 69
  traumatic events, 88
  welfare reform, 52
Welfare reform, 50–54
  evaluation of, 53–54
Welfare-to-work, 52–53
Whole person, 127–129, 145, 155
World Health Organization, 38
World view, 84